SURGERY - PROCEDURES, COMPLICATIONS, AND RESULTS

THE ROLE OF IMAGING TECHNOLOGY IN CURRENT SURGICAL PRACTICE

SURGERY - PROCEDURES, COMPLICATIONS, AND RESULTS

Additional books in this series can be found on Nova's website under the Series tab.

Additional e-books in this series can be found on Nova's website under the e-book tab.

SURGERY - PROCEDURES, COMPLICATIONS, AND RESULTS

THE ROLE OF IMAGING TECHNOLOGY IN CURRENT SURGICAL PRACTICE

GEORGIOS TSOULFAS
EDITOR

New York

Library of Congress Cataloging-in-Publication Data

ISBN: 978-1-63483-490-2
Library of Congress Control Number: 2015946398

Published by Nova Science Publishers, Inc. † New York

CONTENTS

PREFACE

This book represents an effort to document the experience of a carefully-chosen group of international surgeons, regarding the use of imaging technology in their everyday practice.

The aim of this book is to help medical students and surgeons at all levels of training and practice to understand the basics of the more common imaging techniques (CT, MRI, MRCP, US, XR, radionuclide scan, etc.), including their advantages and disadvantages and their optimal use and limitations. Following that, the application of these imaging modalities, including the most current developments, in the different fields and subspecialties of surgical practice (including but not limited to surgical oncology, neurosurgery, endocrine surgery breast surgery, hepatobiliary surgery, pancreatic surgery, transplantation, urology etc.) is presented in detail.

What is important about this book is that it is written by an international group of surgeons who are experts in their respective fields and who offer us here their wisdom and experience, regarding what the communication between the surgeon and the radiologist should be, in order to provide these complex patients with the best possible care. Apart from the radiological and imaging tools commonly used in current practice, in all the chapters we can see the future prospects and challenges regarding how imaging technology can increase surgical efficiency in the future. The overall goal is to help surgeons in today's technology-driven environment, have a proper understanding of the use and limitations of modern imaging techniques.

Chapter 1 - The role of imaging in Vascular Surgery. Vascular imaging has seen a revolution over the last two decades since the introduction of endovascular surgery, which has gradually become routine practice, and the development of advanced cross-sectional imaging modalities with higher fidelity and accuracy. Duplex ultrasound (US), computed tomography (CT), magnetic resonance imaging (MRI), and conventional digital subtraction angiography (DSA) are currently the main imaging modalities in the armamentarium of vascular surgery. Given the recent advances in software and imaging devices, DSA is now typically reserved for intervention rather than diagnosis. The modern vascular surgeon needs to be aware of the limitations and advantages of each imaging modality, and should be able to diagnose and plan therapeutic procedures, involving either open or endovascular reconstruction, independently. This chapter covers the basics behind the main imaging methods in contemporary vascular practice with an aim to aid diagnosis and management of the relevant pathologies.

Chapter 2 - The role of imaging in Colorectal Surgery. Colorectal surgery manages diseases of the small and large bowel, rectum, anal canal and pelvic floor. The colorectal surgeon undertakes a large array of minor and major, elective and emergency procedures. One of the main instruments in his quiver, aiding in the diagnostics of various diseases and conditions, are the radiological investigations. Plain radiographs have been used for many decades to assess patients with abdominal symptoms, but they have been replaced in the last years by more advanced techniques, such as computed tomographies, magnetic resonance imaging and nuclear tests.

This chapter aims to introduce the reader to most radiological tests available to the colorectal surgeon today; some very specialized/specific tests will not be mentioned, as the authors believe that they are outside the aim of the book. Furthermore, we will look at specific diseases and pathologies and how radiological findings aid in their management and treatment.

Chapter 3 – The role of imaging in Breast Surgery. Over the past decades, there has been significant improvement in the equipment and image-recording systems for breast diseases and for investigation of the axilla. In addition to providing better images, these developments have resulted in a significant reduction in radiation dose. Screening mammography is used to detect unexpected breast cancer in asymptomatic women since the 1960s. Specific mammographic features that suggest a diagnosis of breast cancer include a solid mass with or without stellate features, clustered microcalcifications, and asymmetric thickening of breast tissues. Imaging of the breast has evolved from mammography alone to mammography with adjunctive modalities that primarily include ultrasound and magnetic resonance imaging (MRI scan). Until recently, ultrasound and MRI have functioned as problem-solving tools and have been used to help to diagnose a mammographically and/or clinically detected abnormality such as a breast mass or nipple discharge. As these modalities have improved technologically and immense clinical experience has been acquired, so have their roles expanded from diagnostic tools to potential screening tools as well. Ultrasound has many uses that relate to the evaluation of breast masses. Sonographic guidance is used frequently for the direction of percutaneous breast biopsies and to investigate the status of axillary lymph nodes in breast carcinoma. MRI was initially used for the evaluation of implants, but it now has a variety of roles associated with the evaluation of tumors. With a dedicated breast coil and contrast enhancement, MRI has been of great value in identifying the extent of breast carcinoma and contributing to better patient management plan. A breast positron emission tomography (PET) scan is another imaging modality of the breast that uses a radioactive substance (F-18-fluoro-2-deoxy-D-glucose -FDG). Whole-body FDG-PET can detect distant metastatic disease to the lymph nodes, the soft tissues, viscera, and bone. PET scan is also used to assess whether metastatic breast cancer is responding to treatment. After breast biopsy, scarring and distortion of breast tissue occur, making subsequent evaluation by mammography difficult. Thus, other imaging techniques, such as MRI, and PET, are being increasingly used for characterizing lesions in the breast. All imaging techniques now used in breast surgery continue to be modified and improved to maintain optimum image quality that enhances interpretation skills of the clinicians and radiologists.

Chapter 4 - The role of imaging in Neurosurgery. Sir Godfrey N. Hounsfield (28 August 1919 – 12 August 2004) was an electrical engineer who in 1979, together with Allan McLeod Cormack, received the Nobel Prize in Physiology or Medicine for developing the diagnostic technique of X-ray computed tomography (CT). The first CT scanners were designed exclusively for brain CT, and in 1972 a female with a suspected brain tumor was the first patient examined using CT scanning. In the next year, the first publication of brain CT imaging was true. Early CT scans were of limited quality and demanded long scanning and processing times. Nevertheless, the following development of CT scanning provided neuroradiology with much better brain tumor images and revolutionized neurosurgical practice. A new era in modern neurosurgery had commenced. The MRI on the other side has literally transformed the status of neuroimaging by bringing most of the structural details of the brain and spinal cord in front of our eyes. The most important applications of the modern neuroimaging modalities in neurosurgical practice are presented in this chapter.

Chapter 5 - The role of imaging in Parathyroid Surgery. Primary hyperthyroidism (PHPT) is mainly caused by a parathyroid adenoma. The localization of this parathyroid lesion is essential for the surgical treatment of the disease. Various invasive and non-invasive localizing tests are available for evaluating PHPT. The traditional non-invasive imaging modalities include ultrasonography, scintigraphy, computed tomography and magnetic resonance imaging. In the era of minimally invasive parathyroidectomy (MIP), the utilization of SPECT and SPECT/CT in radioimaging, the 4D CT and various combinations of individual visualization techniques have established parathyroid imaging as an essential supplement to parathyroid surgery.

Chapter 6 – The role of imaging in Adrenal Surgery. The adrenal glands constitute indispensable components of normal physiology. In terms of fundamental anatomy, the adrenal is divided in an outer layer, known as the cortex and in an inner layer, the medulla. Each gland weighs approximately 2-4 grams. Being of significant interest in surgical practice, their blood supply can arise from several different vessels including the aorta, the celiac trunk, the inferior phrenic or the renal arteries. The adrenal cortex secretes glucocorticoids, mineralocorticoids and sex hormones, while the adrenal medulla secretes catecholamines (epinephrine and norepinephrine and dopamine). From an embryology perspective, the adrenal cortex tissue stems from the intermediate mesoderm, whilst the medulla is derived from neural crest cells through a complex migration process. Indeed, understanding the basis of embryonic adrenal development is a key aspect of deciphering certain pathology of this gland.

To begin with, lesions affecting the adrenal cortex have a higher prevalence than lesions located in the gland's medulla. Further classification is focused on determining whether the lesion is primary or metastatic. Notably, primary adrenal lesions are metabolically functional in several cases leading to the clinical manifestations of hormone excess (e.g., Cushing syndrome, Conn syndrome, pheochromocytoma etc.). This is rare with metastatic adrenal tumors. In respect to lege artis medicine, Radiologic Imaging proves to be indispensable in diagnosis and staging. Predominantly, adrenal imaging can be accomplished with Computed Tomography (CT), Magnetic Resonance Imaging (MRI), Ultrasonography (US), nuclear imaging and angiography which are implemented with regard to current guidelines and the surgical team's judgment.

Chapter 7 – The role of imaging in Hepatobiliary Surgery. The increasing complexity of hepatobiliary diseases, benign or malignant, that a surgeon is called to treat, has led to a deeper understanding of the importance of a multidisciplinary approach. Imaging, with its various modalities, plays a central role in the diagnosis and management of hepatobiliary malignancies. An integral part of this remains the communication between the surgeon and the radiologist regarding the exact findings, as well as the different types of management, ranging from surgery to interventional radiology. The goal remains to find the best treatment for the patient. This chapter will present the existing preferences regarding the diagnosis and management of one of the main primary hepatobiliary malignancies, which is hepatocellular carcinoma (HCC). Additionally, we will examine certain special cases (such as the imaging of the early lesion or standardization of imaging reporting), as well as report on the possibilities offered by newer imaging developments. Finally, we will also address the identification and management of a focal hepatic lesion. Overall, the goal is for this chapter to be part of the interplay and the dialogue between the surgeon and the radiologist, in terms of information that needs to be communicated and the best way to do that.

Chapter 8 – The role of imaging in Pancreatic Surgery. The pancreas is a retroperitoneal organ that lies in an oblique position, sloping upward from the C-loop of the duodenum to the splenic hilum. In an adult, the pancreas weighs 75 to 100 g and is about 15 to 20cm long. The fact that the pancreas is situated so deeply in the abdomen and is sealed in the retroperitoneum explains the poorly localized and sometimes ill-defined nature with which pancreatic pathology presents. In this chapter we start with a brief overview of basic pancreatic anatomy and then we present thirteen common pancreatic conditions that may require surgical intervention and analyze the role of the various imaging modalities in the diagnosis and planning for surgery. All images used in this chapter originate from the authors' personal archives.

Chapter 9 – The role of imaging in Esophageal Surgery. The different types of imaging used in the diagnosis and treatment of the diverse esophageal pathologies are presented in this chapter with an emphasis on future challenges.

Chapter 10 – The role of imaging in Gastric Surgery. There is a great number of different gastric pathologies, whether malignant or not. This chapter presents the key points of the use of imaging technology in the current surgical practice, in an effort to help us understand their advantages, as well as their limitations.

Chapter 11 - The role of imaging in Urology. In this chapter, we examine the various imaging modalities used to evaluate the genitourinary (GU) tract. Advances in imaging technology have improved the clinical practice of urology and continue to be an active area of growth. Imaging modalities used by urologists include plain film radiography, ultrasonography (US), computed tomography (CT), magnetic resonance imaging (MRI), radionuclide studies, and positron emission tomography (PET). Each modality plays an important role in the diagnosis and management of urologic diseases and when used appropriately, should provide cost-effective care. This chapter explores indications for these modalities and their optimal use.

Chapter 12 - The role of Imaging in Plastic Surgery. From the era that Röntgen discovered X-rays, imaging studies have been a significant adjunct in the clinicians' armamentarium. The rapid development of modern imaging techniques, as well as the increased accessibility to sophisticated imaging techniques, has allowed physicians to have access to detailed anatomical and functional information. Plastic surgery, being one of the surgical specialties that use the most up-to-date technologies in both diagnosis and treatment, is a field that modern imaging techniques have had a significant impact on. Current applications of imaging in plastic surgery range from staging of melanoma patients to preoperative submillimeter-scale planning of perforator flaps. Nearly all currently available imaging techniques, including X-rays, Ultrasound, Computed Tomography, Magnetic Resonance Imaging, and Positron Emission Tomography, are being used as adjuncts in the diagnosis and/or staging of plastic surgical conditions and diseases. Furthermore, as accurate preoperative planning of plastic and reconstructive surgical procedures has been shown to be of high importance for both the patient as well as the health system by improving the surgical outcomes, imaging techniques, and more specifically CT – and MRI – based studies, have emerged as the outstanding gold standard techniques.

Chapter 13 – Wrist fractures in adults: what should a medical student know? Wrist fractures are common fractures and are seen frequently in the emergency department. They mainly occur in the elderly as a result of a fall on an outstretched hand. Wrist fractures are also seen in high-energy mechanism injuries such as road traffic accidents or a fall from a height. Those fractures are always accompanied with other injuries.

The ability to detect the different types of wrist fractures requires an adequate understanding of the anatomy of the wrist, the mechanism that causes that type of injury, and the accurate interpretation of different imaging processes of the bony and articular structures of the wrist. Therefore, appropriate evaluation of the radiological x-rays is important for therapeutic intervention, surgical or conservative, and for the complete restoration of normal wrist function after an injury.

Dr. Georgios Tsoulfas, MD, PhD, FICS, FACS
Assistant Professor of Surgery
Aristotle University of Thessaloniki, Greece
Tel: (30) 6971895190
Email: tsoulfasg@gmail.com

In: The Role of Imaging Technology …
Editor: Georgios Tsoulfas

ISBN: 978-1-63483-490-2

Chapter 1

VASCULAR IMAGING

Athanasios Saratzis*, MBBS, MRCS, PhD
NIHR Academic Clinical Lecturer in Vascular Surgery,
Department of Cardiovascular Sciences
and NIHR Cardiovascular Biomedical Research Unit,
University of Leicester, UK

ABSTRACT

Vascular imaging has seen a revolution over the last two decades, since the introduction of endovascular surgery, which has gradually become routine practice, and the development of advanced cross-sectional imaging modalities with higher fidelity and accuracy. Duplex ultrasound (US), computed tomography (CT), magnetic resonance imaging (MRI), and conventional digital subtraction angiography (DSA) are currently the main imaging modalities in the armamentarium of vascular surgery. Given the recent advances in software and imaging devices, DSA is now typically reserved for intervention rather than diagnosis. The modern vascular surgeon needs to be aware of the limitations and advantages of each imaging modality, and should be able to diagnose and plan therapeutic procedures, involving either open or endovascular reconstruction, independently. This chapter covers the basics behind the main imaging methods in contemporary vascular practice with an aim to aid diagnosis and management of the relevant pathologies.

INTRODUCTION

Vascular imaging has seen a revolution over the last two decades, since the introduction of endovascular surgery, which has gradually become routine practice, and the development of advanced cross-sectional imaging modalities with higher fidelity and accuracy [1]. Duplex ultrasound (US), computed tomography (CT), magnetic resonance imaging (MRI), and

* Corresponding author: Athanasios Saratzis, Robert Kilpatrick Building, Leicester Royal Infirmary, LE15WW, as875@le.ac.uk, (0044) 0 75431418104

conventional digital subtraction angiography (DSA) are currently the main imaging modalities in the armamentarium of vascular surgery. Given the recent advances in software and imaging devices, DSA is now typically reserved for intervention rather than diagnosis. The modern vascular surgeon needs to be aware of the limitations and advantages of each imaging modality, and should be able to diagnose and plan therapeutic procedures, involving either open or endovascular reconstruction, independently [2]. This chapter covers the basics behind the main imaging methods in contemporary vascular practice with an aim to aid diagnosis and management of the relevant pathologies.

Contrast in Vascular Imaging

The majority of the imaging modalities in vascular surgery require the administration of intra-arterial or intra-venous contrast agents to adequately picture the vasculature. Even ultrasound is now aided by the administration of contrast, to depict more complex anatomies, such as after endovascular interventions [3]. There are certain limitations and challenges associated with contrast administration that need to be discussed.

Several types of contrast media are available, based on the imaging modalities where they are used. Contrast media also differ in terms of molecular function and properties. Iodinated media are typically used in vascular imaging, and they may be either ionic or non-ionic. Non-ionic contrast is currently the most widely used medium, given the reduced risk for adverse reactions. Additionally, the vast majority of media used today are low or iso-osmolar, again due to reduced risk for anaphylaxis and nephropathy [4]. Any form of angiography, either CT or MR generated or conventional DSA, requires the administration of a contrast agent. That may lead to contrast induced nephropathy (CIN), which is an acute deterioration in renal function due to direct damage to the kidney, which happens at the level of the renal tubule [5]. CIN has conventionally been defined as an acute rise in serum creatinine levels of at least 25% compared to baseline and is associated with short and long term adverse outcomes [6-8]. Other definitions of acute kidney injury (AKI) have also been made available over the last decade, but are more applicable to interventions, such as endovascular aneurysm repair (EVAR), rather than diagnostic imaging modalities [5, 9]. Patients at increased risk for CIN or AKI after contrast administration include those with diabetes, hypertension, current smoking habit, critical limb ischaemia (especially in the case of existent tissue loss) and those with a baseline estimated glomerular filtration rate of less than 45ml/min/1.73m [5, 10]. The prevention of CIN and AKI in these patient groups is challenging and there are several proposed interventions with variable results, including the use of iso-osmolar contrast agents, adequate patient hydration using normal saline with or without sodium bicarbonate, premedication with N-acetylcysteine, ischaemic preconditioning, or angiography based on carbon dioxide contrast agents [5, 9]. Reno-protection should be guided by pre-existing risk-factors and most definitely contrast use should be avoided if possible. Gadolinium, a non-iodinate medium which is the contrast of choice in MR imaging, is less nephrotoxic but can also lead to a deterioration in renal function as well as interstitial nephritis and a rare type of nephropathy, gadolinium-induced nephrogenic systemic fibrosis, in high-risk patients – especially these with chronic kidney disease stage 3 and above at baseline [11-13]. MR-based angiography also requires fairly small doses of gadolinium (0.1mmol/kg), which may also explain the less pronounced impact on renal function. Carbon dioxide (CO2) is an alternative contrast agent useful in both diagnostic and therapeutic procedures. Catheter-directed injection of CO2 results in a negative contrast image within the target vessel [14]; CO2 is rapidly absorbed and is not nephrotoxic. However, it is very challenging to image below the knee lesions adequately [15] and most centres are not yet familiar with its use [14, 16]. Interestingly, several case-series of EVAR using CO2 as a contrast medium have recently been made available [17, 18].

Several ultrasound contrast media are currently available, most in the form of "micro-bubbles" and various are under developments, hopefully with less nephrotoxic properties. These agents typically consist of micro-bubbles encased in a biodegradable-shell. These are injected whilst an ultrasound probe is used to visualize the vessel in question. The subsequent risk of nephropathy is less. There are no large studies available with regards to usage of contrast-based Duplex ultrasonography in the diagnostic assessment of the peripheral vasculature; however, this modality has shown promising results in post-EVAR follow-up for endoleak [19, 20].

Digital Subtraction Angiography

Conventional angiography involved the selective catheterisation of a target vessel or territory with an angiographic catheter, typically through a femoral (percutaneous) approach. Radiographic images are taken after contrast injection. Digital subtraction angiography (DSA) is almost always employed, which allows the subtraction of background tissue to provide a better picture of the vasculature, using simple software. DSA has been the gold standard for imaging the arterial and venous tree, but is currently being replaced in routine practice by more contemporary cross-sectional modalities that are less invasive and labour intensive. Given its invasive nature, DSA can be associated with access-related complications, such as haematoma, pseudoaneurysm formation, or inadvertent cannulation of an adjacent vessel [21]. To limit these, most interventionists will perform vessel-punctures under ultrasound guidance in contemporary practice. Other complications secondary to DSA include damage to the target vasculature, including dissection, thrombosis, vasospasm, and peripheral embolization or even rupture of the target vessel. Finally, there is an increased risk of CIN given that iodinated contrast is injected intra-arterially [5]. Given these risks, DSA is usually reserved for intervention or imaging of challenging anatomy, such as below the knee lesions or heavily calcified lesions where CT angiography and MR angiography may not be as sensitive. Additionally, DSA yields physiologic information, such as the measurement of pressure gradients across lesions and the ability to observe the flow of contrast through a vessel in real-time. This may particularly helpful in below the knee lesions and in patients where a low cardiac output does not allow adequate imaging with non-invasive modalities.

Computed Tomography (CT)

Angiography based on images obtained by computed tomography (CT) has seen significant advances over the last three decades. The current modality of choice when using

CT to image the vasculature is multi-detector CT angiography (MDCTA). Using intravenous contrast medium, multiple detectors travel in a helical orientation around the patient and collect volumetric data (together with cross-sectional images), which are then displayed using relevant software. Typically, the volume of contrast required is 50 to 150 ml, depending on the patient's respiratory status, left ventricular function, localization of the disease, and the degree of anatomical detail that is necessary. Retrospective or prospective ECG synchronisation can be applied as well, which may be applicable especially when imaging the proximal aorta and dissections. The main differences between conventional spiral CT and MDCTA include the rapid acquisition speed for MDCTA and the fact that volumetric data are obtained, which allow in-depth analyses of the anatomy of the vessels. Reconstruction of the cross-sectional slices together with the volumetric data obtained via MDCTA is performed with relevant software using the following protocols: maximum intensity projection (MIP), vessel density ratio (VDR), and multi-planar reconstruction (MPR) [22]. Maximum intensity projection can provide pictures very similar to DSA but may exaggerate the degree of stenosis in the case of significant calcification; MPR cannot follow the tortuous course of certain arteries but it can very accurately depict intraluminal thrombus. Several solutions are being investigated to overcome these technical problems including curved MPR and digital subtraction imaging. Additionally, the latest generation devices provide even more detailed scanning and the subsequent quality of the images obtained is very similar to DSA. Another important advantage of MDCTA over DSA is the fact that the cross-sectional slices provide important information about the surrounding anatomy, which could not have been obtained using conventional angiography. Overall, MDCTA is a rapid and safe mode of imaging the vasculature. It has become the preferred method of imaging patients before EVAR (instead of DSA) [23] in order to plan the procedure and has largely replaced DSA as a diagnostic modality for peripheral arterial disease [24].

It has long been shown that EVAR can be safely planned using measurements obtained from reconstructed MDCTA images without the need for DSA. A typical EVAR protocol MDCTA scan includes acquisition of unenhanced, arterial contrast, and delayed post-contrast images. Unenhanced images provide a baseline examination against which apparent abnormalities in the arterial phase can be judged. Delayed images allow for the evaluation of slow endoleaks, especially type 2 endoleaks. MDCTA is in fact very accurate at depicting endoleaks, migration and other device-associated or anatomical complications following EVAR [25, 26]. Further classification with DSA may be necessary in the case of an endoleak, as up to 10% of endoleaks may not be classifiable based on CT reconstruction alone. However, most centres now employ MDCTA as the "gold-standard" in imaging endoleaks, at least at the first instance. Regarding routine post-EVAR follow-up, ultrasound has replaced MDCTA as the preferred modality for device surveillance given the as it is less expensive and does not involve contrast or radiation exposure. A recent meta-analysis has shown that unenhanced ultrasound has rather poor sensitivity for endoleak detection; however CEUS is highly sensitive [25].

MDCTA is also useful in the assessment and planning of peripheral arterial disease (PAD). In the evaluation of severe peripheral lesions, MDCTA has a sensitivity of 92% and a specificity of 97% when compared with DSA [27, 28]. When used after ultrasound imaging before intervention, it may lead to a change in the initial treatment strategy in up to 25% of cases. However, in contemporary practice, given the increasing accuracy of ultrasonography, planning of intervention based on ultrasound alone is acceptable in the majority of cases.

MDCTA is associated with lower radiation dose than DSA, and consistency in treatment recommendations based on MDCTA is excellent [28]. Regarding carotid artery disease, MDCTA is a useful adjunct to ultrasonography. It bears a negative predictive value of almost 100% for stenoses between 50% and 70% [29]. All the carotid trials have used ultrasonography as the "gold-standard" for imaging; MDCTA should be reserved for recurrent disease (re-stenosis), and plaques that have significant distal extension, as part of pre operative assessment and planning.

Finally, coronary CTA has recently emerged as a promising non-invasive method for the detection and coronary artery disease (CAD). A recent randomized trial confirmed multidetector MDCTA as a modality that has equal clinical applicability as conventional DSA in diagnosing and planning treatment for CAD [30].

Magnetic Resonance Imaging (MRI)

Angiography can be performed with or without contrast (intravenous) agents using MRI technology. MR-angiography (MRA) without contrast can be performed by imaging the intrinsic motion of protons in flowing blood using time-of-flight (TOF) sequences. However, the resolution is not optimal and the procedure is timely. Gadolinium can be administered intravenously to obtain better resolution pictures. Similar to MDCTA sequences, post-capture reconstruction can take place using maximum intensity projection (MIP), vessel density ratio (VDR), and multi-planar reconstruction (MPR). Gadolinium-enhanced MRA is mainly used to image peripheral arterial disease (PAD), renal artery disease (RAD) and carotid artery disease (CAD) in contemporary practice.

MRA and Peripheral Arterial Disease (PAD)

MRA is becoming an increasingly common modality in PAD to image, mainly, infrainguinal and infrapopliteral disease; MRA reconstructed images using MIP predicted have a sensitivity of 97%–100% and a specificity of 95%–99% compared to DSA in PAD. However, MRA may significantly over-estimate stenoses in the peripheral vasculature, more so than MDCTA, and is associated with increased cost. Interestingly, MRA for preoperative planning has been associated with a higher surgical re-intervention rate when compared with MDCTA.

MRA and Carotid Artery Stenosis (CAS)

Carotid disease is frequently assessed with MRA reconstructed images, mostly in lesions where a stenosis has already been shown using Duplex ultrasonography. Generally, in CAS MDCTA may underestimate clinically relevant grades of stenosis and is mostly helpful in assessing carotid occlusion as suggested by ultrasonography, whilst MRA is more comparable to conventional DSA, even though it may still give rise to a 5.0% overestimation of stenosis [31]. Overall, MRA is a useful, non-invasive modality for assessment of CAS with a more than 70% stenosis [31], even though it cannot be recommended as first line imaging modality in assessing patients with cerebral events, mostly due to cost (compared to ultrasonography). Interestingly, a meta-analysis suggested that MRA has a better discriminatory power compared with ultrasonography in diagnosing 70% to 99% stenosis and is as sensitive and specific as DSA in the evaluation of CAS [32].

MRA and Renal Artery Disease (RAD)

MRA has been used extensively in evaluating patients with RAD. Previously, most patients had to undergo gadolinium enhanced MR imaging, which had a good diagnostic accuracy, but was limited due to cost and use of contrast, especially given that this population is more likely to present with renal dysfunction. More recent MR imaging protocols, such as non-contrast balanced steady-state free precession MRA have been assessed in patients with RAD, and a meta-analysis of 10 high-quality studies comparing this technique with gadolinium enhanced MRA or MDCTA has shown a pooled sensitivity of 0.88 (95% CI, 0.83-0.91) and a pooled specificity of 0.94 (95% CI, 0.93-0.95) [33]. Another type of MR imaging, time-spatial labeling inversion pulse (time-SLIP) MRA has also recently been assess in imaging of RAD without contrast, showing a specificity of 93% and accuracy of 90% compared to contrast-enhanced MDCTA [34]. Overall, MRA is becoming increasingly the study of choice in imaging the renal arteries, with or without gadolinium, depending on local availability and expertise.

Duplex Ultrasonography

Pulse-wave Doppler ultrasound and grey-scale ultrasound imaging are obtained and combined to provide cross-sectional imaging of the vasculature with real-time information regarding blood-flow in duplex ultrasonography (DU). Colour Doppler may be used as well to further augment assessment of blood flow. This non-invasive and dynamic method of imaging the vasculature has found several applications in vascular medicine and vascular surgery. DU is currently the imaging modality of choice in the initial assessment of patients with peripheral arterial disease (PAD), venous disease (VD), surveillance of both grafts and endovascular devices after endovascular aneurysm repair, as well as carotid artery stenosis (CAS). DU is also used more frequently in the assessment of abdominal vasculature as the experience of the operators and imaging capacity of the devices are expanding. Finally, DU is the imaging study of choice in screening the general population for abdominal aortic aneurysm. Clinical studies have shown that the quality of DU depends on the user's level of experience and that some arterial segments may be visualised more readily than others. However, it does not involve radiation or the use of contrast media and is relatively cheap, especially compared to modalities such as MDCTA and MRA. The main patient-associated limitations of DU include: heavily calcified vessels, very low flow (such as in the case of a low cardiac output), significant tissue oedema, obesity and presence of ulceration.

DU in Peripheral Arterial Disease

Ultrasound is now routinely used in the assessment of the vast majority of patients with peripheral arterial disease (PAD). It has been shown to be accurate in assessing stenoses of the vasculature in the upper and lower limbs [35, 36]. More specifically, several studies have looked at DU in isolation in planning peripheral bypass reconstruction in an emergency or semi-elective setting [37-40]. One year patency rates after bypass to the popliteal segment using DU as the sole pre-operative imaging modality are similar to those when using DSA or MDCTA reconstruction [37, 40]. Even infra-popliteal disease can be accurately assessed to allow planning for distal bypasses using DU, with similar patency rates compared to procedures planned with DSA [39, 41].

Besides baseline assessment and planning, DU is an acceptable imaging modality for surveillance of bypass conduits. Interestingly, a recent randomized controlled trial with 594 participants undergoing peripheral bypass demonstrated that intensive surveillance with DU did not show any additional benefit in terms of limb salvage rates for patients undergoing vein bypass graft operations, but it did incur additional costs [42]. If an imaging-guided surveillance programmed is in place, DU is usually the modality of choice, especially given that it performs very similarly to MDCTA or MRA [43, 44]. Testing frequency should be individualized to the patient, type of bypass, and degree of stenosis if one is indeed depicted. Graft surveillance should focus on the identification and repair of critical stenosis (peak systolic velocity exceeding 300 cm/s, and peak systolic velocity ratio across the stenosis exceeding 3.5) correlating with more than 70% diameter-reducing stenosis [43]. A graft surveillance program should result in a graft failure rate of less than 3% per year [43].

DU in Carotid Artery Disease

A large analysis of patients with carotid artery stenosis (CAS) who underwent DU imaging and DSA concluded that DU is similar to DSA in assessing high-grade CAS; however, it tends to lead to an overestimation of the degree of stenosis. Exclusion of 70%-99% angiographic stenosis with DU alone can be achieved with a sensitivity of 98% [45]. DU has been the procedure of choice in screening for CAS in the majority of the carotid trials to date [46]. Relevant diagnostic criteria and cut-offs for intervention have been reported by these trials with the NASCET and ECST criteria representing the most commonly used [47]. The recommended criteria, at least for the United Kingdom, are based on the NASCET method of grading carotid bulb disease. Key recommendations include recording peak systolic velocity (PSV) and end-diastolic velocity (EDV) in both internal and distal common carotid arteries; measuring all velocities at a Doppler angle of 45-60 degrees; the use of internal carotid PSV of >1.25 ms (-1) and >2.3 ms (-1) and a Peak Systolic Velocity Ratio of >2 and >4 to indicate >50% and >70% stenosis respectively; and the use of the St Mary's Ratio to grade >50% stenoses in deciles [47]. Regarding post-surgery or stenting stenoses, DU is also excellent in detecting recurrent disease with a sensitivity and specificity of greater than 95% compared to DSA [48]. The main advantage in using DU in assessing patients with CAS is the fact that it provides a dynamic image of the carotid plaque. High-risk plaques from symptomatic patients have been shown to demonstrate characteristics such as intraplaque hemorrhage, higher lipid content, larger lipid core, less distance between lipid core and flow lumen, and less calcium compared to plaques from asymptomatic patients [49].

DU in Post-EVAR Surveillance and Endoleak Assessment

The role of DU in surveillance after endovascular aneurysm repair (EVAR) and the assessment of possible endoleak remains controversial [50]. EVAR offers the advantage of lower perioperative mortality and morbidity [51] but carries the cost of device-related complications such as endoleak, graft migration, graft thrombosis, and structural graft failure [52]. These mandate a lifelong surveillance. A low sensitivity of DU in detecting endoleak has previously been reported, in the range of 25% to 42% [53-56]. However, one study has reported that DU is better at determining the subsequent intervention strategy than CT alone in the case of endoleak [57]. Overall, studies comparing CDU with CT scan for investigation of post-EVAR complications have produced mixed results [25]. Newer DU imaging modalities aided by the administration of contrast may be more accurate at depicting endoleak, avoiding the need for radiation (MDCTA). A recent meta-analysis of plain and contrast enhanced DU including 25 studies (3,975 paired scans) compared DU with CT for all types of endoleak after EVAR. The pooled sensitivity was 74% and the pooled specificity was 94% for all endoleaks. Thirteen studies (2,650 paired scans) reported detection of types 1 and 3 endoleak by DU; the pooled sensitivity was 83% and the pooled specificity was 100%. The pooled sensitivity of contrast endhanced DU was 96% with a specificity of 85% (all endoleaks). For type 1 and 3 endoleaks the sensititivity and specificity of contrast enhanced DU were 99% and 100% respectively [25]. Current practices among centres vary; however, given the results of the aforementioned recent meta-analysis a surveillance programme using radiographs (serially) to assess for migration and DU with or without contrast can be considered as safe and is employed by several centres.

References

[1] Perry JT, Statler JD. Advances in vascular imaging. *Surg. Clin. North Am.* 2007;87 (5):975-93, vii.

[2] Fitridge R, Quigley F, Vicaretti M. Should we develop a core international curriculum for Vascular and Endovascular Surgery? *Eur. J. Vasc. Endovasc. Surg.* 2010;39 Suppl 1:S10-4.

[3] Staub D, Partovi S, Imfeld S, Uthoff H, Baldi T, Aschwanden M, et al. Novel applications of contrast-enhanced ultrasound imaging in vascular medicine. *Vasa.* 2013;42 (1):17-31.

[4] Tepel M. Preventing nephropathy induced by contrast medium. *N. Engl. J. Med.* 2006;354 (17):1853-5; author reply -5.

[5] Saratzis AN, Goodyear S, Sur H, Saedon M, Imray C, Mahmood A. Acute kidney injury after endovascular repair of abdominal aortic aneurysm. *J. Endovasc. Ther.* 2013;20 (3):315-30.

[6] Walsh SR, Tang T, Gaunt ME, Boyle JR. Contrast-induced nephropathy. *J. Endovasc. Ther.* 2007;14 (1):92-100.

[7] Stacul F, van der Molen AJ, Reimer P, Webb JA, Thomsen HS, Morcos SK, et al. Contrast induced nephropathy: updated ESUR Contrast Media Safety Committee guidelines. *Eur. Radiol.* 2011;21 (12):2527-41.

[8] Saratzis A, Sarafidis P, Melas N, Saratzis N, Kitas G. Impaired renal function is associated with mortality and morbidity after endovascular abdominal aortic aneurysm repair. *J. Vasc. Surg.* 2013;58 (4):879-85.

[9] Hypertension: The Clinical Management of Primary Hypertension in Adults: Update of Clinical Guidelines 18 and 34. National Institute for Health and Clinical Excellence: Guidance. London2011.

[10] Eckardt KU, Kasiske BL. Kidney disease: improving global outcomes. *Nature reviews Nephrology.* 2009;5 (11):650-7.

[11] Prince MR, Arnoldus C, Frisoli JK. Nephrotoxicity of high-dose gadolinium compared with iodinated contrast. *J. Magn Reson Imaging.* 1996;6 (1):162-6.

[12] Ergun I, Keven K, Uruc I, Ekmekci Y, Canbakan B, Erden I, et al. The safety of gadolinium in patients with stage 3 and 4 renal failure. *Nephrol. Dial Transplant.* 2006;21 (3):697-700.

[13] Hellman RN. Gadolinium-induced nephrogenic systemic fibrosis. *Semin. Nephrol.* 2011;31 (3):310-6.

[14] Patel BN, Kapoor BS, Borghei P, Shah NA, Lockhart ME. Carbon dioxide as an intravascular imaging agent: review. *Curr. Probl. Diagn Radiol.* 2011;40 (5):208-17.

[15] Spinosa DJ, Angle JF, Hagspiel KD, Kern JA, Hartwell GD, Matsumoto AH. Lower extremity arteriography with use of iodinated contrast material or gadodiamide to supplement CO2 angiography in patients with renal insufficiency. *J. Vasc. Interv. Radiol.* 2000;11 (1):35-43.

[16] Lee AD, Hall RG. An evaluation of the use of carbon dioxide angiography in endovascular aortic aneurysm repair. *Vasc. Endovascular Surg.* 2010;44 (5):341-4.

[17] Criado E, Kabbani L, Cho K. Catheter-less angiography for endovascular aortic aneurysm repair: a new application of carbon dioxide as a contrast agent. *J. Vasc. Surg.* 2008;48 (3):527-34.

[18] Criado E, Upchurch GR, Jr., Young K, Rectenwald JE, Coleman DM, Eliason JL, et al. Endovascular aortic aneurysm repair with carbon dioxide-guided angiography in patients with renal insufficiency. *J. Vasc. Surg.* 2012;55 (6):1570-5.

[19] Cantisani V, Ricci P, Grazhdani H, Napoli A, Fanelli F, Catalano C, et al. Prospective comparative analysis of colour-Doppler ultrasound, contrast-enhanced ultrasound, computed tomography and magnetic resonance in detecting endoleak after endovascular abdominal aortic aneurysm repair. *Eur. J. Vasc. Endovasc. Surg.* 2011;41 (2):186-92.

[20] Giannoni MF, Citone M, Rossini M, Speziale F, David V. Role of contrast-enhanced ultrasound in the follow-up of endo-vascular aortic aneurysm repair: an effective and safe surveillance method. *Current pharmaceutical design.* 2012;18 (15):2214-22.

[21] Melas N, Saratzis A, Saratzis N, Kiskinis D. Endovascular repair of inadvertent subclavian artery perforation during cannulation for dialysis access: case report and review of the literature. *Eur. J. Emerg. Med.* 2009;16 (6):323-6.

[22] Heo YC, Lee HK, Yang HJ, Cho JH. Analysis of enlarged images using time-of-flight magnetic resonance angiography, computed tomography, and conventional angiography. *Journal of medical systems*. 2014;38 (12):146.

[23] Pua U, Tan K. Radiology of advanced EVAR techniques in complex abdominal aortic aneurysms. *Eur. Radiol*. 2012;22 (2):387-97.

[24] Ohana M, Georg Y, Lejay A, Girsowicz E, Gaertner S, Labani A, et al. Current optimal morphological evaluation of peripheral arterial diseases. *J. Cardiovasc. Surg*. (Torino). 2015;56 (2):287-97.

[25] Karthikesalingam A, Al-Jundi W, Jackson D, Boyle JR, Beard JD, Holt PJ, et al. Systematic review and meta-analysis of duplex ultrasonography, contrast-enhanced ultrasonography or computed tomography for surveillance after endovascular aneurysm repair. *Br. J. Surg*. 2012;99 (11):1514-23.

[26] Nordon IM, Karthikesalingam A, Hinchliffe RJ, Holt PJ, Loftus IM, Thompson MM. Secondary interventions following endovascular aneurysm repair (EVAR) and the enduring value of graft surveillance. *Eur. J. Vasc. Endovasc. Surg*. 2010;39 (5):547-54.

[27] Swanberg J, Nyman R, Magnusson A, Wanhainen A. Selective intra-arterial dual-energy CT angiography (s-CTA) in lower extremity arterial occlusive disease. *Eur. J. Vasc. Endovasc. Surg*. 2014;48 (3):325-9.

[28] Shareghi S, Gopal A, Gul K, Matchinson JC, Wong CB, Weinberg N, et al. Diagnostic accuracy of 64 multidetector computed tomographic angiography in peripheral vascular disease. *Catheter Cardiovasc Interv*. 2010;75 (1):23-31.

[29] Cinat ME, Casalme C, Wilson SE, Pham H, Anderson P. Computed tomography angiography validates duplex sonographic evaluation of carotid artery stenosis. *Am. Surg*. 2003;69 (10):842-7.

[30] Kock MC, Adriaensen ME, Pattynama PM, van Sambeek MR, van Urk H, Stijnen T, et al. DSA versus multi-detector row CT angiography in peripheral arterial disease: randomized controlled trial. *Radiology*. 2005;237 (2):727-37.

[31] Magarelli N, Scarabino T, Simeone AL, Florio F, Carriero A, Salvolini U, et al. Carotid stenosis: a comparison between MR and spiral CT angiography. *Neuroradiology*. 1998;40 (6):367-73.

[32] Nederkoorn PJ, van der Graaf Y, Hunink MG. Duplex ultrasound and magnetic resonance angiography compared with digital subtraction angiography in carotid artery stenosis: a systematic review. *Stroke*. 2003;34 (5):1324-32.

[33] Tao W, Shen Y, Guo L, Bo G. Role of non-contrast balanced steady-state free precession megnetic resonance angiography compared to contrast-enhanced megnetic resonance angiography in diagnosing renal artery stenosis: a meta-analysis. *Chin. Med. J. (Engl)*. 2014;127 (19):3483-90.

[34] Albert TS, Akahane M, Parienty I, Yellin N, Catala V, Alomar X, et al. An international multicenter comparison of time-SLIP unenhanced MR angiography and contrast-enhanced CT angiography for assessing renal artery stenosis: the renal artery contrast-free trial. *AJR Am. J. Roentgenol*. 2015;204 (1):182-8.

[35] Eiberg JP, Gronvall Rasmussen JB, Hansen MA, Schroeder TV. Duplex ultrasound scanning of peripheral arterial disease of the lower limb. *Eur. J. Vasc. Endovasc. Surg*. 2010;40 (4):507-12.

[36] Kakkos SK, Tsolakis IA. Is duplex ultrasound scanning for peripheral arterial disease of the lower limb a non-invasive alternative or an adjunct to angiography? *Eur. J. Vasc. Endovasc. Surg*. 2010;40 (4):513-4.

[37] Ascher E, Hingorani A, Markevich N, Costa T, Kallakuri S, Khanimoy Y. Lower extremity revascularization without preoperative contrast arteriography: experience with duplex ultrasound arterial mapping in 485 cases. *Ann. Vasc. Surg*. 2002;16 (1):108-14.

[38] Ascher E, Hingorani A, Markevich N, Schutzer R, Kallakuri S. Acute lower limb ischemia: the value of duplex ultrasound arterial mapping (DUAM) as the sole preoperative imaging technique. *Ann. Vasc. Surg*. 2003;17 (3):284-9.

[39] Ascher E, Mazzariol F, Hingorani A, Salles-Cunha S, Gade P. The use of duplex ultrasound arterial mapping as an alternative to conventional arteriography for primary and secondary infrapopliteal bypasses. *Am. J. Surg*. 1999;178 (2):162-5.

[40] Mazzariol F, Ascher E, Hingorani A, Gunduz Y, Yorkovich W, Salles-Cunha S. Lower-extremity revascularisation without preoperative contrast arteriography in 185 cases: lessons learned with duplex ultrasound arterial mapping. *Eur. J. Vasc. Endovasc. Surg*. 2000;19 (5):509-15.

[41] Grassbaugh JA, Nelson PR, Rzucidlo EM, Schermerhorn ML, Fillinger MF, Powell RJ, et al. Blinded comparison of preoperative duplex ultrasound scanning and contrast arteriography for planning revascularization at the level of the tibia. *J. Vasc. Surg*. 2003;37 (6):1186-90.

[42] Mills JL, Sr. Is duplex surveillance of value after leg vein bypass grafting? Principal results of the Vein Graft Surveillance Randomised Trial (VGST). *Perspect Vasc. Surg. Endovasc. Ther*. 2006;18 (2):194-6.

[43] Bandyk DF. Surveillance after lower extremity arterial bypass. *Perspect Vasc.Surg. Endovasc. Ther*. 2007;19 (4):376-83; discussion 84-5.

[44] Willmann JK, Mayer D, Banyai M, Desbiolles LM, Verdun FR, Seifert B, et al. Evaluation of peripheral arterial bypass grafts with multi-detector row CT angiography: comparison with duplex US and digital subtraction angiography. *Radiology*. 2003;229 (2):465-74.

[45] Sabeti S, Schillinger M, Mlekusch W, Willfort A, Haumer M, Nachtmann T, et al. Quantification of internal carotid artery stenosis with duplex US: comparative analysis of different flow velocity criteria. *Radiology*. 2004;232 (2):431-9.

[46] Yavin D, Roberts DJ, Tso M, Sutherland GR, Eliasziw M, Wong JH. Carotid endarterectomy versus stenting: a meta-analysis of randomized trials. *The Canadian journal of neurological sciences Le journal canadien des sciences neurologiques*. 2011;38 (2):230-5.

[47] Oates CP, Naylor AR, Hartshorne T, Charles SM, Fail T, Humphries K, et al. Joint recommendations for reporting carotid ultrasound investigations in the United Kingdom. *Eur. J. Vasc. Endovasc. Surg*. 2009;37 (3):251 61.

[48] Telman G, Kouperberg E, Sprecher E, Gruberg L, Beyar R, Hoffman A, et al. Duplex ultrasound verified by angiography in patients with severe primary and restenosis of internal carotid artery. *Ann. Vasc. Surg*. 2006;20 (4):478-81.

[49] Mayor I, Momjian S, Lalive P, Sztajzel R. Carotid plaque: comparison between visual and grey-scale median analysis. *Ultrasound Med. Biol*. 2003;29 (7):961-6.

[50] Karanikola E, Dalainas I, Karaolanis G, Zografos G, Filis K. Duplex Ultrasound versus Computed Tomography for the Postoperative Follow-Up of Endovascular Abdominal Aortic Aneurysm Repair. Where Do We Stand Now? *The International journal of angiology : official publication of the International College of Angiology*, Inc. 2014;23 (3):155-64.

[51] Sadat U, Boyle JR, Walsh SR, Tang T, Varty K, Hayes PD. Endovascular vs open repair of acute abdominal aortic aneurysms--a systematic review and meta-analysis. *J. Vasc. Surg*. 2008;48 (1):227-36.

[52] Melas N, Saratzis A, Saratzis N, Lazaridis J, Psaroulis D, Trygonis K, et al. Aortic and iliac fixation of seven endografts for abdominal-aortic aneurysm repair in an experimental model using human cadaveric aortas. *Eur. J. Vasc. Endovasc. Surg*. 2010;40 (4):429-35.

[53] Bakken AM, Illig KA. Long-term follow-up after endovascular aneurysm repair: is ultrasound alone enough? *Perspect Vasc. Surg. Endovasc. Ther.* 2010;22 (3):145-51.

[54] Clevert DA, Minaifar N, Weckbach S, Kopp R, Meimarakis G, Clevert DA, et al. Color duplex ultrasound and contrast-enhanced ultrasound in comparison to MS-CT in the detection of endoleak following endovascular aneurysm repair. *Clin. Hemorheol. Microcirc. 2008*;39 (1-4):121-32.

[55] Elkouri S, Panneton JM, Andrews JC, Lewis BD, McKusick MA, Noel AA, et al. Computed tomography and ultrasound in follow-up of patients after endovascular repair of abdominal aortic aneurysm. *Ann. Vasc. Surg*. 2004;18 (3):271-9.

[56] Sandford RM, Bown MJ, Fishwick G, Murphy F, Naylor M, Sensier Y, et al. Duplex ultrasound scanning is reliable in the detection of endoleak following endovascular aneurysm repair. *Eur. J. Vasc. Endovasc. Surg*. 2006;32 (5):537-41.

[57] Schmieder GC, Stout CL, Stokes GK, Parent FN, Panneton JM. Endoleak after endovascular aneurysm repair: duplex ultrasound imaging is better than computed tomography at determining the need for intervention. *J. Vasc. Surg*. 2009;50 (5):1012-7; discussion 7-8.

In: The Role of Imaging Technology …
Editor: Georgios Tsoulfas ISBN: 978-1-63483-490-2

Chapter 2

THE ROLE OF IMAGING IN COLORECTAL SURGERY

M. G. Pramateftakis*[*,1], A. Kalogera-Fountzila[2], K. Sapalidis[1] and E. Kotidis[1]

[1]3rd Surgical Department, AHEPA Hospital,
Aristotle University of Thessaloniki, Greece
[2]Department of Radiology, AHEPA Hospital,
Aristotle University of Thessaloniki, Greece

ABSTRACT

Colorectal surgery manages diseases of the small and large bowel, rectum, anal canal and pelvic floor. The colorectal surgeon undertakes a large array of minor and major, elective and emergency procedures. One of the main instruments in his quiver, aiding in the diagnostics of various diseases and conditions, are the radiological investigations. Plain radiographs have been used for many decades to assess patients with abdominal symptoms, but they have been replaced in the last years by more advanced techniques, such as computed topographies, magnetic resonance imaging and nuclear tests.

This chapter aims to introduce the reader to most of the radiological tests available to the colorectal surgeon today; some very specialized/specific tests will not be mentioned, as the authors believe that they are outside the aim of the book. Furthermore, we will look at specific diseases and pathologies and how radiological findings aid in their management and treatment.

ANATOMY OF THE COLON AND RECTUM

The colon frames the abdomen and is surrounded by fat. It has five distinguished portions: the cecum, the ascending, transverse, descending and sigmoid colon and the rectum, with a length of 1.5 m from the ileocecal valve to the distal rectum. Three longitudinal bands, the teniae, approximately 8 mm wide, run the length of the colon on its outer surface and

[*] Corresponding author: M.G. Pramateftakis, Department of Surgery, Aristotle University of Thessaloniki, Email: mpramateftakis@hotmail.com

merge in the appendicocecal and the rectosigmoid junction. Between the teniae, prominent saculations are formed known as the haustrae. Along the teniae run epiploic appendices, which are small packets of fat. Their size depends on the nutritional status of the individual. The calibre of the colon varies from a 9 cm diameter in the cecum, to 6 cm in the transverse colon and with a slightly smaller diameter in the descending and sigmoid colon, with a large variation in the caliber of the rectum. The thickness of the wall is less than 3 mm; when the bowel is distended it is barely seen.

The rectum is bound by the sigmoid colon and the anus, extending 12 cm above the anal verge. Its proximal portion is located in the peritoneal cavity while the distal portion is extraperitoneal. The dentate line, extending for 5-10 mm in the anal canal, separates the rectal columnar epithelium from the anal squamous epithelium. At the rectosigmoid junction, the confluence of the taenia coli muscles form a surgically recognized line, at the level of the sacral promontory and the peritoneal reflection. The rectum is supplied by the inferior mesenteric and the superior and middle hemorrhoidal arteries. The proximal part is drained by the inferior mesenteric vein via the portal vein, while the distal part is drained by the internal ileac veins via the inferior vena cava. This venous drainage explains why cancers of the distal rectum usually form metastases in the lung, whereas proximal rectal cancers usually metastasize to the liver. Hemorrhoidal venous plexi, internal and external, are located on either side of the dentate line, causing hemorrhoids when dilated. Three valves of Houston project into the lumen, being normal folds in the mucosa, run up the length of the rectum in a spiral way. The internal anal sphincter is the thickening and continuation of the circular muscle layer of the rectum. The external sphincter is composed by the inferior portion of the levator ani muscle, the puborectalis muscle and the deep, superficial and subcutaneous external sphincter muscles. The wall of the rectum consists of five layers—the mucosa, the muscularis mucosa, the submucosa, the muscularis propria and the serosa—that are easily recognized in T2 weighted images at magnetic resonance imaging (MRI). On the MRI, one can also recognize the mesorectal fat and the fascia surrounding the rectum [1-4].

IMAGING

Plain Radiographs

Plain radiographs have always been a quick tool for assessment of bowel symptoms. 3 views are usually taken: The supine, which contrasts intra-abdominal organs and shows retroperitoneal air. The decubitus, which displays gas distribution in the bowel loops.

The erect chest radiograph, which detects extraluminal intra-abdominal air, presenting as free air under the diaphragm. Plain radiographs of the abdomen in these three positions can reveal signs of obstructive or paralytic ileus with air fluid levels and bowel distention (Figure 1), free peritoneal or retroperitoneal air (Figure 2), as well as stones (such as appendicoliths), calcifications and foreign bodies. Furthermore, it can aid in the diagnosis of pseudo-obstruction, volvulus or colitis.

The best indication for a plain abdominal x-ray is a patient with symptoms of bowel obstruction, and it aids in the differentiation between small and large bowel obstruction. As a rule of thumb, the more distal the obstruction, the more dilated loops of small bowel can be seen. In case of large bowel obstruction, the appearance and gas distribution may be similar to the one of small bowel. Small bowel loops have plicae circulares, which traverse the whole lumen diameter, whereas colon shows haustral markings that do not reach the opposite wall.

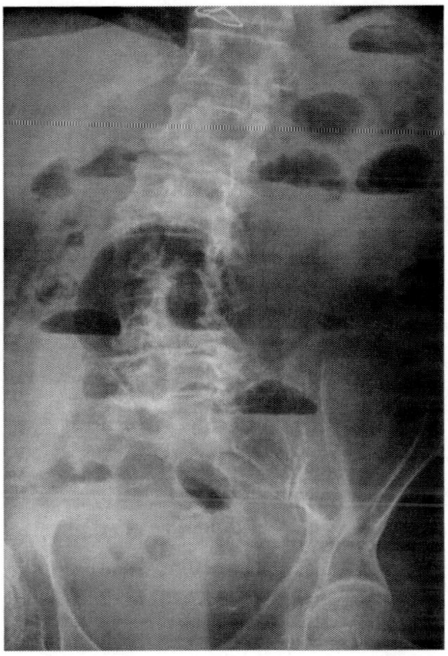

Figure 1. Abdominal x-ray showing typical air-fluid levels of small bowel loops in the central and lower abdomen, suggestive of small bowel obstruction.

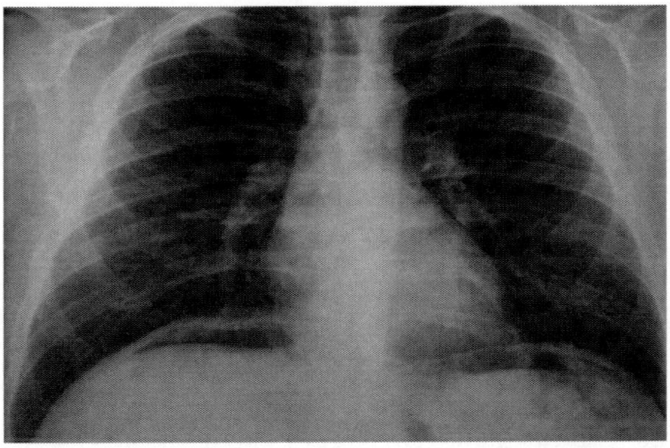

Figure 2. Erect chest radiograph, displaying free intraabdominal air under the diaphragm, suggestive of perforation of intraabdominal viscus.

Contrast Studies

Barium enema or air enema examination has acted as the gold standard examination in diagnosis of large bowel diseases for many years. In recent years, it has been replaced by more advanced techniques such as computed tomography (CT) and MRI. These tests allow a more precise evaluation of mucosal or submucosal, benign or neoplastic lesions, which is of course aided by the use of endoscopy. Cross sectional imaging can show the entire length of the large intestine and the thickness of the bowel wall, with the complementary evaluation of the surrounding tissues, the extent of the disease, the origin and the internal composition of the lesion [3, 4].

Two different forms of contrast agents have been used to visualize colonic abnormalities: Barium studies and water-soluble contrast studies. Furthermore, one can differentiate between single and double contrast studies. Single contrast studies, using one medium to detect colonic lesions, are limited to only lesions of larger size. Double-contrast studies use gas as the second medium, which creates a thin coating on the mucosal surface allowing visualization of smaller lesions. Good bowel preparation is essential for any contrast study.

Double contrast barium enemas are simple and risk-free to perform and can rule out gross pathologies. They are obviously less accurate than endoscopy, as they can miss smaller lesions, there is no direct visualization and no biopsy possibility. Contrast enemas are, nevertheless, extremely useful in case of failed or incomplete colonoscopies, where the patient has undergone bowel preparation already.

In the case of a suspicion of perforation, barium as a contrast needs to be avoided. In this case, a water-soluble contrast such as Gastrografin® or Urografin® has to be used. When given orally, these agents also have a therapeutic effect on small bowel paralytic ileus. Contrast agents can also be used to visualize anastomotic integrity in colorectal or coloanal anastomoses and to visualize ileoanal pouches, giving information about the pouch's form, function and volume [5, 6].

Computed Tomography

Computed tomography (CT) is one of the commonest investigations undertaken by surgeons on a daily basis. CT takes cross-sectional images of the body and the computer software combines them to create tomographic images of the organ / body area of interest. Conventional CT scanning takes images at 1-cm intervals, whereas modern spiral CT scanners produce a continuous image as the camera rotates around the patient. Accurate CT imaging requires the opacification of the gastrointestinal tract and the vessels with the use of contrast medium, which is given as a bolus at the beginning of the investigation. CT is extremely useful in identifying postoperative complications but is also used in the investigation of non-specific abdominal symptoms and the staging of colorectal cancer. Images are obtained in two phases: the hepatic arterial and the portal venous phase. The radiologist analyzes the contrast behavior in various phases and concludes on the presenting pathology. Staging of colorectal cancer using CT includes assessment of the liver, grading of lymphadenopathy and assessment of possible intraperitoneal disease.

CT Colonography

CT colonography is also known as a virtual colonoscopy. Its accuracy is higher than that of the conventional CT, but the patients require full bowel preparation as for colonoscopy. Furthermore, they are exposed to radiation, even though there is no evidence that this radiation induces additional carcinogenesis. It is a good solution in patients too frail or unwell to undergo colonoscopy. The use of faecal tagging (with agents such as meglumine ioxithalamate) coats any residual bowel contents not cleared by the laxatives and allows the radiologist to substract remaining faeces from the images, minimizing the risk of false positive results [7, 8].

Magnetic Resonance Imaging

MRI scanners use magnetic fields to acquire images of the body. Water molecules in tissues are used to create signals, translated into images. The radio-frequency emitted by the hydrogen atoms is measured by receiving coils. The contrast between various tissues is determined by the rate the hydrogen atoms return to their state of equilibrium. Contrast agents are given orally or intravenously.

Image contrast can be weighted to demonstrate different anatomical structures. Tissues return to their equilibrium states by the independent processes of T1 or T2 relaxation. T1-weighted images are better for assessing morphological information, whereas T2-weighted images are useful in detecting oedema and inflammation. MR Diffusion Weighted Imaging (DWI) measures the diffusivity of extracellular water. This is a very rapid acquisition which can identify active inflammation in inflammatory conditions of the colon and rectum, being equivalent to contrast enhanced MRI [9-11].

MRI is a very important tool for the management of anorectal diseases, the two most important being low rectal cancers and perianal fistulas. MRI is used for the accurate staging of rectal cancer, leading to tailored case-guided treatment protocols. Similarly, the topography of complex perianal fistulas can be very well assessed by MRI, showing the exact location of tracts and abscesses, which can map the surgical exploration.

Scintigraphy (Radionuclide Imaging)

For scintigraphy, an isotope is administered within the body or a specific organ. A gamma-camera (also called a scintillation camera) picks up the radiation emitted by the isotope. Depending on the organ being scanned, the physician can choose a specific isotope. For example, thalium is preferred for cardiac stress tests, whereas technetium99m-sestamibi is used to detect parathyroid adenomas. In colorectal practice, GI bleeding can be detected by tagging red blood cells with Technetium99m and re-injecting them into the patient.

Positron Emission Tomography

Positron emission tomography (PET) produces a three-dimensional image of functional body processes. It studies metabolic activity in tissues. A low-dose radionuclide (tracer) is coupled with glucose and injected intravenously. The PET scanning system measures the photon emission of the tracer within the body and constructs a 3D-image. Because malignant tumors consume glucose faster than normal tissue, this can be displayed as a dynamic image. PET-CT is a hybrid technique utilizing the strengths of PET and CT. It is powerful in detecting disease recurrence and has become established in assessing response to oncological treatment [E].

Defecography

Defecography is a traditional imaging technique, evaluating the functional aspects of the anorectal region. Even though it can be used to define various pathologies, its main strength lies in the understanding of postoperative conditions. Following formation of an ileo-anal pouch, a low colo-anal anastomosis for a low rectal tumor or a stapled resection of a rectal doughnut during a STARR procedure, the defecogram can give answers to the new anatomical configuration and the efficiency of the pelvic floor work during defecation. After insertion of radiopaque contrast (most commonly paste) in the rectum, a patient is asked to defecate. This test will pick up poor emptying, poor contrast retention, rectal pockets and rectoceles, giving also the possibility of measuring their size. Furthermore, it can identify sinus tracts, strictures and ulcerations.

Colorectal Diagnostics

There are a number of mucosal and submucosal lesions, neoplastic or non-neoplastic, that can be identified and have to be differentiated in the wall of the colon and rectum. Neoplastic lesions include adenocarcinomas, dysplastic or carcinomatoid polyps, lipomas, carcinoid tumors, lymphomas, hemangiomas, gastrointestinal stromal tumors, metastases, as well as direct bowel invasion of extracolonic tumor and peritoneal carcinomatosis. Non-neoplastic lesions include lymphoid polyps and hyperplasia, vascular lesions, cystic lesions, hematomas, endometriosis, extrinsic impressions, and pre-sacral lesions. Imaging studies play an important role in differentiating neoplastic or non-neoplastic lesions, as well as in the evaluation of patients for screening and staging of colorectal cancer. Below we are mentioning the most common colorectal conditions a surgeon is faced with, and the radiological tests he has available, to aid him to the correct diagnosis.

Infective / Inflammatory Conditions of the Colon and Rectum

Appendicitis

Inflammation of the appendix vermiformis results in the commonest acute abdominal presentation in hospitals nowadays, namely appendicitis, which is expressed with right lower quadrant pain, fever and nausea/vomiting. Appendiceal lumen occlusion results in accumulation of fluid in the appendix with lumen dilatation (>6 mm), inflammation and ischemia with wall thickening of more than 2 mm. Furthermore, it can lead to stranding of the pericaecal fat, perforation and abscess formation (Figure 3). An appendicolith (a calcified deposit within the appendix) is detected in 25% to 40% of cases. CT is routinely used as the initial imaging modality in adults with suspicion of appendicitis, with high accuracy rates, while ultrasonography (US) is preferably used in children, young adults and pregnant women. At MRI, STIR (short tau inversion recovery) images and single shot T2 images can easily reveal fluid in the periappendicular fat and wall thickening respectively, whereas strong contrast enhancement and restricted diffusion is indicative of appendicitis. The latter can also provide information about abscess formation [2, 13-15].

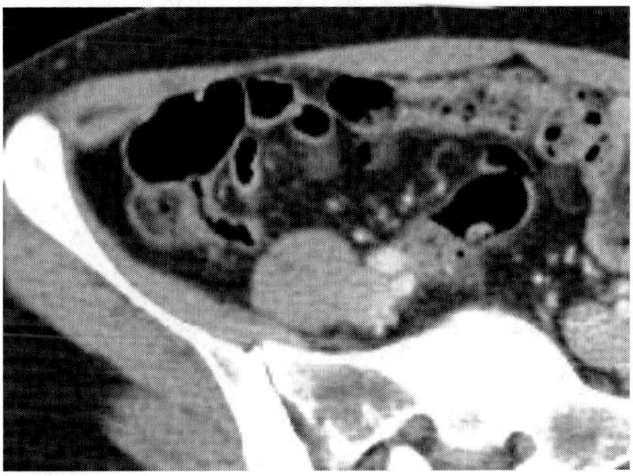

Figure 3. 38 year old female with right lower abdominal pain and leucocytosis. CT shows appendiceal wall thickening, lumen dilatation, inflammation and stranding of the pericecal fat, suggestive of appendicitis.

Epiploic Appendagitis

Torsion or venous thrombosis of one of the appendices epiploicae can result in inflammation or ischemia of the appendix, with sudden focal abdominal pain. An oval, up to 4 cm, fatty paracolic lesion accompanied by mesenteric inflammation is seen on CT, with a central dot corresponding to the thrombosed vein [2, 15].

Typhlitis

Typhlitis, also known as neutropenic enterocolitis, describes the inflammation and often necrosis of the cecum, ascending colon and terminal ileum. It can lead to edema, wall thickening and subsequent perforation. Clinical symptoms include fever, diarrhea and pain in the right lower quadrant. It is most often seen in neutropenic patients usually due to chemotherapy for leukemia or lymphoma, in patients with aplastic anemia, AIDS, or following kidney transplantation. Ischemia, cytomegalovirus infection and neoplastic infiltration are the probable mechanisms of the inflammation. In CT, hypodense wall thickening due to submural edema and sometimes intramural air is seen, as well as fat stranding and intraperitoneal free fluid or air [2, 15] (Figure 4).

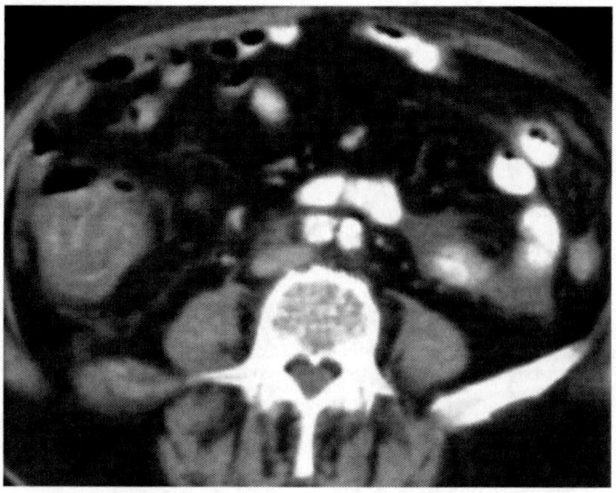

Figure 4. CT of a neutropenic patient following chemotherapy for leukemia. Ischemia of the cecum, hypodense wall thickening due to submural edema as well as fat stranding, suggestive of typhlitis.

Diverticulitis

Diverticulae represent small pouches of the colonic mucosa and submucosa through the muscular layers of the colonic wall, where the vessels pierce the muscularis, between the mesenteric and antimesenteric teniae. Diverticulosis corresponds to the presence of multiple diverticulae seen as air filled pouches, measuring from 2-3 mm to 2 cm. They are most commonly located in the sigmoid colon. Diverticulosis is a very common condition nowadays, mostly related to modern diet and lifestyle. Occlusion of the neck of the diverticulum results in inflammation, called diverticulitis. Findings of diverticulitis are very well seen in contrast enhanced CT, with or without oral contrast medium (Figures 5, 6a, 6b).

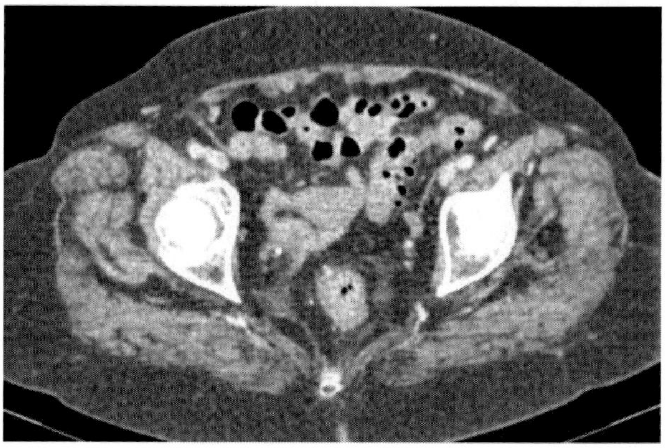

Figure 5. Diverticulosis. Non-inflammed pouches of the transverse and sigmoid colon.

Diverticulitis can lead to localised perforation, pericolic inflammation with fat stranding and presence of free air in the peritoneal cavity or retroperitoneum. Differential diagnosis of right colon diverticulitis, even though uncommon, can be made from appendicitis with careful analysis of CT images. In a study by Padidar et al, CT differentiation is made between acute diverticulitis and colonic cancer. Diverticulitis causes fluid in the root of the sigmoid mesentery as well as engorgement of mesenteric vasculature, whereas in colon cancer enlarged pericolic lymphnodes are found. Coronal STIR MRI and axial T2 images, as well as contrast enhanced and diffusion images, can also diagnose diverticulitis and its complications [2, 7, 15, 16-20].

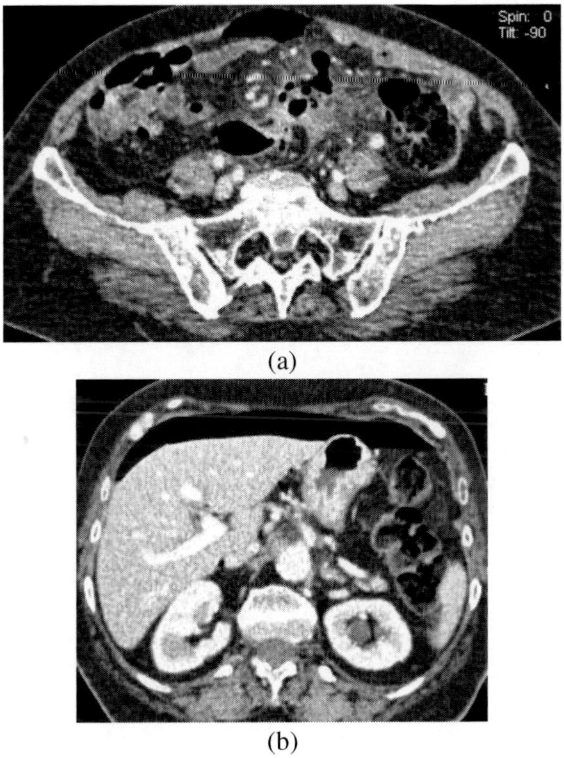

Figure 6. CT scan of a patient with diverticulitis. Inflammatory pericolic fat stranding and enhancement, with perforation and presence of free air locally in the peritoneal cavity (6a) with excessive air in the subphrenic space (6b).

Radiation Colitis

Following radiotherapy, any part of the colon can be affected, with acute findings of wall thickening and fat stranding. Chronic radiation injury causes strictures and fistulas, and can present with increased pelvic fat and thickening of perirectal fibrous tissue. All findings are best appreciated on CT images [2].

Ischemic Colitis

Ischemic Colitis is a cause of abdominal pain most commonly in the elderly. Causative factors can be colonic hypoperfusion, trauma, tumor invasion and mesenteric vascular occlusion by thrombus or embolus. When hypovolaemia is the etiologic factor, ischemic changes can be seen in the border of main vascular territories, such as in the splenic flexure and the rectosigmoid.

When ischemia is suspected, CT evaluation of the colon can reveal diffuse or segmental circumferential, symmetric wall thickening with fold enlargement. The double halo or target sign, which can be seen in the thickened bowel wall, is due to hypodense submural edema and hyperdense intramural hemorrhage (Figures 7a, 7b). Thrombosis or embolic disease can easily be delineated by CT (Figures 8a, 8b), as well as the presence of intramular air or air in the mesenteric and portal veins (Figures 9a, 9b), a finding suggestive of bowel necrosis. Imaging of thrombosis or embolic disease, vasoconstriction, as well as aortic dissection relies mainly on CT or MRI angiographic techniques. MRI coronal STIR images can reveal the area of ischemic bowel with thickening of the wall and infiltration of the surrounding fat, while axial T2 images can be unremarkable. Patchy bowel enhancement in contrast enhanced MR images show the disturbed perfusion of the bowel wall. In conservatively treated patients, the colon can sometimes return to normal, with development of strictures of the involved segment [2, 16].

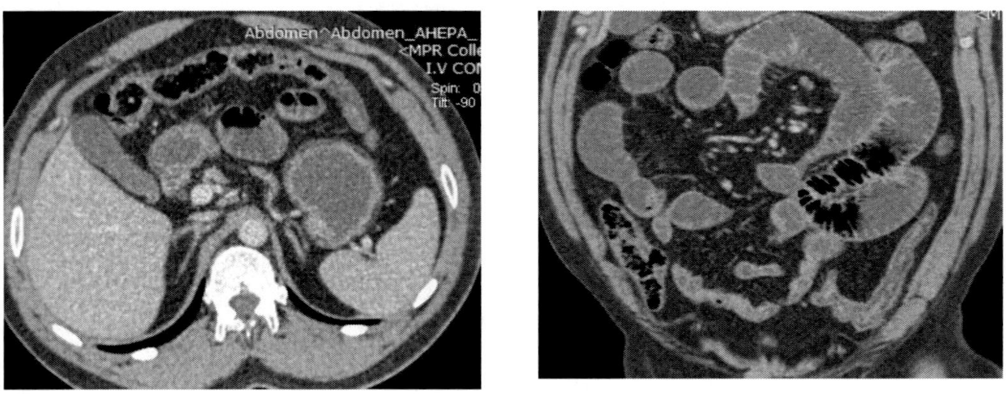

(a) (b)

Figure 7. Axial (7a) and coronal (7b) reformation in a patient with hypovolemia and ischemic changes in the small and large bowel. Symmetric wall thickening, double halo or target sign (hypodense submural edema and hyperdense intramural hemorrhage) that can be seen in the thickened wall.

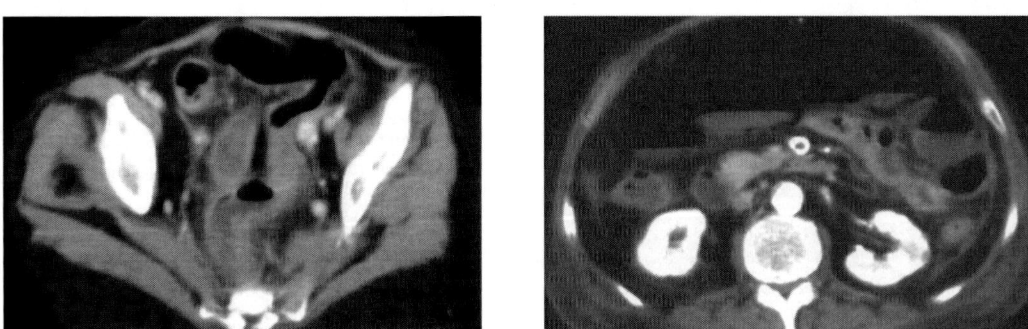

(a) (b)

Figure 8. Necrosis of the rectum and the sigmoid colon (8a) in an 80 years old man due to embolic disease in IMA, that is shown non-enhanced with extensive wall calcifications in 8b.

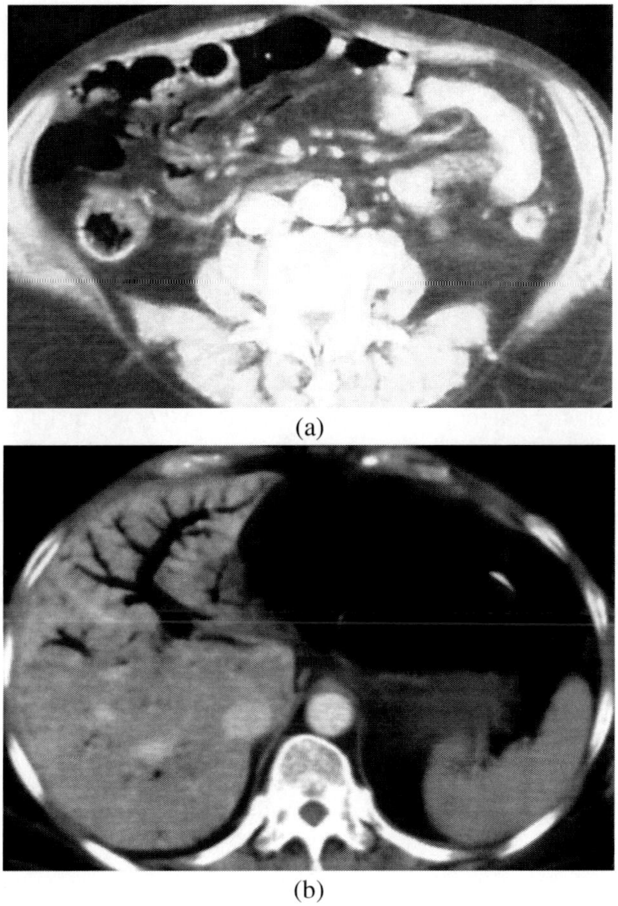

Figure 9. Presence of air in the mesenteric veins (9a) and portal vein (9b) due to bowel necrosis in a 79 years old patient.

Infectious Colitis

Bacteria, fungi and viruses can cause infectious colitis that can affect any portion of the colon. The definitive diagnosis is given mainly by laboratory tests. CT, when utilized, reveals bowel wall thickening with intramural diffuse or segmental edema, depending on the causative microorganism, with presence of pericolic inflammation and ascites [2].

Pseudomembranous Colitis

Antibiotic therapy, hypovolemia, chemotherapy or abdominal surgery can cause overgrowth of clostridium difficile, which results in pseudomembranous colitis (secondary to the production of toxins). Associated symptoms include diarrhea, fever and abdominal pain. On CT, the colon is dilated with wall thickening due to edema and a visible target sign. Significant haustral thickening with oral contrast entrapment can be seen, known as the accordion sign. The wall thickening is irregular and shaggy as well as greater than the thickness observed in other inflammatory bowel conditions. Only in Crohn's disease is the amount of wall thickness as great as it is in pseudomembranous colitis but it is symmetric and homogeneous [2].

INFLAMMATORY BOWEL DISEASES (IBD)

The incidence of inflammatory bowel disease in the Western World has increased in the past 50 years up to 8–14/100,000 patients for ulcerative colitis (UC) and up to 6–15/100,000 patients for Crohn's disease (CD). It is continuing to increase worldwide. The occurrence in the pediatric population is 4.56 per 100,000 children [21-23].

The principal tools for diagnosis and evaluation of suspected inflammatory bowel disease are CT and MRI, although classic barium studies are still used with sometimes equivocal results. CT and MRI have the advantage of visualization of the bowel wall, adjacent structures, extra luminal disease and complications in both diseases. The imaging modalities of choice are CT and/or MRI, with similar sensitivities in diagnosing IBD, with the latter being more sensitive in the detection of strictures and fistulas. MRI is the preferred modality in children and young adults because of lack of ionizing radiation and the potential in differentiation of chronic from acute disease, especially with the use of Diffusion Weighted Imaging. Restricted diffusion correlates with the severity of IBD, being an indicator of severe complications such as bowel perforation and abscess formation [11, 16, 21-23].

Ulcerative Colitis

Ulcerative colitis occurs more frequently in men and it is a typically left sided, diffuse disease (colon and rectum). It rarely involves the right colon only and it extends in a continuous retrograde mode. Wall thickening, with a mean of about 7.8 mm, may be diffuse and symmetric in thickness (Figure 10). A low attenuation ring, like a halo sign, can commonly be seen in the thickened bowel wall, due to deposition of submucosal fat [2, 11, 21].

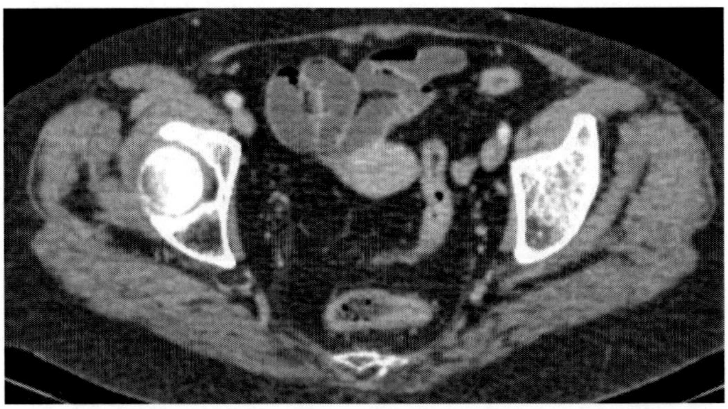

Figure 10. Ulcerative colitis: Diffuse and symmetric sigmoid wall thickening.

Crohn's Disease

CD occurs more frequently in women and it usually involves the right colon and small intestine with a mean wall thickening of about 11–13 mm that may be eccentric and segmental with skip regions. The thickened edematous bowel wall enhances strongly and homogeneously and it is accompanied by proliferation of mesenteric fat and mesenteric lymphadenopathy. (Figures 11, 12) Fibrofatty proliferation can also be seen in UC and in other inflammatory conditions of the bowel wall.

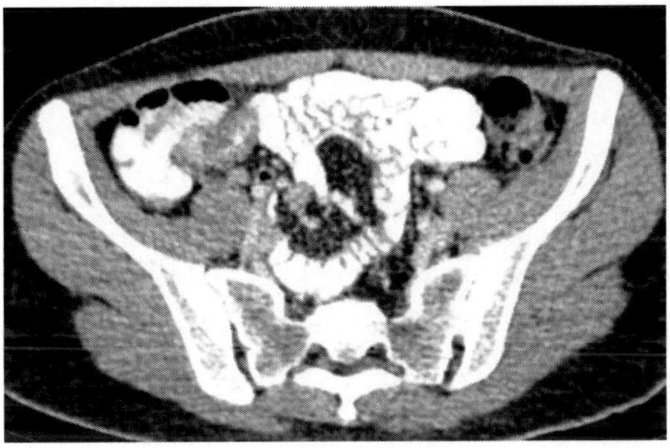

Figure 11. Transverse CT image of a young patient with Crohn's disease. Thickened and edematous bowel wall at the ileocecal valve and terminal ileum.

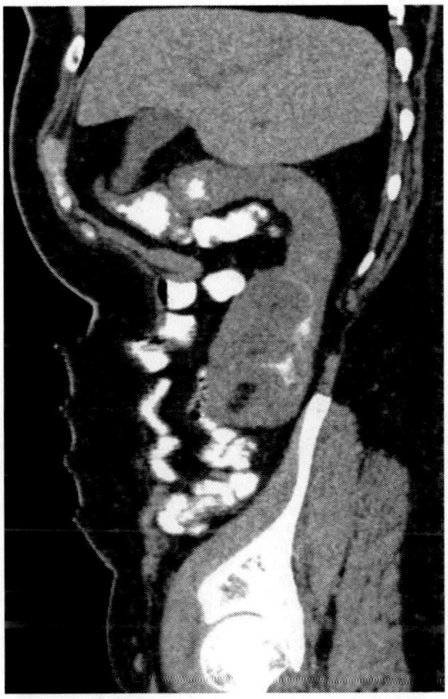

Figure 12. Saggital reformative CT image of a patient with Crohn's disease in the ileocecal valve, cecum and ascending colon with asymmetrically thickened wall.

CT and MRI can visualize abscesses, strictures and fistulas as complications of CD. Abscesses can be confined to the bowel wall and pericolic fat, or can involve adjacent structures that can be drained under CT or US guidance. CD begins with apthous ulcers that develop into strictures and fistulas. Fistulas can be enteroenteric, enterocutaneous, enterovesical, rectovaginal or perianal. They can be evaluated with MRI, as well as with CT performed after oral or rectal contrast administration. Fistulas are more frequent in patients with terminal ileal disease. Large bowel Crohn's disease can remain uncomplicated for years. The diagnosis of terminal ileitis mainly relies on MRI, coronal STIR and axial T2 images. Lymphadenopathy is easily depicted with DWI [2, 11, 15, 19-23].

Colorectal Cancer

Computed Tomography

CT enterography and CT colonography provides important information about TNM staging in preoperative assessment of colon cancer, as well as information about vascular anatomy. Standard colon window settings should be used, with a width of 1,500 Hounsfield Units (HU) and a level of -200 HU, as well as abdominal window settings with a width of 440 HU and a level of 20 HU.

The ability of CT colonography to demonstrate lesions >10 mm is very good. On the contrary small polyps, adenomas or lipomas < 5mm are impossible to be demonstrated, while lesions of 6-9 mm are demonstrated with less sensitivity compared to the larger ones. Colorectal carcinogenesis occurs after a series of mutations, as a polyp progresses from adenoma to adenocarcinoma. Larger polyps more likely harbor dysplasia or malignancy compared to sessile polyps, whereas pedunculated lesions do not usually harbor malignancies. An attempt should be made for lesions 6-9 mm to be removed colonoscopically. Larger polyps may be removed endoscopically but may require surgery, given the technical difficulties due to their size.

Flat colorectal lesions are difficult to identify at CT colonography, as are small or larger lesions that are hidden behind folds. Large carcinomas are either fungating masses or areas of mucosal irregularity homogeneously enhanced, that in a 5% of cases can be accompanied by a synchronous carcinoma elsewhere in the colon (Figure 13).

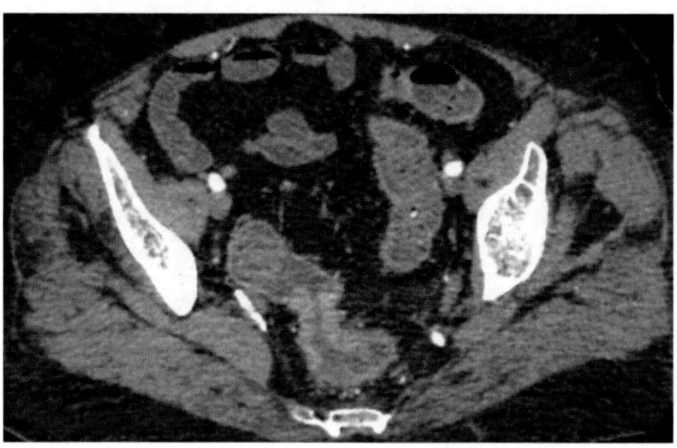

Figure 13. Sigmoid cancer: Mucosal irregular thickening of the sigmoid colon and stranding of the pericolic fat.

Lymphnode metastases from colorectal cancer often present with calcifications, as do liver metastases in about 10%-30% of cases.

Liver metastases are hypoattenuating lesions in non-enhanced CT scans, with rim enhancement in the arterial phase and heterogeneous enhancement in portal venous phase. Most of the lesions depicted in the lung are benign unless they are multiple and the primary tumor is located in the distal part of the rectum [3, 24, 25].

Magnetic Resonance Imaging

MRI, MR enterography and MR colonography with the use of DWI and T2 imaging can also give important information about TNM staging in colon but especially in rectal cancer. MRI has proven to be priceless in the analysis of rectal cancers, where one can evaluate intraluminal and extraluminal extent, mesorectal involvement, and assessment of tissues beyond the mesorectal fascia.

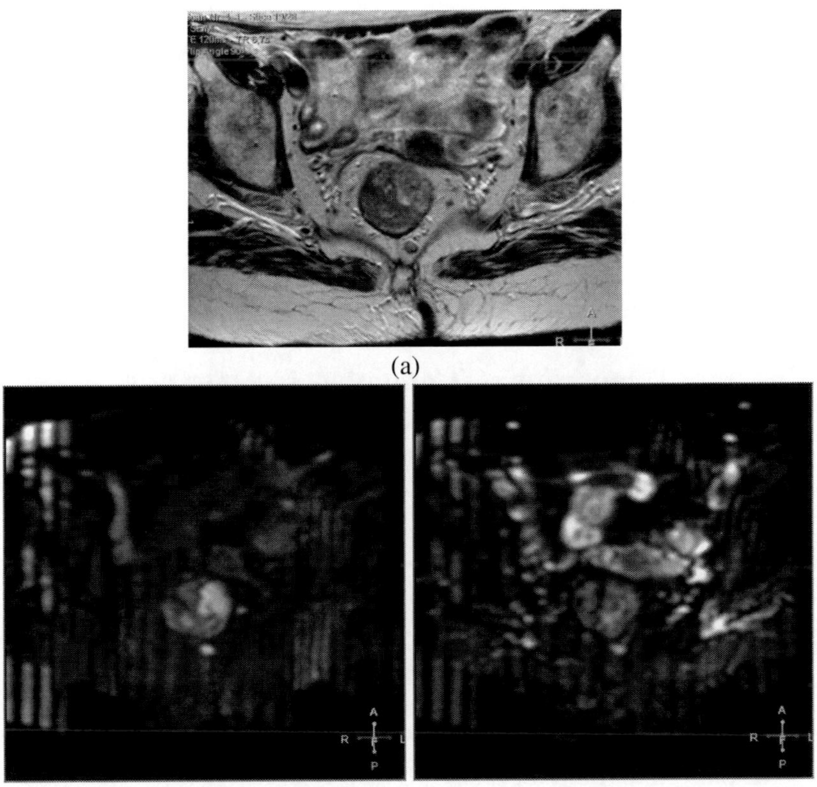

(a)

(b) (c)

Figure 14. MRI of a rectal carcinoma shown in 14a with intermediate signal intensity on T2 weighted image, that infiltrates the mesorectal fat (shown with high signal) and its distance from mesorectal fascia (shown with low signal) is more than 5 mm. It is accompanied by two enlarged round lymphnodes with an intermediate signal intensity. The primary tumor and the metastatic lymphnodes show restricted diffusion on DWI with high signal intensity in image 14b with low apparent diffusion coefficient values and low signal intensity shown in image 14c (ADC values of the primary tumor and the metastatic lymphnodes of about 0.98 × 10-3 sec/mm2).

MRI can evaluate the integrity of rectal wall layers, as they are very well delineated on T2WI, with visualization of the rectal mucosa and muscularis propria by low signal intensity, the submucosa and mesorectum by high signal intensity and the mesorectal fascia by linear low signal intensity, with a high accuracy in T staging.

It is very important for the mesorectal fascia to be intact, as it determines the circumferential resection margin for a total mesorectal excision. The frequency of recurrence is 19%-22% in patients with positive circumferential resection margin, compared to 3%-5% in patients with negative circumferential resection margin. It is also frequently associated with distant metastatic disease.

Diffusion weighted imaging has high accuracy in depicting colorectal cancer, with a 90.9% sensitivity and 100% specificity. The cellularity of malignant tumors is greater than that of normal tissue and appears hyperintense in DWI with restricted diffusion, and hypointense in apparent diffusion coefficient (ADC) maps with low values (Figures 14a-14c). Possible fibrotic and desmoplastic tissue can be differentiated from tumor infiltration with low signal intensity in both DWI and ADC maps.

Criteria in predicting nodal involvement is a cutoff in size of 10 mm of a round lymphnode as well as the border irregularity, mixed signal intensity and T2* low signal of ultra-small iron particle uptake from the metastatic lymph node. Metastatic lymphnodes show restricted diffusion on MRI DWI with low ADC values (ADC values by using a threshold of $1.0\text{-}1.38 \times 10^{-3}$ sec/mm^2), that is a good indicator of cancer cell viability and it is also used to show changes before and after chemo-radiation therapy in the assessment of the primary tumor and the lymphnodes [4, 25-28].

Recurrence of rectal cancer is best appreciated with MRI, being the modality of choice for follow up, evaluating recurrence patterns and findings of un-resectability [27].

Positron Emission Tomography – Computed Tomography

PET-CT better delineates primary, lymphnode and metastatic disease in colorectal cancer for preoperative staging, and it is recommended for identification of recurrent disease. PET-CT colonography is recommended in patients with obstructive colorectal cancers [20].

Most of the times, a combination of CT, MRI and PET-CT is needed for accurate preoperative tumor staging.

References

[1] Gray's Anatomy, 39th Edition, *Churchill Livingstone* 2005, Elsevier.

[2] Horton KM, Frank M, Elliot K et al. CT Evaluation of the Colon: Inflammatory Disease. *RadioGraphics* 2000; 20: 399–418.

[3] Silva AC et al. Evaluation of Benign and Malignant Rectal Lesions with CT Colonography and Endoscopic Correlation. *RadioGraphics* 2006; 26: 1085–1099.

[4] Kaur H, Choi H, You YN et al. MR Imaging for Preoperative Evaluation of Primary Rectal Cancer: Practical Considerations. *RadioGraphics* 2012; 32: 389–409.

[5] Branco BC, Barmparas G, Schnueriger B, et al. Systematic review and meta-analysis of the diagnostic and therapeutic role of water-soluble contrast agent in adhesive small bowel obstruction. *Br. J. Surg* 2010; 97: 470-478.

[6] Kalady MF, Mantyh CR, Petrofski J, et al. Routine contrast imaging of low pelvic anastomosis prior to closure of defunctioning ileostomy: is it necessary? *J. Gastrointest. Surg.* 2008; 12: 1227-1231.

[7] Veerappan GR, Ally MR, Choi JH, et al. Extracolonic findings on CT colonography increases yield of colorectal cancer screening. *AJR Am. J. Roentgenol.* 2010; 195: 677-686.

[8] Laghi A, Iafrate F, Rengo M, et al. Colorectal cancer screening: the role of CT colonography. *World J. Gastroenterol.* 2010; 16: 3987-3994.

[9] Pickhardt PJ, Kim DH, Menias CO, et al. Evaluation of submucosal lesions of the large intestine part 1. Neoplasms. *RadioGraphics* 2007; 27: 1681–1692.

[10] Pickhardt PJ, Kim DH, Menias CO, et al. Evaluation of submucosal lesions of the large intestine part 2. Non-neoplastic Causes. *RadioGraphics* 2007; 27: 1693–1703.

[11] Neubauer H, Pabst T, Dick A, et al. Small-bowel MRI in children and young adults with Crohn's disease: retrospective head-to-head comparison of contrast-enhanced and diffusion-weighted MRI. *Pediatr Radiol.* 2013; 43(1): 103–114.

[12] Chowdhury FU, Shah N, Scarsbrook Af, et al. [18F]FDG PET/CT imaging of colorectal cancer: a pictorial review. *Postgrad. Med. J.* 2010; 86: 174-82.

[13] Lee SS, Kim AY, Yang SK, et al. Crohn's disease of the small bowel: comparison of CT enterography, MR enterography, and small-bowel follow-through as diagnostic techniques. *Radiology* 2009; 251(3): 751–761.

[14] Balthazar EJ, Megibow AJ, Hulnick D, et al. CT of appendicitis. *AJR Am. J. Roentgenol.* 1986; 147: 705–710.

[15] Purysko AS, Remer EM, Filho HM, et al. Beyond Appendicitis: Common and Uncommon Gastrointestinal Causes of Right Lower Quadrant Abdominal Pain at Multidetector CT. *RadioGraphics* 2011; 31: 927- 947.

[16] Heverhagen JT, Klose KJ. MR Imaging for Acute Lower Abdominal and Pelvic Pain. *RadioGraphics* 2009; 29: 1781-1796.

[17] Labs JD, Sarr MG, Fishman EK, et al. Complications of acute diverticulitis of the colon: improved early diagnosis with computerized tomography. *Am. J. Surg.* 1988; 155: 331-336.

[18] Hulnick DH, Megibow AJ, Balthazar EJ, et al. Computed tomography in the evaluation of diverticulitis. *Radiology* 1984; 152: 491–495.

[19] Padidar AM, Jeffrey RB Jr, Mindelzun RE, Dolph JF. Differentiating sigmoid diverticulitis from carcinoma on CT scans: mesenteric inflammation suggests diverticulitis. *AJR Am. J. Roentgenol.* 1994; 163: 81–83.

[20] Chintapalli KN, Esola CC, Chopra S, et al. Pericolic mesenteric lymph nodes: an aid in distinguishing diverticulitis from cancer of the colon. *AJR Am. J. Roentgenol.* 1997; 169: 1253–1255.

[21] Tontini GE, Vecchi M, Pastorelli L, et al. Differential diagnosis in inflammatory bowel disease colitis: State of the art and future perspectives. *World J. Gastroenterol.* 2015 January 7; 21(1): 21-46.

[22] Cosnes J, Gower-Rousseau C, Seksik P, et al. Epidemiology and Natural History of Inflammatory Bowel Diseases. *Gastroenterology* 2011; 140: 1785–1794.

[23] Towbin AJ, Sullivan J, Denson LA, et al. CT and MR Enterography in Children and Adolescents with Inflammatory Bowel Disease. *RadioGraphics* 2013; 33: 1843–1860.

[24] Macari M, Bini EJ, Jacobs SL, et al. Filling defects at CT colonography: pseudo- and diminutive lesions (the good), polyps (the bad), flat lesions, masses and carcinomas (the ugly). *RadioGraphics* 2003; 23: 1073-1091.

[25] Kijima S, Sasaki T, Nagata K, et al. Preoperative evaluation of colorectal cancer using CT colonography, MRI and PET-CT. *World J. Gastoenterol.* 2014; 20(45): 16964-16975.

[26] Sinha R, Rajiah P, Ramachandran I, et al. Diffusion-weighted MR Imaging of the gastrointestinal tract: technique, indications and imaging findings. *RadioGraphics* 2013; 33: 655-676.

[27] Sinaei M, Swallow C, Moghaddam PA, et al. Patterns of signal intensity characteristics of pelvic recurrence of rectal cancer at MR Imaging. *RadioGraphics* 2013; 33: E171-E187.

[28] Nagtegaal ID, Quirke P. What is the role for circumferential margin in the modern treatment of rectal cancer? *J. Clin. Oncol.* 2008; 26: 303-312.

In: The Role of Imaging Technology …
Editor: Georgios Tsoulfas
ISBN: 978-1-63483-490-2

Chapter 3

THE ROLE OF IMAGING IN BREAST SURGERY

Vasileios N. Papadopoulos**, MD, PhD, FACS
Associate Professor of Surgery
1st Surgical Propedeutic Department
Medical School of Aristotle's University of Thessaloniki, Greece

ABSTRACT

During the past decades, there has been significant improvement in the equipment and image-recording systems for breast diseases and for investigation of the axilla. In addition to providing better images, these developments have resulted in a significant reduction in radiation dose. Screening mammography is used to detect unexpected breast cancer in asymptomatic women since the 1960s. Specific mammographic features that suggest a diagnosis of breast cancer include a solid mass with or without stellate features, clustered microcalcifications, and asymmetric thickening of breast tissues. Imaging of the breast has evolved from mammography alone to mammography with adjunctive modalities that primarily include ultrasound and magnetic resonance imaging (MRI scan). Until recently, ultrasound and MRI have functioned as problem-solving tools and have been used to help to diagnose a mammographically and/or clinically detected abnormality such as a breast mass or nipple discharge. As these modalities have improved technologically and immense clinical experience has been acquired, so have their roles expanded from diagnostic tools to potential screening tools as well. Ultrasound has many uses that relate to the evaluation of breast masses. Sonographic guidance is used frequently for the direction of percutaneous breast biopsies and to investigate the status of axillary lymph nodes in breast carcinoma. MRI was initially used for the evaluation of implants, but it now has a variety of roles associated with the evaluation of tumors. With a dedicated breast coil and contrast enhancement, MRI has been of great value in identifying the extent of breast carcinoma and contributing to better patient management plan. A breast positron emission tomography (PET) scan is another imaging modality of the breast that uses a radioactive substance (F-18-fluoro-2-deoxy-D-glucose - FDG). Whole-body FDG-PET can detect distant metastatic disease to the lymph nodes, the soft tissues, viscera, and bone. PET scan is also used to assess whether metastatic breast cancer is responding to treatment. After breast biopsy, scarring and distortion of

* Corresponding author - email: bnpap@med.auth.gr

breast tissue occur, making subsequent evaluation by mammography difficult. Thus, other imaging techniques, such as MRI, and PET, are being increasingly used for characterizing lesions in the breast. All imaging techniques now used in breast surgery continue to be modified and improved to maintain optimum image quality that enhances interpretation skills of the clinicians and radiologists.

INTRODUCTION

Over the past decades the use of breast imaging has increased, with more emphasis being placed on ultrasound (US) and magnetic resonance imaging (MRI) than ever before. While mammography remains the front line in screening and first-time diagnosis, US and MRI allow a more accurate characterization of lesions and symptomatic findings [1, 2]. The number of breast cancer detections has increased, as have the instances of surgical breast interventions. In order to detect the abnormal changes in the breast, breast surgeons and breast imagers must be also familiar with the normal findings of the postsurgical breast. The techniques of biopsy, implantation, and reconstruction have also evolved, changing the breast imaging findings as well [1-4].

The progress of technology has enabled control of the status of breast and axillary lymph nodes with many imaging methods. The main methods currently used are:

i) Ultrasonography
ii) Mammography
iii) MRI
iv) CT scan
v) Pet scan
vi) Scintimammography

I. ULTRASONOGRAPHY (US)

In breast US, sound waves are emitted into the breast, and an image is created by the returning sound waves received by the ultrasound detector. As there is no ionizing radiation, it is useful in young and pregnant women. Advantages of breast ultrasound include the ability to better characterize the composition of breast parenchyma, and to investigate the presence of lesions - nodules and easily recognize compact or cystic texture and the size, shape, perfusion, elements that distinguish and characterize a lesion as benign or malignant. In suspected lesions enable biopsy under the guidance of ultrasound. In axillary cavity status information of nodes there is substantial and ultrasound also checks outside of the lymph nodes status of vessels (arteries, veins) (Figure 1), nerves, connective tissue and sometimes ectopic mammary gland. The axillary lymph nodes are divided into three levels based on their anatomic relationship to the pectoralis minor muscle: level I nodes are inferior to the pectoralis minor muscle, level II nodes are posterior to the muscle, and level III nodes are medial to the muscle [5].

The main groups of axillary lymph nodes include: The group of axillary vein lymph nodes, the group of scapular, the central group, the lymph nodes of Rotter (between the pectoral muscles) the team of the pectoralis major muscle, and the group of subclavicular lymph nodes. Skandalakis JE et al., [6], report that the axillary drainage of the breast includes an average number of 35.3 nodes in 6 groups.

Group 1. External mammary nodes (average number of 1.7 nodes), also called the anterior pectoral nodes. These lie along the lateral edge of the pectoralis minor, deep to the pectoralis major muscle, along the medial side of the axilla following the course of the lateral thoracic artery on the chest wall from the second to the sixth rib. Deep to the areola there is an extensive network of lymphatic vessels, the so-called subareolar plexus of Sappey. In the circumareolar region, large lateral and medial trunks receive much of the lymph from the breast parenchyma. The lateral trunk receives collaterals from the upper half of the breast and the internal trunk drains the lower part of the breast. These vessels pass around the lateral border of the pectoralis major muscle to reach the external mammary nodes.

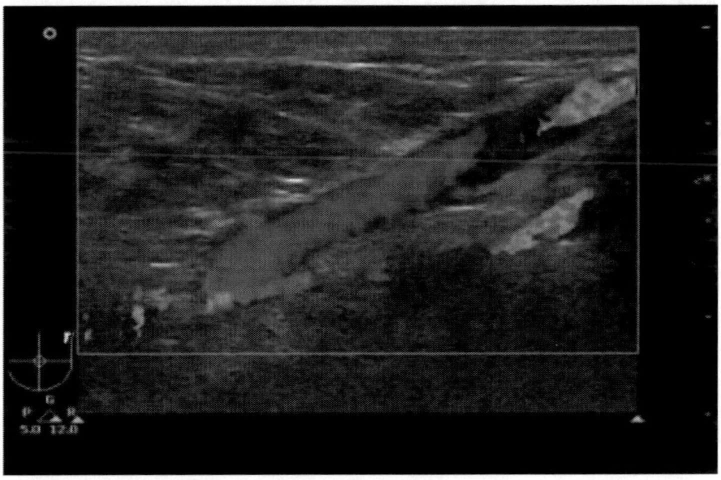

Figure 1. Axillary vessels in color US.

Group 2. Scapular nodes (average number of 5.8 nodes). These lie on the subscapular vessels and their thoracodorsal branches. Lymphatics from these intercommunicate with intercostal lymphatic vessels.

Group 3. Central nodes (average number of 12.1 nodes). This is the largest group of lymph nodes; they are the nodes most easily palpated in the axilla, because they are generally larger in size. They are embedded in fat in the center of the axilla. When these nodes enlarge, they can compress the intercostobrachial nerve, the lateral cutaneous branch of the second or third thoracic nerve, causing accompanying pain.

Group 4. Interpectoral nodes (Rotter's nodes) (average number of 1.4 nodes). These lie between the pectoralis major and minor muscles. Often there is a single node. They are the smallest group of axillary nodes and will not be found unless the pectoralis major is removed.

Group 5. Axillary vein nodes (average number of 10.7 nodes). This is the second largest group of lymph nodes in the axilla. They lie on the caudal and ventral surfaces of the lateral part of the axillary vein.

Group 6. Subclavicular nodes (average number of 3.5 nodes). These lie on the caudal and ventral surfaces of the medial part of the axillary vein [6].

Second only to mammography in frequency of use for breast imaging, ultrasonography is an important method of resolving equivocal mammographic findings, defining cystic masses, demonstrating the echogenic qualities of specific solid abnormalities, and greatly facilitates the recommendations for follow-up or further evaluation of the patient [4].

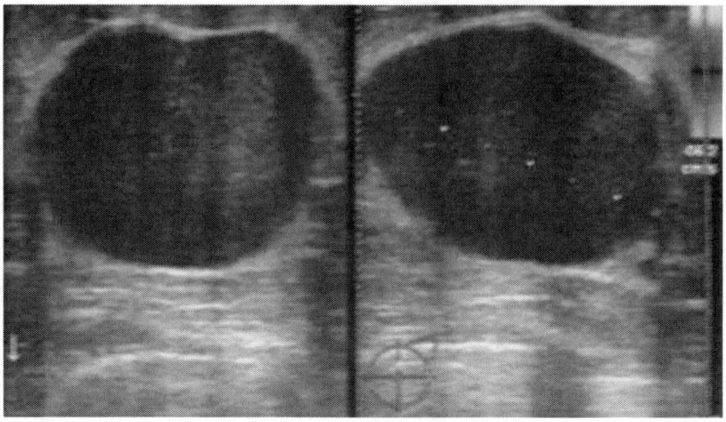

Figure 2. Breast cyst on ultrasound.

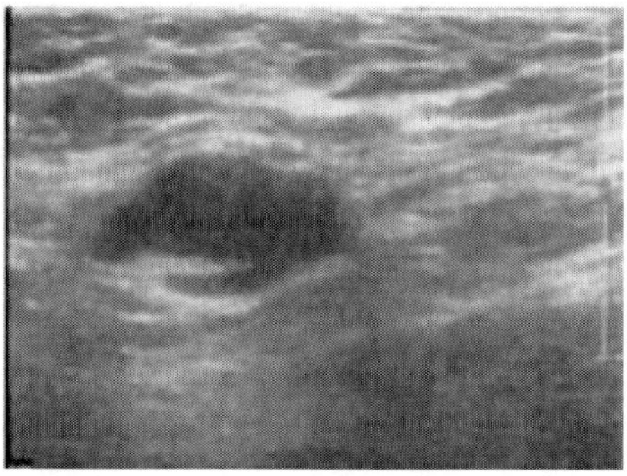

Figure 3. Solid tumor of left breast in US.

On ultrasound examination, breast cysts are well circumscribed, with smooth margins and an echo-free center (Figure 2). Benign breast masses usually show smooth contours, round or oval shapes, weak internal echoes, and well defined anterior and posterior margins. Breast cancer characteristically has irregular walls but may have smooth margins with acoustic enhancement (Figure 3, 4).

Ultrasonography is used to guide fine-needle aspiration biopsy, core-needle biopsy, and needle localization of breast lesions (Figure 5). Its findings are highly reproducible and it has a high patient acceptance rate, but it does not reliably detect lesions that are less than one cm in diameter. In patients with breast cancer, evaluation of axillary lymph nodes (ALNs) is very important, as it is a powerful prognostic indicator and decisive factor for developing a breast cancer treatment plan. Traditionally, axillary lymph node dissection (ALND) has been used for nodal staging, but currently use of sentinel lymph node biopsy (SLNB) has increased in frequency as an alternative procedure for patients with early breast cancer. Importantly, while SLNB has decreased the morbidity of staging by avoiding unnecessary ALND, it is also an invasive method, and it may be an inconvenience for some patients to undergo a two-stage surgical procedure. Therefore, it would be of great clinical benefit if a reliable imaging method or minimally invasive procedure for determining ALN status were available. If there were no evidence of ALN metastasis in preoperative staging, SLNB would be performed. On the other hand, patients with ALN metastasis found on preoperative staging would directly undergo ALND or neoadjuvant chemotherapy [7, 8].

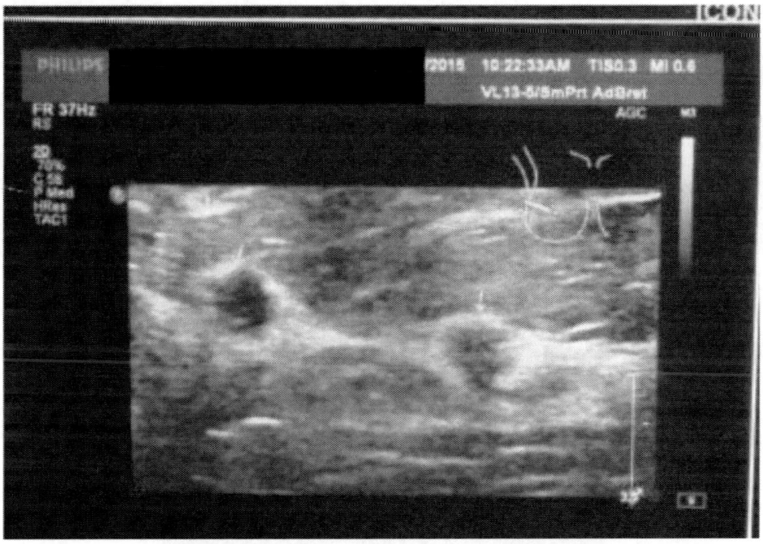

Figure 4. Right breast tumor (BIRADS 5) in US.

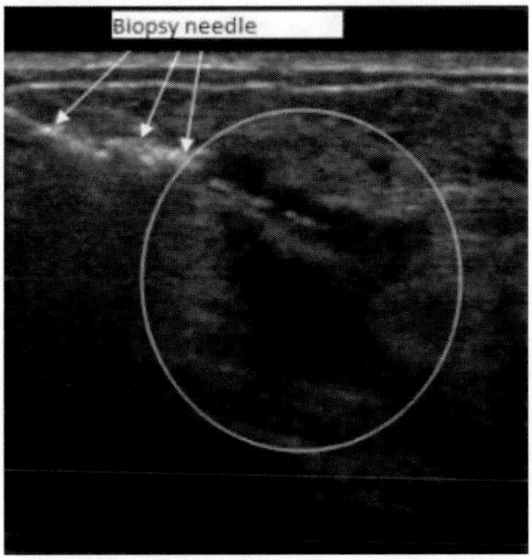

Figure 5. Needle biopsy with US guidance.

In terms of preoperative evaluation for ALN metastasis, physical examination has low sensitivity, between 35 and 82% and specificity ranges from 73% to 97%. Ultrasonography (US) of ALN has superior diagnostic accuracy in many studies when combined with US-guided fine-needle aspiration biopsy (US-FNA) of sonographically suspicious lymph nodes. The sensitivity and specificity of US examination in the evaluation of ALN metastasis have been reported to be 36–92 and 69–100%. Addition of US-FNA to axillary US may increase specificity to 93–100% [7-11].

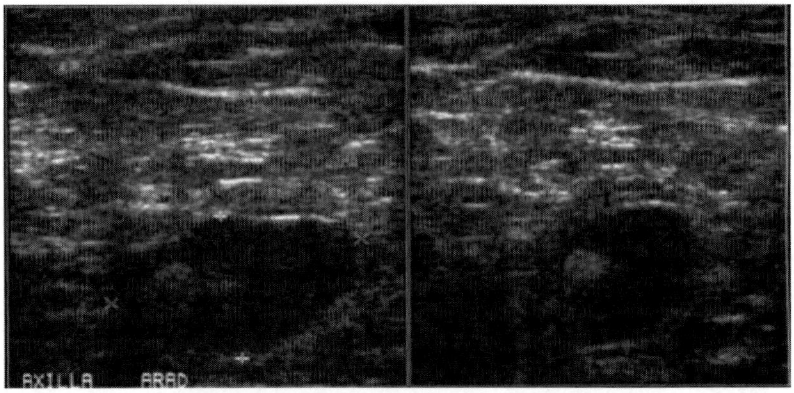

Figure 6. Metastatic axillary lymph node in US.

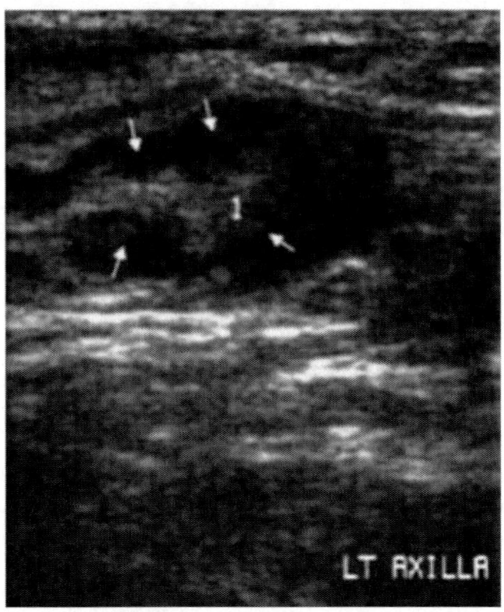

Figure 7. Metastatic axillary lymph node in US.

The combination of axillary US and US-FNA is useful in preoperative work-up of breast cancer patients and is valuable in planning proper management of breast cancer patients.

Ultrasonography can also be utilized to image the regional lymph nodes in patients with breast cancer (Figure 6, 7, 8). On ultrasound, lymph nodes have a characteristic appearance. They are very well defined and oval or lobular with mixed echogenicity (Figure 9). The cortex is hypoechoic, and the fatty hilum is hyperechoic. Abnormal nodes may lose this appearance and be more rounded and poorly marginated. Intramammary lymph nodes have an appearance similar to that of axillary nodes; namely, they are well defined, mixed density or medium to low density, round, ovoid, or reniform nodules with a fatty notch or center. Intramammary nodes can be found throughout the breast but most commonly are located in the middle- to upper-outer aspect of the breasts [12].

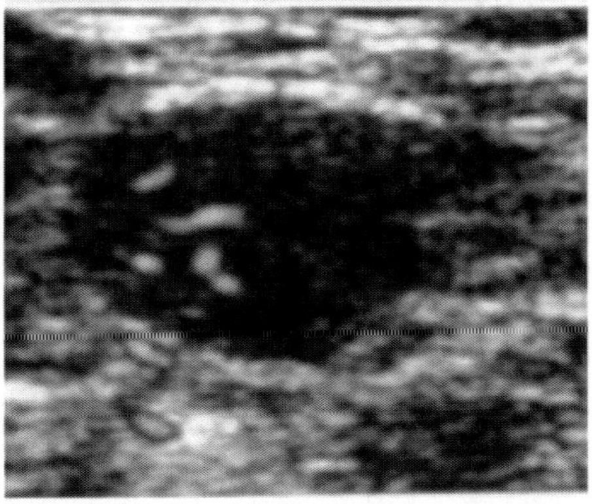

Figure 8. Multiple vessels in metastatic axillary lymph node in US.

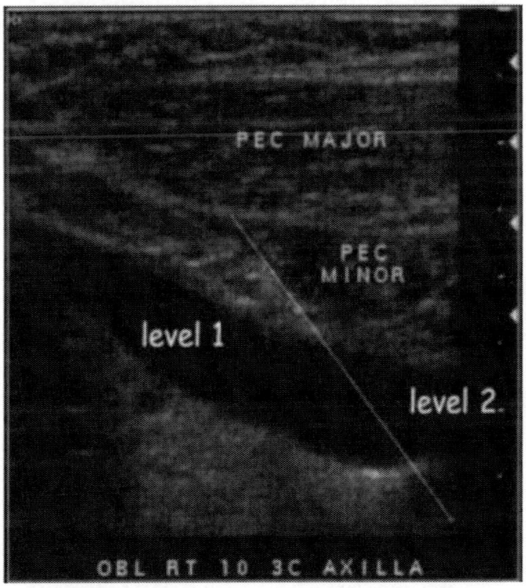

Figure 9. Normal axillary lymph node in US.

Ultrasound is an essential component in the workup of a palpable or mammographically evident lesion. It is also highly specific, relatively inexpensive, and widely available. Sonography can be used for a targeted region of the breast. Poor visualization of microcalcifications, which are often a sign of malignancy, is the ultrasound's main disadvantage. Although sonography cannot definitely differentiate benign from malignant solid masses, the correlation of a circumscribed mass that has not enlarged on mammography and benign sonographic characteristics can be used to follow rather than biopsy a nonpalpable lesion. Malignant sonographic criteria include spiculation, a taller-than-wide shape, angular margins, shadowing, branching pattern, hypoechoicity, duct extension, and microlobulation. The presence of these features, even in the face of a relatively circumscribed mass on mammography, should prompt biopsy [4, 12].

Pneumocystography also may be performed at the time of aspiration to outline the internal aspect of the cyst wall. When sonography demonstrates a complicated cyst (imperceptible wall, acoustic enhancement, and low-level echoes) or a cluster of microcysts, the likelihood of malignancy is very low. Cystic masses with thick walls, thick septae, or an intracystic solid component or predominately solid masses with cystic foci are categorized as complex cysts. Complex cysts may be malignant, and biopsy is warranted. Papillomas and intracystic papillary carcinomas may develop within a cyst. Invasive papillary carcinomas tend to present as multiple, relatively well-defined masses. If a cyst contains an intracystic lesion, lobulation or slight irregularity of the wall may be seen on mammography. On pneumocystography, papillary lesions are seen as a polypoid filling defect within the cyst cavity [12, 13].

US Report Organization

According to the Guidelines of "The American College of Radiology (ACR)" in ACR BI-RADS® Atlas 5, the report should be concise and organized using a structure such as that provided in Table 1.

Table 1. Report organization

	Report Structure
1.	Indication for examination
2.	Statement of scope and technique of breast US examination
3.	Succinct description of the overall breast composition (screening only)
4.	Clear description of any important findings
5.	Comparison to previous examination(s), including correlation with physical, mammography, or MRI findings
6.	Composite reports
7.	Assessment
8.	Management

The indication for examination, relevant clinical history, and pertinent risk factor information should be clearly stated. If the study is performed for follow-up of a specific mass or area of concern, this should be described. The dates of any comparison examinations should be specified. When a specific sonographic finding is documented by recording a complete set of images, the longest horizontal dimension should be reported first, followed by the vertical measurement, and the orthogonal horizontal dimension last. Multiple simple cysts or a combination of multiple simple and complicated cysts need not be reported individually. If any lesions have been biopsied previously, this should be noted together with the prior biopsy results, if known. Correlation of any clinical, mammographic, and MRI findings with the sonographic findings should be specifically stated in the report. For diagnostic evaluations involving US characterization of mammographic abnormalities or confirmation of a mass suspected but not delineated mammographically, a single report integrating the two modalities will clearly communicate a final assessment based on the highest likelihood of malignancy and appropriate management recommendations. Consistent use of BI-RADS® descriptors for US, as for mammography and MRI, helps in lesion assessment and clarifies communication with physicians and patients. Also, structured, software-based reporting should be based on BI-RADS® terminology. For coding and reimbursement, it is considered the advisability of splitting the report combining the findings of two or more concurrently performed imaging modalities or procedures into specific sections or paragraphs, one for each type of examination. However, a single assessment and recommendation for patient management should reflect integration of the findings from all of the imaging studies. It is important that an assessment based on specific findings needing most urgent attention will have the greatest clinical utility.

1. Indication for Examination

The reason for performing the examination should be stated briefly at the beginning of the report. The most common indications for breast US are confirmation and characterization of a palpable mass or mammographic or MRI abnormality, guidance of interventional procedures and as the initial imaging technique for young, pregnant, or lactating patients. Additional applications are listed in the ACR Practice Guideline for the Performance of the Breast Ultrasound Examination and include the extent of disease evaluation supplementing mammography in high-risk women who are not candidates for breast MRI or who have no easy access to MRI, and in breast imaging practices that provide the service, supplementary whole-breast screening in order to increase cancer detection in asymptomatic women with mammographically dense breasts.

2. Statement of Scope and Technique of Breast US Examination

The scope of examination and technique used should be stated, for example, whether the examination was directed or targeted to a specific location, or whether it was performed for supplementary screening. It is important, since US is a real-time examination, to indicate who performed the examination (sonographer, sonographer and physician, physician alone) or whether an automated whole-breast scanning system was used. If a lesion was evaluated with color or power Doppler or with strain or shear-wave elastography, observations relevant to the interpretation should be reported. In certain situations, it may be beneficial to describe the position of the patient during the examination (e.g., "The breasts were imaged in both supine and lateral decubitus position." or "The patient was imaged in seated position, the position in which she feels the left breast thickening best.").

3. Succinct Description of the Overall Breast Composition (Screening Only)

Tissue composition patterns can be estimated more easily in the large field of view (FOV) of automated US scans but can also be discerned in the small FOV of a handheld US scan. The three US descriptors for tissue composition are "homogeneous background echotexture-fat," "homogeneous background echotexture-fibroglandular," and "heterogeneous background echotexture" (Table 2) correspond loosely to the four density descriptors of mammography and the four fibroglandular tissue descriptors of MRI. At US, breast tissue composition is determined by echogenicity. Subcutaneous fat, the tissue relative to which echogenicity is compared, is medium gray and darker than fibroglandular tissue, which is light gray. Heterogeneous breasts show an admixture of hypoechoic and more echogenic areas. Careful real-time scanning will help differentiate a small hypoechoic area of normal tissue from a mass.

Table 2. Breast tissue composition patterns

	Tissue composition
a.	Homogeneous background echotexture-fat
b.	Homogeneous background echotexture-fibroglandular
c.	Heterogenous background echotexture

4. Clear Description of Any Important Findings

The description of important findings should be made, in order of clinical relevance, using lexicon terminology, and should include:

a) Characterization of a mass using the morphological descriptors of shape, margin, and orientation. Note should be made of the lesion's effect on the surrounding tissue, such as architectural distortion. Feature categories, such as posterior features and echogenicity, and techniques, such as color or power Doppler and elastography, may contribute information to the analysis, but only pertinent positives need to be described. Recognition of special case findings, such as simple and complicated cysts, clustered microcysts, intramammary lymph nodes, and foreign bodies, should simplify interpretation. In reporting screening examinations in asymptomatic women, as in mammography, characteristically benign findings may be reported (assessment category 2), but it is not obligatory, and the appropriate assessment would then be negative (assessment category 1).
b) For important findings, lesion size should be given in at least two dimensions; three dimensions are preferable, especially if the volume of a mass is compared with one or more previous examinations. It is not necessary to report the measurements of every small simple cyst, and if numerous cysts are present, especially in both breasts; location and measurements of the largest cyst in each breast will suffice.

If a mass is measured, images should be recorded with and without calipers. Marginal characteristics are one of the most important criteria to be applied in assessing the likelihood of malignancy of a mass, and, particularly with small masses, caliper markings may obscure the margin, hindering analysis.

c) Location of the lesion(s) should be indicated using a consistent and reproducible system, such as clock-face location and distance from the nipple. When more than one mass or abnormality is located in the same scan frame or in the same locale, measurement of the distance from the skin to the center of the mass or its anterior aspect may help to differentiate one lesion from another. This measurement may be particularly useful when one mass is singled out for biopsy and others are depicted in the field.

5. Comparison to Previous Examination(s), Including Correlation with Physical, Mammography, or MRI Findings

Breast US should be correlated with physical findings, mammography, MRI, or other imaging studies, if performed. If no statement of comparison is included in the US report, it will be assumed that no comparison was made. Note that some report templates include a "comparison" heading, in which the word "none" (if appropriate) may be entered. When correlating US findings with those seen at mammography and/or MRI, the operator performing handheld scanning should correlate the size and location of lesions and match the type and arrangement of tissues surrounding the lesion in order to reduce the likelihood of misregistration (identifying a different lesion or lesions at different imaging modalities). In doing this, allowance for positional changes should be made going from upright with mammography and prone with MRI to supine or supine-oblique with US. If it is determined that a sonographic finding corresponds to a palpable abnormality, or to a mammographic or MRI finding, this should be stated explicitly in the US report. If the US finding is new or has no correlate, this should also be stated in the report.

If the US examination was performed as part of a surveillance protocol to assess a previously identified finding, or if the finding was reported on a previous examination, the current report should describe any changes. An increase of 20% or more in the longest dimension of a probably benign solid mass within 6 months may prompt biopsy. An increase of only 1–2 mm in lesion size may be related to differences in scanning technique or patient positioning.

6. Composite Reports

When more than one type of examination is performed concurrently (on the same day), it is preferable that the examinations be reported together. The findings for each examination should be described in separate paragraphs with an overall assessment and management recommendations for the combined examinations.

In general, when the assessments for two examinations differ, the overall assessment (and concordant management recommendations) should reflect the more abnormal of the individual assessments (whatever management is expected to come first, supplemented by likelihood of malignancy), according to the following hierarchy of increasing abnormality: category 1, 2, 3, 6, 0, 4, 5 (Table 3.).

Table 3. Abnormality Hierarchy

BI-RANDS Assessment category	Degree of Abnormality
1	Lowest
2	↓
3	
6	
0	
4	
5	Highest

Exceptions to this rule occur when the characteristically benign features of a given imaging finding on one examination supersede the less specifically benign features of the same finding on the other examination. An example is that of a partially circumscribed, non-calcified mass at mammography, superseded by simple cyst at US.

7. Assessment

The report should conclude with a concise summary of pertinent US findings with a final assessment using BI-RADS® US categories 1–6 and the phrases associated with them.

If report of a US examination is integrated with that of a concurrently performed mammography examination, the combined final assessment should reflect the highest likelihood of malignancy assessed at the two examinations. Clear and consistent communication is a goal that can be achieved for breast US by using the same assessment categories and similar wording described in the BI-RADS® Mammography section (Table 4).

In some cases, the interpreting physician may render an incomplete assessment (category 0) in order to request additional examination(s), such as mammography, comparison with previous but currently unavailable examinations, or additional physican-performed real-time scanning after either a sonographer-produced, real-time or automated whole-breast screening US examination.

Table 4. BI-RADS® Classification

BI-RADS® Category	Descriptive Recommendation
0	Incomplete - Needs further evaluation (Additional views, ultrasound, comparison with old films)
1	Negative - Routine annual screening
2	Benign - Routine annual screening
3	Probably benign - Short interval follow-up mammography
4	Suspicious - Biopsy should be considered
5	Highly suspicious - Appropriate action/biopsy
6	Proven malignancy - Appropriate action

8. Management

Management recommendations should be included in every report. Clear recommendations should be made as to the next course of action. Recommendations may include routine age-appropriate screening, surveillance imaging for a probably benign mass, annual follow-up after percutaneous or surgical biopsy, and clinical management. If an imaging-guided interventional procedure is recommended, the type of imaging for the procedure might also be suggested, for example, stereotactic, US, or MRI guidance.

II. MAMMOGRAPHY

During the last decades convincing evidence has emerged that mammographic screening has contributed to a significant reduction in breast cancer mortality. Mammographic screening is especially important in the diagnosis of early-stage breast cancer, which relies primarily on nonpalpable mammographic abnormalities for detection (Figure 10, 11, 12). Ductal carcinoma in situ (DCIS) now accounts for approximately 20–30% of mammographically detected cancers. Current US Preventive Services Task Force (USPSTF) guidelines recommend against routine screening mammography in women aged 40–49 years [14].

Mammography has evolved from more dedicated equipment and industrial film, through dedicated film-screen mammography, and now to full-field digital mammography. Factors that affect the image quality include equipment, image-recording system, processing, compression of the breast, and the technologist's skill in positioning the patient. Adherence to strict quality assurance guidelines is critical in mammography to maintain optimum image quality.

Once the mammographic images are presented to the radiologist for interpretation, an approach to the analysis and interpretation defines how lesions are identified and how they are described and managed. The assessment and description of the mammographic findings are defined in a standardized method known as the Breast Imaging Reporting and Data System (BI-RADS®) (Table 4).

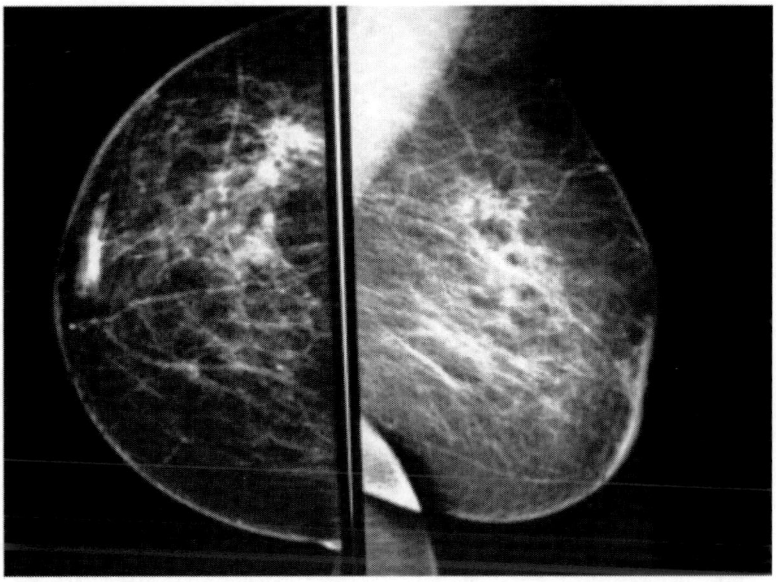

Figure 10. Right breast tumor in mammography.

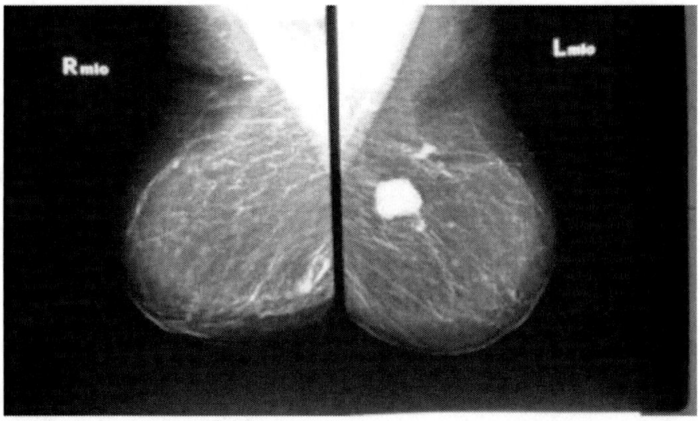

Figure 11. Left breast tumor in mammography.

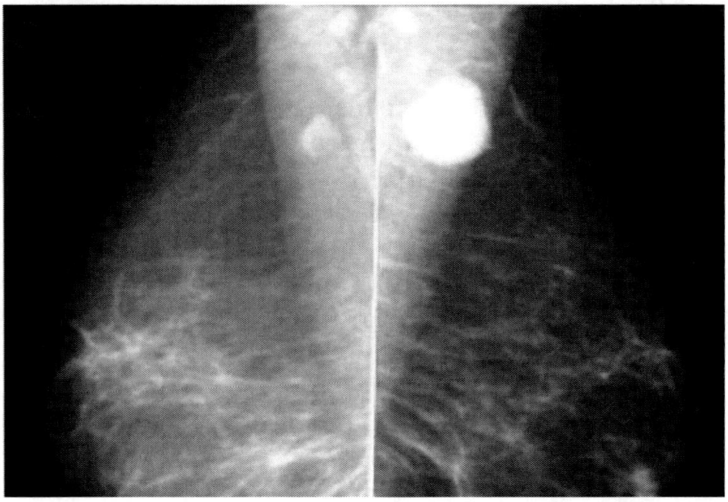

Figure 12. Metastatic axillary lymph nodes in mammography with no evidence of primary breast cancer.

BI-RADS® was developed by the American College of Radiology in the mid-1990s and includes a nomenclature for lesion description and overall assessment. BI-RADS® incorporates three basic components: (a) a description of the parenchymal density, (b) specific lesion descriptions for masses, calcifications, and other findings, and (c) an overall assessment or management recommendation for the patient. The use of this lexicon is ideal: The terms are standardized, and the correct use of the terms to describe an abnormality is helpful to the radiologist to correctly manage each case. The use of the standardized terminology and the requirement for an overall assessment are also very helpful for communication of the findings to the referring surgeon [12].

Mammogram reports will also include an assessment of breast density. BI-RADS® classify breast density into 4 groups:

1. The breasts are almost entirely fatty (Figure 13). The breasts contain little fibrous and glandular tissue, which means the mammogram would likely detect anything abnormal.

2. There are scattered areas of fibroglandular density (Figure 14). There are a few areas of fibrous and glandular tissue in the breast.
3. The breasts are heterogeneously dense, which may obscure small masses (Figure 15). The breast has more areas of fibrous and glandular tissue that are found throughout the breast. This can make it hard to see small masses.
4. The breasts are extremely dense, which lowers the sensitivity of mammography (Figure 16). The breast has a lot of fibrous and glandular tissue. This may make it harder to find a cancer that may be present, as it can blend in with normal breast tissue.

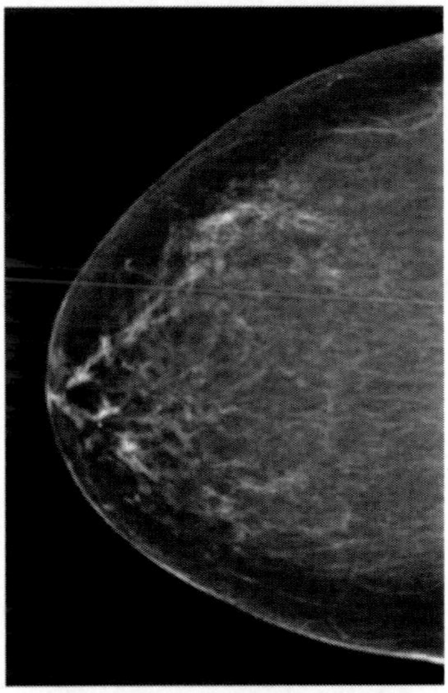

Figure 13. The breast is almost entirely fatty containing little fibrous and glandular tissue (Group 1).

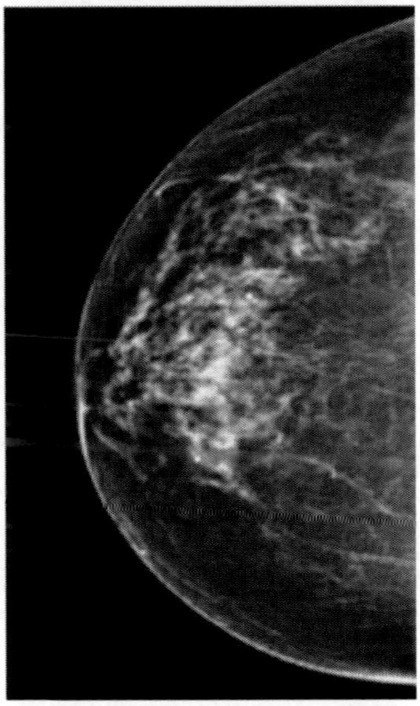

Figure 14. There are scattered areas of fibroglandular density (Group 2.).

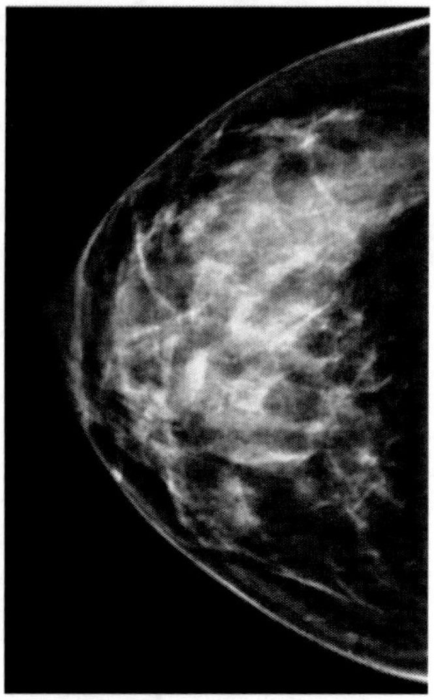

Figure 15. The breast is heterogeneously dense, which may obscure small masses (Group 3.).

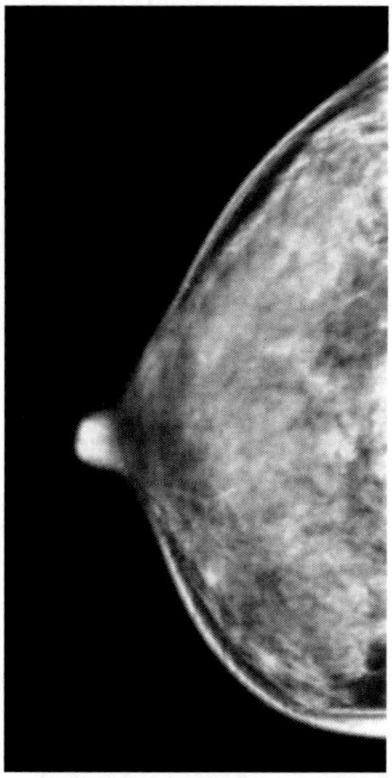

Figure 16. The breast is extremely dense, which lowers the sensitivity of mammography (Group 4.).

The fourth edition of BI-RADS®, unlike previous editions, indicated quartile ranges of percentage dense tissue (increments of 25% density) for each of the four density categories, with the expectation that the assignment of breast density would be distributed more evenly across categories than the historical distribution of 10% fatty, 40% scattered, 40% heterogeneously, and 10% extremely dense. However, it has since been demonstrated in clinical practice that there has been essentially no change in this historical distribution across density categories, despite the 2003 guidance provided in the BI-RADS® Atlas. The absence of change in clinical practice of the assignment of breast density across categories may reflect the reality that a few coalescent areas of dense tissue may be present in breasts with as little as

10% dense tissue, whereas primarily fatty areas may be present in breasts with as much as 90% dense tissue. The fifth edition of BI-RADS® no longer indicates ranges of percentage dense tissue for the four density categories. This is done to emphasize the text descriptions of breast density, which reflect the masking effect of dense fibroglandular tissue on mammographic depiction of non-calcified lesions, because the Committee on BI-RADS® concludes that the association of subjectively estimated breast density with changes in the sensitivity of mammography is clinically more important than the relatively smaller effect of percentage breast density as an indicator for breast cancer risk.

The Committee on BI-RADS® indeed is aware of recent and continuing investigations of percent-age breast density as an indicator for breast cancer risk, and by eliminating percentage ranges they do not intend to compromise or impede any such research. They simply recognize the reality that interpreting physicians will continue to use density categories in mammography reports as they have done over the past years, independent of BI-RADS® guidance on percentage breast density. They further recognize that both subjective estimates and planimetry measurements of breast density based on area as depicted on (2-D) mammograms are imprecise indicators of the volume of dense tissue, which may be measured using (3-D) cross-sectional breast imaging modalities. They await publication of robust volume-based breast density data, using validated percentage cut points (not necessarily quartiles) that are readily and reproducibly determined at imaging, before again indicating percentage ranges for BI-RADS® density categories. They also urge avoidance of numbers to classify breast density instead of BI-RADS® terminology in order to avoid confusion with BI-RADS® assessment categories, which are numbered. Some breasts may appear more or less dense when imaged using full-field digital mammography compared to screen-film mammography. Superior depiction of the skin line by digital mammography provides the observer with a more accurate (and usually larger) estimate of the extent of the subcutaneous fat. However, no change in the distribution across density categories has been observed when comparing full-field digital mammography with screen-film mammography.

Screening mammography is used to detect unexpected breast cancer in asymptomatic women, supplementing history taking and physical examination. Standard mammographic views include craniocaudal (CC) and mediolateral oblique (MLO) views. The MLO view images the greatest volume of breast tissue, including the upper outer quadrant and the axillary tail of Spence. Compared with the MLO view, the CC view provides better visualization of the medial aspect of the breast and permits greater breast compression. The 90-degree lateral view is used along with the CC view to triangulate the exact location of an abnormality. Spot compression may be done in any projection by using a small compression device, which is placed directly over a mammographic abnormality that is obscured by overlying tissues. The compression device minimizes motion artifact, improves definition, separates overlying tissues, and decreases the radiation dose needed to penetrate the breast. Magnification techniques (×1.5) often are combined with spot compression to better resolve calcifications and the margins of masses [12 18].

The most important findings on mammography (that are either of concern at screening, inherently suspicious, new, or seen to be larger or more extensive when compared to previous examination) are:

a. Mass: size, morphology (shape, margin), density, associated calcifications, associated features, location.
b. Calcifications: morphology, description of typically benign type or description of the shape of particles, distribution (may not be appropriate for typically benign calcifications), associated features, location.
c. Architectural distortion: associated calcifications, associated features, location.
d. Asymmetries (asymmetry, global asymmetry, focal asymmetry, developing asymmetry): associated calcifications, associated features, location.
e. Intramammary lymph node (rarely important): location.
f. Skin lesion: location.
g. Solitary dilated duct (rarely present): location.

Comparison to previous examination may assume importance if the finding of concern requires an evaluation of change or stability. Comparison is not important when a finding has unequivocally benign features. Comparison may be irrelevant when the finding is inherently suspicious for malignancy.

All final assessments (BI-RADS® categories 1, 2, 3, 4, 5, and 6 should be based on thorough evaluation of the mammographic features of concern or after determination that an examination is negative or benign.

An incomplete (category 0) assessment is usually given for screening examinations when additional imaging evaluation is recommended before it is appropriate to render a final assessment. There may be rare situations in the screening setting in which a category 4 or 5 assessment is used, but this practice is discouraged because it may compromise some aspects of outcome analysis. A recall (category 0) assessment should include specific suggestions for the next course of action (spot-compression magnification views, US, etc.)

In most circumstances and when feasible, if a mammography examination is not assessed as negative or benign, the current examination should be compared with prior examination(s). The interpreting physician should use judgment on how vigorously to attempt obtaining prior examinations, given the likelihood of success of such an endeavor and the likelihood that comparison will affect the final assessment. In this context, it is important to note that comparison with previous examination(s) may be irrelevant when a finding is inherently suspicious for malignancy.

Category 0 should be used for prior image comparison only when such comparison is required to make a final assessment. When category 0 is used in the context of awaiting prior examinations for comparison, there should be in place a tracking procedure guaranteeing with 100% reliability that a final assessment will be made within 30 days (preferably sooner) even if prior examinations do not become available. Some mammography practices may reasonably choose never to use category 0 in the context of awaiting prior examinations simply because they do not have a 100% reliable tracking procedure. If a mammography examination is assessed as category 0 in the context of awaiting prior examinations and then the prior examinations do become available, an addendum to the initial mammography report should be issued, including a revised assessment.

Category 1: Negative. This is a normal examination.

Category 2: Benign. Like category 1, this is a normal assessment, but here the interpreter chooses to describe a benign finding in the mammography report. Involuting calcified fibroadenomas, skin calcifications, metallic foreign bodies (such as core biopsy and surgical clips), and fat-containing lesions (such as oil cysts, lipomas, galactoceles, and mixed-density hamartomas) all have characteristically benign appearances and may be described with confidence. The interpreter may also choose to describe intramammary lymph nodes, vascular calcification, implants, or architectural distortion clearly related to prior surgery while still concluding that there is no mammographic evidence of malignancy. On the other hand, the interpreter may choose not to describe such findings, in which case the examination should be assessed as negative (category 1). Note that both category 1 and category 2 assessments indicate that there is no mammographic evidence of malignancy. Both should be followed by the management recommendation for routine mammography screening. The difference is that category 2 should be used when describing one or more specific benign mammographic findings in the report, whereas category 1 should be used when no such findings are described (even if such findings are present).

Category 3: Probably Benign. A finding assessed using this category should have a ≤ 2% likelihood of malignancy, but greater than the essentially 0% likelihood of malignancy of a characteristically benign finding. A probably benign finding is not expected to change over the suggested period of imaging surveillance, but the interpreting physician prefers to establish stability of the finding before recommending management limited to routine mammography screening.

There are several prospective clinical studies demonstrating the safety and efficacy of periodic mammographic surveillance instead of biopsy for specific mammographic findings. Three specific findings are validated as being probably benign (non-calcified circumscribed solid mass, focal asymmetry, and solitary group of punctate calcifications). All the previously cited studies emphasize the need to conduct a complete diagnostic imaging evaluation before making a probably benign (category 3) assessment; hence, it is recommended not to render such an assessment in interpreting a screening mammography examination. The practice of rendering category 3 assessments directly from screening examination also has been shown to result in adverse outcomes: 1) unnecessary follow-up of many lesions that could have been promptly assessed as benign, and 2) delayed diagnosis of a small number of cancers that otherwise may have been smaller in size and less likely to be advanced in stage. Also, all the previously cited studies exclude palpable lesions, so the use of a probably benign assessment for a palpable lesion is not supported by robust scientific data, although there are two single-institution studies that do report successful outcomes for palpable lesions.

Finally, because evidence from previously cited studies indicates the need for biopsy rather than continued surveillance when a probably benign finding increases in size or extent, it is not prudent to render a category 3 assessment when a finding that otherwise meets "probably benign" imaging criteria is either new or has increased in size or extent.

Category 4: Suspicious. This category is reserved for findings that do not have the classic appearance of malignancy but are sufficiently suspicious to justify a recommendation for biopsy. The ceiling for category 3 assessment is a 2% likelihood of malignancy and the floor for category 5 assessment is 95%, so category 4 assessments cover the wide range of likelihood of malignancy in between. Thus, almost all recommendations for breast interventional procedures will come from assessments made using this category.

Category 5: Highly Suggestive of Malignancy. These assessments carry a very high probability (≥ 95%) of malignancy. This category initially was established to involve lesions for which 1-stage surgical treatment was considered without preliminary biopsy, in an era when preoperative wire localization was the primary breast interventional procedure.

Nowadays, given the widespread acceptance of imaging-guided percutaneous biopsy, 1-stage surgery is rarely, if ever, performed. Rather, current oncologic management almost always involves tissue diagnosis of malignancy via percutaneous tissue sampling to facilitate treatment options, such as when sentinel node biopsy is included in surgical management or when neoadjuvant chemotherapy is administered prior to surgery. Therefore, the current rationale for using a category 5 assessment is to identify lesions for which any non-malignant percutaneous tissue diagnosis is automatically considered discordant, resulting in the recommendation for repeat (usually surgical) biopsy.

Category 6: Known Biopsy-Proven Malignancy. This category is reserved for examinations performed after biopsy proof of malignancy (imaging performed after percutaneous biopsy but prior to complete surgical excision), in which there are no mammographic abnormalities other than the known cancer that might need additional evaluation.

Digital mammography was developed to allow the observer to manipulate the degree of contrast in the image. Digital mammography captures x-ray information after it passes through the breast in a digital format—without a film—that can be viewed, edited, and transferred electronically to viewing stations and picture archiving and communications systems viewers. This is especially useful in women with dense breasts and women less than 50 years of age. The use of digital breast tomosynthesis with 3D images has been introduced as an alternative to standard 2D mammography imaging that is limited by superimposition of breast parenchyma and breast density. The STORM trial reported that in 7,292 women screened, 3D mammography had a higher cancer detection rate and fewer false-positive recalls than the standard 2D imaging [19].

Specific mammographic features that suggest a diagnosis of breast cancer include a solid mass with or without stellate features, asymmetric thickening of breast tissues or architectural distortion, and clustered microcalcifications. The presence of fine, stippled calcium in and around a suspicious lesion is suggestive of breast cancer and occurs in as many as 50% of nonpalpable cancers. These microcalcifications are an especially important sign of cancer in younger women, in whom it may be the only mammographic abnormality.

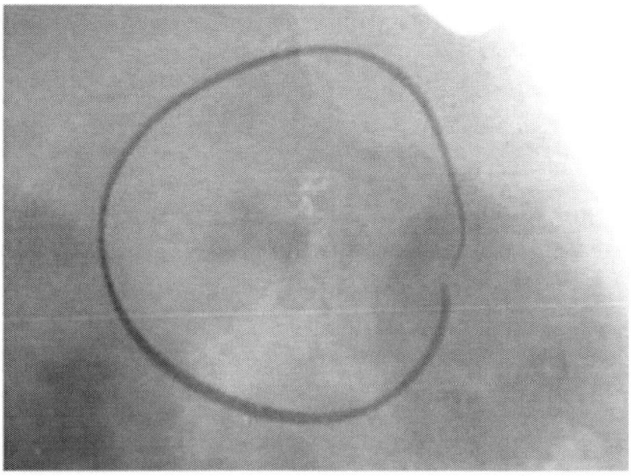

Figure 17. Microcalcifications in mammography.

The usual approach to the evaluation of a well-defined mass on mammography includes an assessment of the shape, size, margins, density, orientation, presence of a fatty halo, and presence of other findings (i.e., calcifications, Figure 17). Benign lesions tend to be isodense or less dense than the parenchyma and to have very circumscribed margins, whereas malignant masses are more often of greater density and have fine irregularity or micronodularity on their borders (Figure 18). A microlobulated margin appears as fine nodularity or undulation of the edge of the lesion and implies a more malignant nature.

The shapes of masses that are circumscribed may be oval, round, or lobular. The margination that is described as circumscribed allows one to visualize a fine, clear edge around the entire mass (i.e., cyst, Figure 19). Often masses that are circumscribed may be overlapped by parenchyma in some areas. These are described as obscured or partially circumscribed.

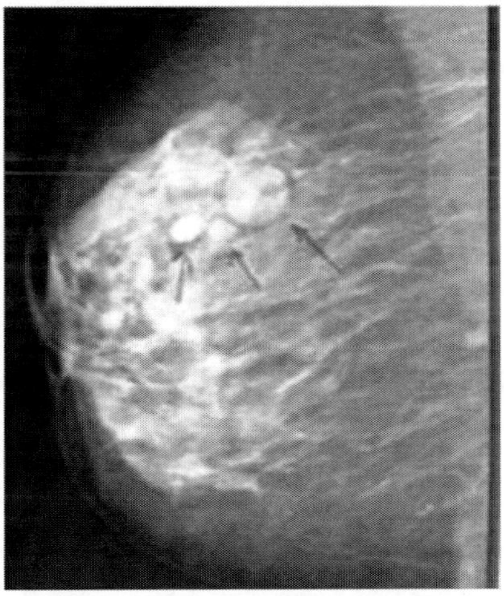

Figure 18. Fibroadenomas in mammography (arrows).

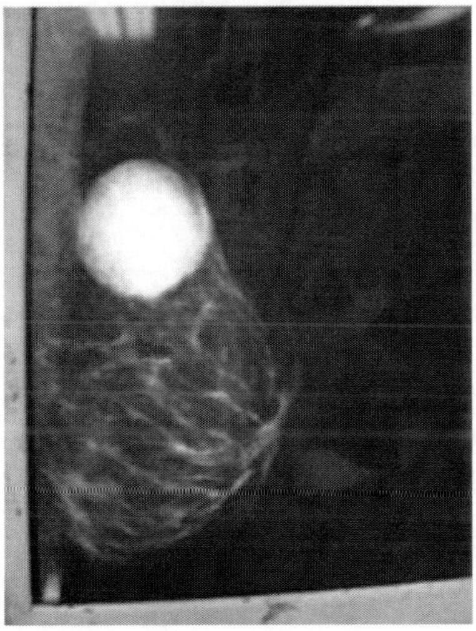

Figure 19. Breast cyst in mammography.

A basic division of well-circumscribed masses based on their density is of help in determining possible etiologies of and approach to such lesions. Masses that are fatty such as lipomas, oil cysts, and galactoceles and circumscribed masses that are mixed density are characteristically benign. Isodense circumscribed masses include benign and malignant lesions, and an evaluation of the borders is critical to help differentiate these etiologies. Masses that are of high density, particularly for their size, are of concern for malignancies. However, in a study of radiologists' interpretations of mass density, Jackson et al., [20] found that the assessment of mammographic density of masses was quite variable among different readers; in addition, the density assessment was of limited value in the prediction of benign versus malignant for noncalcified breast masses.

The mammographic feature of greatest importance in assessing a relatively circumscribed isodense mass is its margination. Any waviness, notching, or indistinctness of the margins of a mass should be regarded with suspicion. The presence of a halo sign, i.e., a fine radiolucent ring surrounding a well-defined mass, has long been considered to be a mammographic sign of benignancy. The halo may be due to compression of fat by the mass or to Mach effect. Swann et al. [21] have, however, described 25 malignant lesions from approximately 1,000 breast cancers in which a halo sign was present. The presence of a halo suggests but does not guarantee a benign process. Certainly, the presence of a partially circumscribed margin and a partially indistinct margin is suspicious, and biopsy is indicated in this situation.

Stability in size from prior mammography is an important factor that suggests that a circumscribed non-cystic mass is benign. The growth rates of breast cancers are quite variable. In two series, the mean doubling times for mammary carcinoma have been found to be 212 and 325 days, respectively [22, 23]. The lack of interval change suggests that a well-defined lesion is more likely benign, but this is not confirmatory. Meyer and Kopans [24] reported five cases of occult cancers that did not change in size on follow-up mammography over a minimum of 2 years and a maximum of 4.5 years from the original study. Therefore, if a nodule is followed and there is no interval change in the size at 6 months or 1 year, continued follow-up is necessary. In addition, the other features of density and margination are used to decide whether to follow or biopsy a circumscribed mass.

Small solid breast lesions that are radiologically indeterminate sometimes yield an indeterminate histopathological assessment following a radiologically guided biopsy.

Although some centers may wish to just follow these lesions up, increasingly these are being treated using radiological wire localization followed by open surgery in the form of a wide local excision (Figure 20, 21, 22). However many of these are subsequently benign on final surgical pathology.

Important step is the marking of the specimen with two sutures in order to assist the pathologist for better orientation on specimen findings (Figure 23). More recently there has been alternative radiological management to excise biopsy proven benign lesions, usually fibroadenomas, in women wishing to have them removed. This has been with vacuum assisted biopsy devices, such as the mammotome™ (Johnson and Johnson Ethicon Endo-Surgery Inc, Cincinnati, Ohio, USA), Encor™ (C.R.Bard, New York, USA) and Suros ATEC™(Suros Surgical Systems Inc, Indianapolis, USA). The advantages of these minimally invasive approaches to many women made this technique increasingly popular. They can be performed usually in less than 30 min, with only local anaesthetic and a minimal scar. Complication rates are very low, and the procedures are extremely well tolerated. These procedures are particularly suitable for young women where risk of the lesion being non benign is very low, and cosmesis is premium. The obvious limitation of this technique however, is that as it is only able to remove lesions in a "piecemeal" fashion. Such excisions are unable to provide an assessment of margins of the excision, thus there is no way of determining completeness of excision and whether any residual lesion is left behind. While this may not be particularly relevant if the lesions excised are fibroadenomas, or other such similar benign lesions, it will however obviate the vacuum assisted excision from being utilised for many other more "border- line" lesions where completeness of excision and a full margin status is desirable or essential [1, 4, 12].

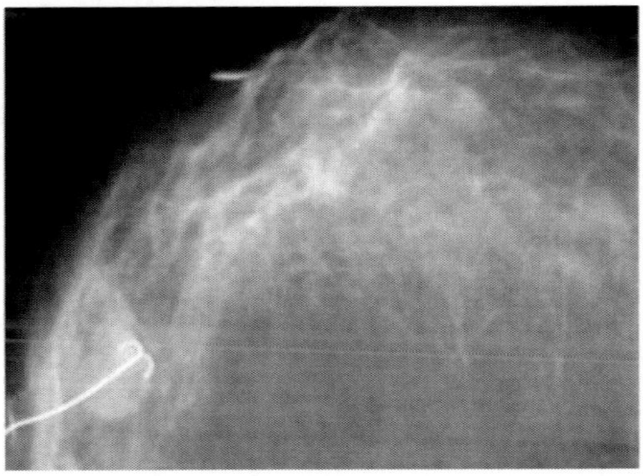

Figure 20. Radiological wire localization of breast lesion.

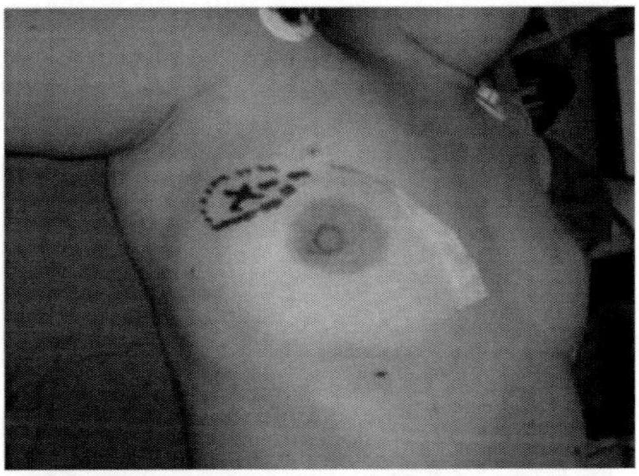

Figure 21. Radiological wire localization followed by open surgery in the form of a wide local excision.

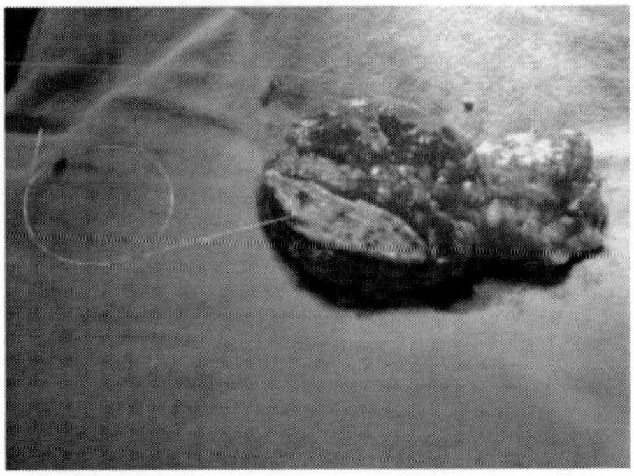

Figure 22. Specimen of open biopsy after Kopans wire used in needle localization.

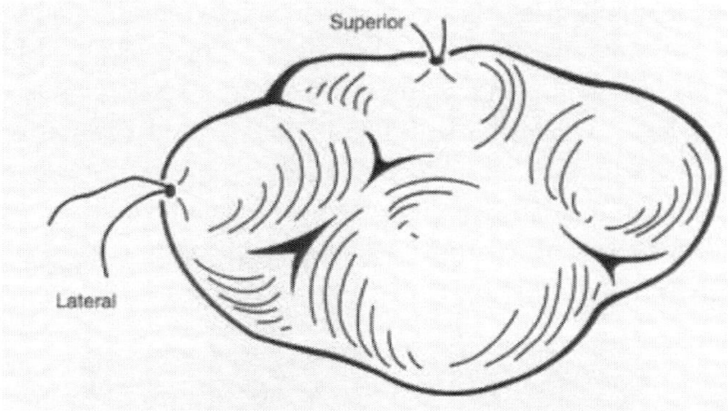

Figure 23. Important step is that of marking the specimen with two sutures (Long suture for Lateral, and Short suture for Superior).

Since 2001 the breast lesion excision system (BLES, Intact Medical, Framingham, USA), has been used as an alternative large biopsy device to other vacuum assisted biopsy devices in over 50,000 cases in the USA. It has been well validated as a safe and efficacious biopsy procedure. It however has the unique feature of using radiofrequency cautery to excise a small but whole sample in one piece with intact architecture and clear margins, as a swift local anaesthetic outpatient procedure [25].

The BLES biopsy is an efficacious technique at excising small indeterminate breast lesions with a complete margin without the need for follow-up diagnostic surgery in the majority (Figures 24, 25, 26).

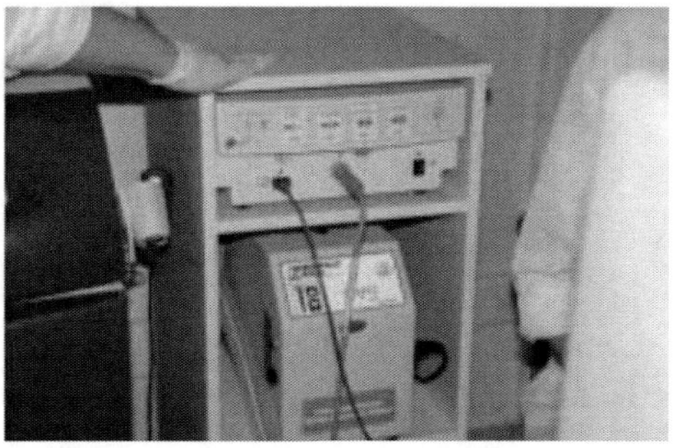

Figure 24. Breast Lesion Excision System.

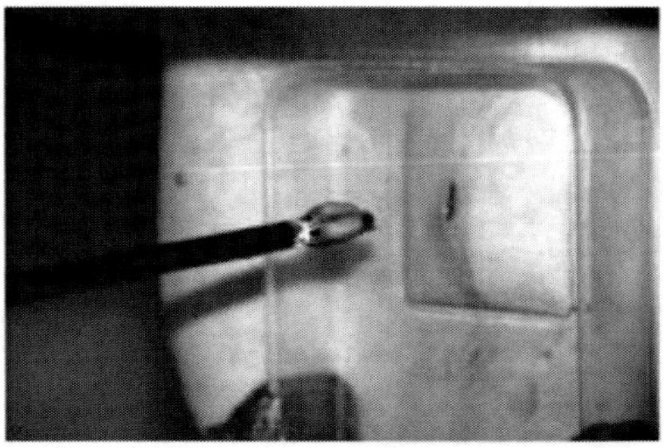

Figure 25. Removing suspicious breast area using BLES.

Post–core biopsy mammographic changes are few and very uncommon. In cases of clip placement, a small metallic clip should be visible at the biopsy site (Figure 27). Clips may demonstrate some migration from the area of initial placement [1, 26, 27].

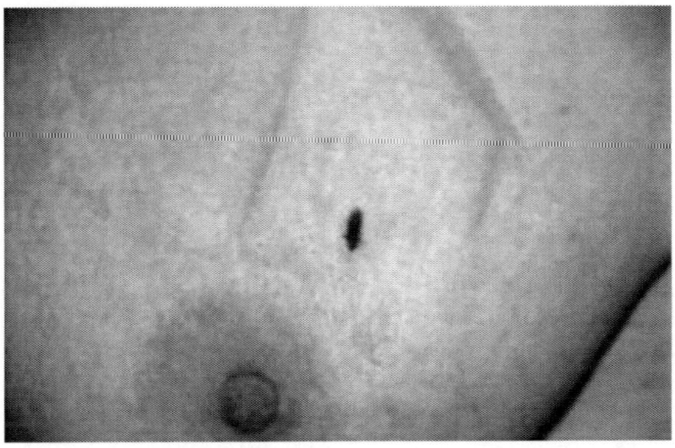

Figure 26. Post excision trauma after BLES.

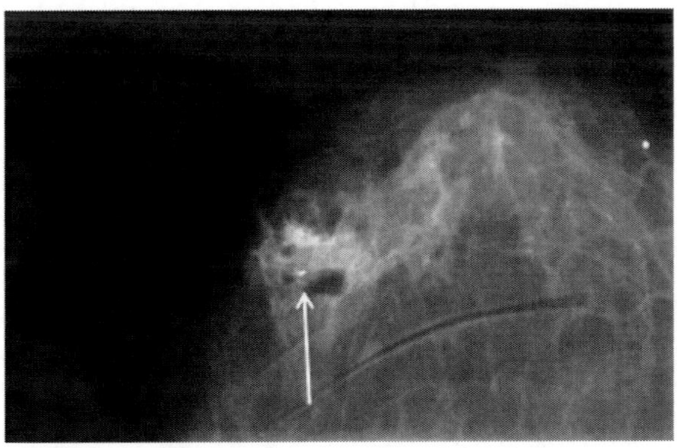

Figure 27. Clip placement after biopsy.

In cases with post biopsy parenchymal hemorrhage, a localized area of increased density corresponding to increased fluid and blood may be seen. Needle tracts may be noted as subtle, cylindrical mammographic densities in a projection parallel to the biopsy tract with 11-gauge needles. Fourteen gauge needles have not been shown to produce any detectable abnormality. Following vacuum-assisted core biopsy, gas pockets and hematomas are common, but they resolve within 2 to 4 weeks [28]. Overall, post–core biopsy changes should not be recognized on mammography after approximately 6 months; any density after this period likely represents an abnormality and should be further evaluated [29].

Post excisional breast biopsies, which involve the removal of a larger amount of breast tissue, demonstrate significantly more imaging findings. Fifty percent of benign excisional breast biopsies show some mammographic change [30].

Postsurgical mammograms are ideally performed at about 3 to 6 months after surgery and serve as new baseline views. Benign pathologies, however, may not prompt postsurgical imaging unless there is a need to confirm successful removal of a lesion or evaluate for postoperative complications.

In a postsurgical mammogram, a thin metallic marker is placed on the surgical skin scar to indicate its location on the images. The most commonly viewed post excisional change is architectural parenchymal distortion, followed by overlying focal skin thickening. These changes are seen mostly in the first 6 months after surgery. Other findings include calcifications or fat necrosis. Occasionally, 6 or more months after the procedure, calcifications form in the post excisional bed. Most are dystrophic in nature or associated with fat necrosis or oil cysts. Small irregular calcifications mimicking malignancy may also be seen and should be closely monitored for malignancy [31].

Ductography

Breast ductography (also known as galactography) is an imaging technique which is used to evaluate lesions causing nipple discharge. It helps in precisely locating the mass within breast tissue and gives useful information for surgical approach and planning.

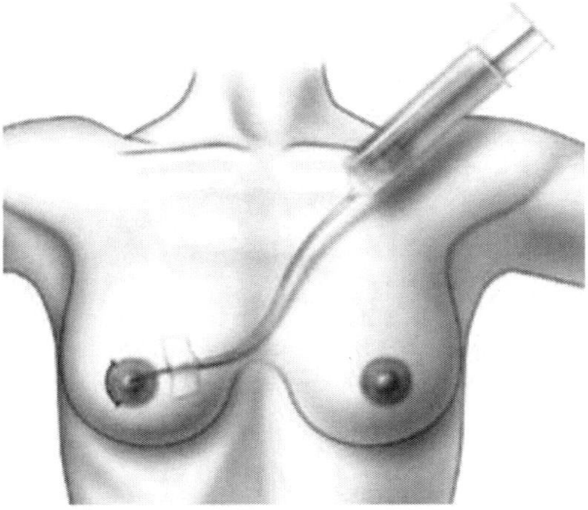

Figure 28. Ductography.

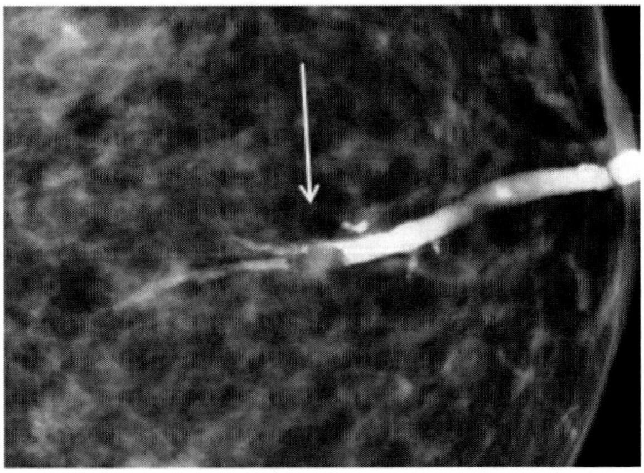

Figure 29. Intraductal papillomas are seen as small filling defects surrounded by contrast media.

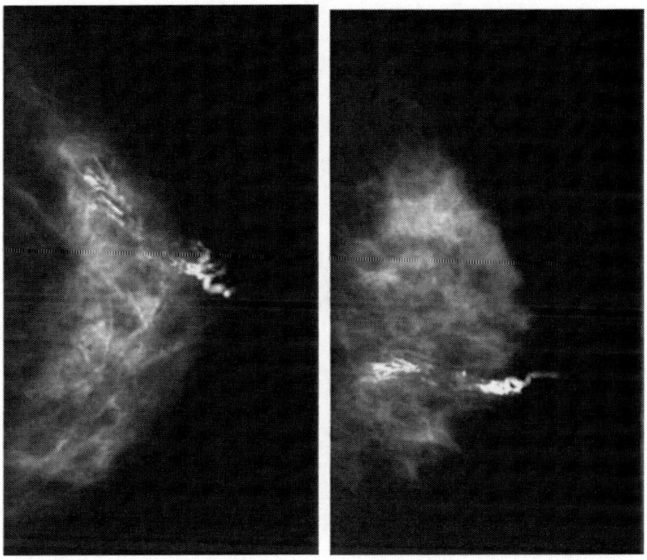

Figure 30. Cancers may appear as irregular masses or as multiple intraluminal filling defects.

The primary indication for ductography is nipple discharge, particularly when the fluid contains blood. Radiopaque contrast media is injected into one or more of the major ducts and mammography is performed (Figure 28). A duct is gently enlarged with a dilator and then a small, blunt cannula (sialogram needle of 30 gauge) is inserted under sterile conditions into the nipple ampulla. With the patient in a supine position, 0.1 to 0.2 mL of dilute contrast media is injected and a standard two view mammography (CC and MLO projections) are obtained without compression. Intraductal papillomas are seen as small filling defects surrounded by contrast media (Figure 29). Cancers may appear as irregular masses or as multiple intraluminal filling defects (Figure 30) [4, 12].

The majority of the lesions found in ducts are duct papillomas. Current practice holds that these lesions should be excised to exclude a malignant lesion. If the duct lesion is large enough, ultrasound guided percutaneous biopsy can make the diagnosis of a papilloma quite successfully. The duct is excised after it is filled carefully with dye.

III. Magnetic Resonance Imaging (MRI)

In the process of evaluating magnetic resonance imaging (MRI) as a means of characterizing mammographic abnormalities, additional breast lesions have been detected. However, in the circumstance of negative findings on both mammography and physical examination, the probability of a breast cancer being diagnosed by MRI is extremely low. Contrast enhanced breast MRI indications include (a) evaluation of the extension of known breast cancer, (b) detection of contralateral breast cancer in women with newly diagnosed breast cancer, (c) screening for women who are at high risk and/or positive for BRCA1 and BRCA2, (d) assessment of neoadjuvant chemotherapy response, (e) evaluation of chest wall invasion or mastectomy site for recurrence, and (f) detection of breast cancer in women with axillary metastases and a normal mammogram [1, 32, 33, 34].

The patient receives an intravenous line and is given gadolinium for contrast enhancement. Then 20 minutes of motionless scan time follows [35]. There are three different patterns of dynamic enhancement. The type 1 pattern (persistent) shows slow, progressive contrast uptake over time and is suggestive of benignity. The type II contrast pattern (plateau) shows a rapid uptake in contrast and then a leveling off of uptake. This pattern is suggestive of malignancy. The type III pattern (washout) is indicative of malignancy [36]. The diagnostic evaluation must also include the assessment of lesion morphology, which requires high-resolution imaging. The border of the lesion is the most important feature. Spiculated and irregular margins have a positive predictive value of malignancy ranging from 76% to 91%. Most benign masses have a smooth border with a negative predictive value for malignancy of 90% [36, 37]. DCIS is suggested by small, clumped foci that are within a segment or duct [38].

The use of dedicated breast coils is mandatory in the MRI imaging of the breast. A BIRADS lexicon is assigned to each examination and an abnormality noted on MRI that is not seen on mammography requires a focused ultrasound examination for further assessment. If the abnormality is not seen on corresponding mammogram or ultrasound then MRI guided biopsy is necessary. Some clinical scenarios where MRI may be useful include the evaluation of a patient who presents with nodal metastasis from breast cancer without an identifiable primary tumor; to assess response to therapy in the setting of neoadjuvant systemic treatment; to select patients for partial breast irradiation techniques; and evaluation of the treated breast for tumor recurrence.

There is current interest in the use of MRI to screen breasts of high-risk women and of women with a newly diagnosed breast cancer. In the first case, women who have a strong family history of breast cancer or who carry known genetic mutations require screening at an early age, because mammographic evaluation is limited due to the increased breast density in younger women [4].

In the second case, an MRI study of the contralateral breast in women with a known breast cancer has shown a contralateral breast cancer in 5.7% of these women. MRI can also detect additional tumors in the index breast (multifocal or multicentric disease) that may be missed on routine breast imaging and this may alter surgical decision making. In fact, MRI has been advocated by some for routine use in surgical treatment planning based on the fact that additional disease can be identified with this advanced imaging modality and the extent of disease may be more accurately assessed [4].

Preoperative imaging can change the case management approach in a significant number of cases: 18% using US and 11% to 30% using MRI [8, 39, 40]. US and MRI are generally more sensitive than mammography for invasive carcinomas, especially in dense and heterogeneous breasts. MRI is commonly used for the detection of multicentric and multifocal diseases once cancer is diagnosed [1].

A randomized trial performed in the United Kingdom (COMICE trial)[41] which enrolled 1,623 women did not show a decrease in rates of reoperation in those women randomized to undergo MRI in addition to mammography and ultrasonography (19%) compared to those undergoing standard breast imaging without MRI (19%). Houssami et al., [42] performed a meta-analysis including 2 randomized trials and 7 comparative cohort studies to examine the effect of preoperative MRI compared to standard preoperative evaluation on surgical outcomes. They reported that the use of MRI was associated with increased mastectomy rates. This is problematic since there is no evidence that the additional disease detected by MRI is of clinical or biologic significance, particularly in light of the low local-regional failure rates currently reported in patients undergoing breast conserving surgery who receive whole breast irradiation and systemic therapies [4, 42].

The manifestation of an isolated metastatic axillary lymph node without any clinical and radiologic evidence of primary breast cancer is uncommon, but this disease most commonly originates from breast cancer in women. For these cases, the traditional therapy has been upper outer quadrantectomy or blind mastectomy with axillary lymph node dissection, with or without radiation. However, 30 to 40% of the upper outer quadrantectomy or blind mastectomy specimens show no histologic evidence of carcinoma, and the survival rate of patients who undergo blind mastectomy with axillary dissection is similar to those who undergo axillary dissection only [43]. Breast MRI techniques have improved significantly in recent years, and MRI with dynamic enhancement has been established as an important imaging modality for evaluating breast cancer with the highest sensitivity.

A Korean study [44] investigated the ability of breast MR imaging to identify the primary malignant focuses in patients with metastatic axillary lymph nodes and initially negative mammography and sonography, and correlated the results with the conventional imaging. The authors concluded that the high sensitivity of contrast-enhanced breast MRI played an essential role in evaluating occult breast cancer in patients who presented with a metastatic axillary lymph node with an unknown primary malignancy, and contrast-enhanced breast MRI also played an essential role for determining the therapeutic plan. In 90% of their cases, histologic work-up for the lesions detected on the breast MRI was practically feasible with successful localization being achieved under MR-guided, second-look US, or MR-correlated mammography.

With its recent technical advances, contrast-enhanced MRI plays an important role in identifying primary breast cancer, for defining the extent of tumor and for helping decide the therapeutic plans. While mammography is the primary imaging modality used to evaluate breast lesions, the false negative rate for mammography has been reported to be about 30% [45, 46]. The sensitivity of mammography is especially limited when the lesion is within dense breast parenchyma, and it is often as low as 45% [8]. Among mammography, US and MRI, MRI is the most sensitive method for evaluating breast cancer and it is well recognized that MRI can detect otherwise occult breast cancer [8, 32, 47].

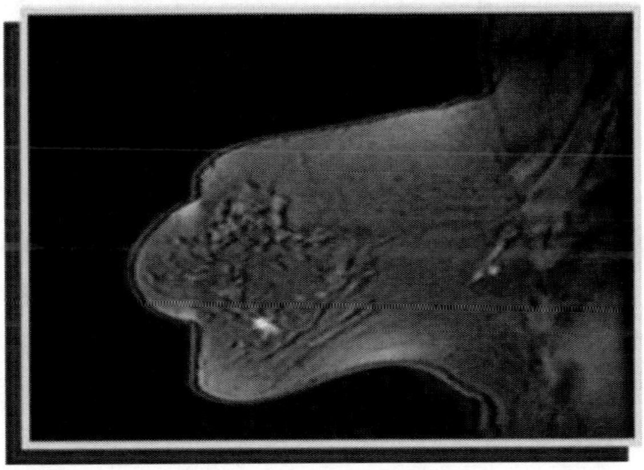

Figure 31. Small breast cancer in MRI.

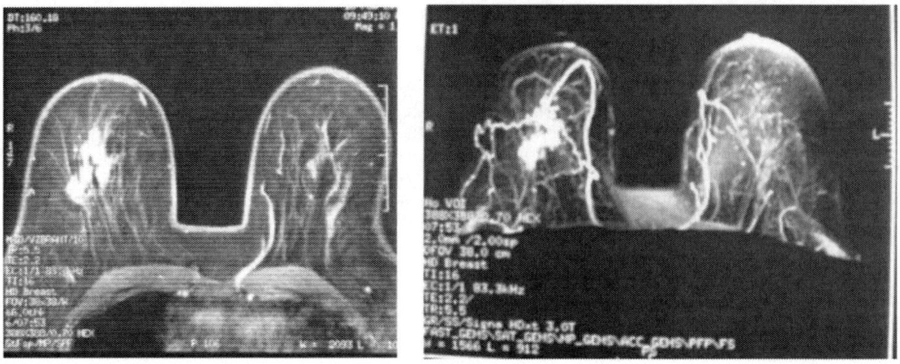

Figure 32. MRI Right breast tumor.

A few previous reports that detailed the MR images of patients with axillary lymph node metastases, and the patients had prior negative clinical and mammography findings, demonstrated 36%, 75% and 86% rates of detecting cancer by breast MRI, respectively [48, 49]. In another previous study [50] on patients with axillary lymph node metastasis and negative clinical, mammographic and US findings, the investigators showed a lesion detection rate of 64% with breast MRI, and 67% of the detected lesions were found to be primary breast cancer [50].

The reported mean size of the lesions visible by breast MRI alone was between 4.8 to 14.6 mm (Figure 31, 32) [44, 51].

Historically, the reported incidence of axillary metastasis in patients with DCIS is 1-2%, but the prevalence of positive lymph nodes in patients with pure DCIS is approximately 2-13% with performing immunohistochemical staining [52, 53].

Many authors suggest that before developing a therapeutic plan, breast MRI must be performed for those patients with axillary lymph node metastasis and who are without evidence of primary breast cancer. Although contrast-enhanced MRI has the highest sensitivity among the many imaging modalities for the breast, the specificity of breast MRI is low [8, 47, 53]. Therefore, preoperative biopsy or localization of the MRI-detected lesion is necessary [54]. Yet MR imaging-guided biopsy or localization requires commercially available MRI guiding equipment. Also, the cost-effectiveness of MRI-guided biopsy or localization has not yet been fully assessed [55]. Even when MRI guiding equipment is available, lesions in the medial breast are difficult to access and small enhancing lesions (around 5 mm) may be difficult to localize due to the transient nature of contrast enhancement and the obscuring that occurs when placing the biopsy needle. MR imaging-guided biopsy or localization is also a time-consuming procedure that lasts as long as 45 to 60 minutes [51, 54, 55].

A few studies have reported excellent performance of MR-guided second-look US localization [48, 56]. Therefore, localization with using MR-correlated mammography or MR-guided second-look US can be a cheaper, practical imaging alternative.

When BI-RADS category 2 or 3 lesions are detected on conventional images, but they do not correlate with the MR findings of the patients with suspicious occult breast cancer, then we should not neglect these lesions.

However, biopsy for all benign-looking lesions is not desirable or even necessarily meaningful [57]. When there is a benign or benign-looking lesion on the conventional images of the patients with metastatic axillary lymph node(s) and an unknown primary malignancy, then the conventional images should first be correlated with MR findings before performing a biopsy of the lesions [44].

MRI Report Organization

According to ACR BI-RADS® atlas the MRI reporting system should be concise and organized. Any pertinent clinical history that may affect scan interpretation, as well as any MRI acquisition techniques (including post-processing information) that may affect the scan interpretation, should be described (Table 5). The breast MRI report should first describe the amount of fibroglandular tissue and the background parenchymal enhancement (BPE -Table 6).

Abnormal enhancement (unique and separate from the BPE) is described based on morphology, distribution, and kinetics. Results from any physiologic or parametric imaging should be described.

An assessment is rendered that includes the degree of concern and any recommendation(s). Benign findings need not be reported, especially if the interpreting physician is concerned that the referring clinician or patient might infer anything other than absolute confidence in benignity.

Table 5. Report Organization

	Report Structure
1.	Indication for examination
2.	MRI technique
3.	Succinct description of overall breast composition
4.	Clear description of any important findings
5.	Comparison to previous examination(s)
6.	Assessment
7.	Management

Table 6. Breast Tissue: Background parenchymal enhancement (BPE)

	Background Parenchymal Enhancement
a.	Minimal
b.	Mild
c.	Moderate
d.	Marked

1. Indication for Examination

Provide a brief description of the indication for examination. For example, this may be high-risk screening, follow-up of a probably benign lesion, follow-up of cancer treated with neoadjuvant chemotherapy, or evaluation of the newly diagnosed cancer patient.

As background parenchymal enhancement can be affected by cyclical hormonal changes, it may be helpful to include menstrual history. If the patient is pre-menopausal, the week of the menstrual cycle may be important information to aid in interpretation. Current therapy (neoadjuvant, adjuvant, hormonal, or radiation therapy) for breast cancer treatment in the pre- or postsurgical setting may be important information and may inform exam interpretation.

The indication for examination should contain a concise description of the patient's clinical history, including:

a. Reason for performing the exam (e.g., screening, staging, problem solving)
b. Clinical abnormalities, including size, location, and duration
   i. Palpable finding
   ii. Nipple discharge
   iii. Other pertinent clinical findings or history

c. Previous biopsies
   i. Biopsy type
   ii. Biopsy location
   iii. Benign or malignant pathology (cytology or histology)

d. Hormonal status if applicable
   i. Pre- or post-menopausal
   ii. ii. Menstrual cycle phase (second week or other) or last menstrual period
   iii. Peripartum
   iv. Exogenous hormone therapy, tamoxifen, aromatase inhibitors, or other hormones or medications/herbs/vitamins that might influence MRI

2. MRI Technique

A detailed description of the technical factors of how the MRI examination was obtained must be given. At a minimum, a bright-fluid sequence of both breasts should be obtained. Pre- and post-gadolinium T1-weighted images should be obtained, preferably with fat suppression, simultaneously of both breasts. Subtraction imaging may be desired as well as other as processing techniques and parametric analysis. Elements of this description routinely include:

a. Right, left, or both breasts
b. Location of markers and their significance (scar, nipple, palpable lesion, etc.)
c. Weighting
   i. T1 weighted
   ii. ii. T2 weighted
   iii. Fat saturation
   iv. Scan orientation and plane
   v. Other pertinent pulse sequence features

d. Contrast dose
   i. Name of contrast agent
   ii. ii. Dosage (mmol/kg) and volume (in cc)
   iii. Injection type: bolus or infusion
   iv. Timing (relationship of bolus injection to scan start time and scan length)

v. If multiple scans: number of post-contrast scans and acquisition techniques of each (how fast, how many slices, and slice thickness)

e. Post-processing techniques as applicable
   i. MPR/MIP (Multiplanar reconstruction / Maximum Intensity Projection)
   ii. ii. Time/signal intensity curves
   iii. Subtraction
   iv. Other techniques

3. Succinct Description of Overall Breast Composition

This should include an overall description of the breast composition, including:

a. The amount of FGT (FibroGlandular breast Tissue) that is present

The four categories of breast composition are defined by the visually estimated content of FGT within the breasts. If the breasts are not of apparently equal amounts of FGT the breast with the most FGT should be used to categorize breast composition. Although there may be considerable variation in visually estimating breast composition, categorizing based on percentages (and specifically into quartiles) is not recommended.

The BIRADS® committee recognizes that quantification of breast FGT volume on MRI may be feasible in the future, but they await publication of robust data before endorsing percentage recommendations. They urge the use of BI-RADS® terminology instead of numbers to classify breast FGT in order to eliminate any possible confusion with the BIRADS® assessment categories, which are numbered.

b. The amount of background parenchymal enhancement in the image

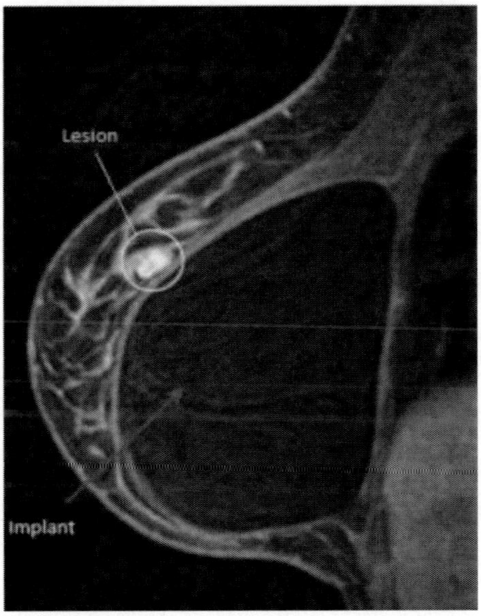

Figure 33. Breast MRI: Lesion over implant.

The four categories of BPE are defined by the visually estimated enhancement of the FGT of the breast(s). If the breasts are not of an apparently equal amount of BPE, the breast with the most BPE should be used to categorize BPE. In the event that treatment has altered BPE in one or both breasts, this can be reported. Although there may be considerable variation in visually estimating BPE, categorizing based on percentages (and specifically into quartiles) is not recommended.

Quantification of BPE volume and intensity on MRI may be feasible in the future, but the BIRADS® committee awaits publication of robust data on that topic before endorsing percentage recommendations.

The committee recognizes that there are variations in BPE distribution and morphology. However, committee defers on recommending descriptions of distribution or morphology until additional data are available. Currently, BPE refers to the volume of enhancement and the intensity of enhancement. On bilateral scans, describe whether the pattern is asymmetric or symmetric, if appropriate. Asymmetric denotes more enhancement in one breast than in the other. Symmetric enhancement is mirror image.

c. Whether implants are present (Figure 33)

If an implant is present, it should be so stated in the report. Information should include its composition (saline, silicone, or other) and the number of lumens (single or multiple).

4. Clear Description of Any Important Findings

Abnormal enhancement is unique and separate from BPE. Its description should indicate the breast in which the abnormal enhancement occurs, the lesion type, and modifiers. The clinical location of the abnormality as extrapolated from the MRI location (based on clock-face position and quadrant location) should be reported. It should be recognized that there may be variation in location of a clinically detected lesion (patient is upright or supine), a mammographically detected lesion (patient is upright and compressed), a sonographically detected lesion (patient is supine or supine oblique), and an MRI-detected lesion (patient is prone) based on positional differences.

A more consistent measurement is the distance from the nipple. It is encouraged that distance from the nipple for a lesion is reported in order to facilitate correlation between modalities, although it should be understood that one should expect some difference in distance from the nipple among the breast imaging modalities. For bilateral axial examinations, the breasts should be pointing up, following the cross-sectional imaging convention.

The descriptors should include techniques, all data, and any findings from MRI listed in Table 6.

Also, it is recognized that other techniques may be used in the evaluation of breast lesions. Newer and evolving techniques are constantly being introduced. Findings from other techniques, such as diffusion-weighted imaging or MR spectroscopy, should be reported if clinically important.

Table 6. Description of all data and any important findings

a. Size
b. Location
i. Right or left
ii. Breast quadrant and clock-face position (or central, retroareolar, and axillary tail descriptors)
iii. Distance from nipple, skin, or chest wall in centimeters (if applicable)
Descriptors for abnormal enhancement:
c. Findings associated with abnormal enhancement include:
i. Artifacts that affect interpretation
ii. Focus: a tiny dot of enhancement that does not clearly represent a space-occupying lesion or mass and does not clearly show a mass on precontrast imaging
iii. Masses: space-occupying lesions, usually spherical or ball-like, may displace or retract surrounding breast tissue
Descriptors - modifiers describing a mass:
(a) Shape: describes the overall morphology of the enhancement
Oval (includes lobulated)
Round
Irregular
(b) Margin: describes the borders
Circumscribed
Not circumscribed
- Irregular
- Spiculated
(c) Internal enhancement characteristics
Homogeneous
Heterogeneous
Rim enhancement
Dark internal septations

iv. Non-mass enhancement (NME): modifiers describing enhancement patterns with a specific MRI pattern
(a) Distribution
- Focal
- Linear
- Segmental
- Regional
- Multiple regions
- Diffuse
(b) Internal enhancement patterns (for all other types)
- Homogenous
- Heterogeneous
- Clumped
- Clustered ring
v. Intramammary lymph node (rarely important)
vi. Skin lesion
vii. Non-enhancing findings
a. Ductal precontrast high signal on T1W
b. Cyst
c. Postoperative collections (hematoma/seroma)
d. Post-therapy skin thickening and trabecular thickening
e. Non-enhancing mass
f. Architectural distortion
g. Signal void from foreign bodies, clips, etc.
viii. Associated features
a. Nipple retraction
b. Nipple invasion
c. Skin retraction
d. Skin thickening
e. Skin invasion (Direct invasion, Inflammatory cancer)
f. Axillary adenopathy
g. Pectoralis muscle invasion
h. Chest wall invasion
i. Architectural distortion

ix. Fat-containing lesions
(a) Lymph nodes
a. Normal
b. Abnormal
(b) Fat necrosis
(c) Hamartoma
(d) Postoperative seroma/hematoma with fat

x. Stability: describe how enhancement changed (if new, stable, or changed in size from previous examination)

xi. Kinetic curve assessment
(a) The fastest enhancing portion of the lesion or the most suspicious washout curve pattern in the lesion should be assessed
- Sample fast enhancing areas

Table 6. (Continued)

- Sample for and report on the worst looking curve shape

(b) Signal intensity/time curve
- Initial enhancement phase-describes the enhancement pattern within the first 2 minutes or when the curve starts to change
  - Slow
  - Medium
  - Fast
- Delayed phase – describe the enhancement pattern after 2 minutes or after the curve starts to change
  - Persistent
  - Plateau
  - Washout

xii. Implants

(a) Implant material and lumen type
- Saline
- Silicone
  - Intact
  - Ruptured
- Other implant material (such as soy oil, polypropylene, polyurethane, and sponges; includes direct injections)
- Lumen type

(b) Implant location
- Rectoglandular
- Retropectoral

(c) Abnormal implant contour
- Focal bulge

(d) Intracapsular silicone findings
- Radial folds
- Subcapsular line
- Keyhole design (teardrop, noose)
- Linguine sign

(e) Extracapsular silicone
- Breast
- Lymph nodes

(f) Water droplets

(g) Peri-impland fluid

5. Comparison to Previous Examination(s)

Include a statement indicating that the current examination has been compared to previous examination(s) with specific date(s). If this is not included, it should be assumed that no comparison has been made; however, it is preferable to indicate explicitly that no comparison was made. Comparison to a previous examination may assume importance if the finding of concern requires an evaluation of change or stability. Comparison is less important when the finding has characteristically benign features. Comparison may be irrelevant if the finding is inherently suspicious for malignancy. Information in this area should include:

a. Previous MRI with the date of examination
b. Other imaging studies (mammogram, US, nuclear medicine examination, other) and date of examination (Figure 34, 35, 36).

6. Assessment

This is a description of an overall summary of MRI findings, including assessment.

Incorporating an assessment category in the overall summary of the breast MRI report is sound medical practice. All final impressions should be complete with each lesion fully categorized.

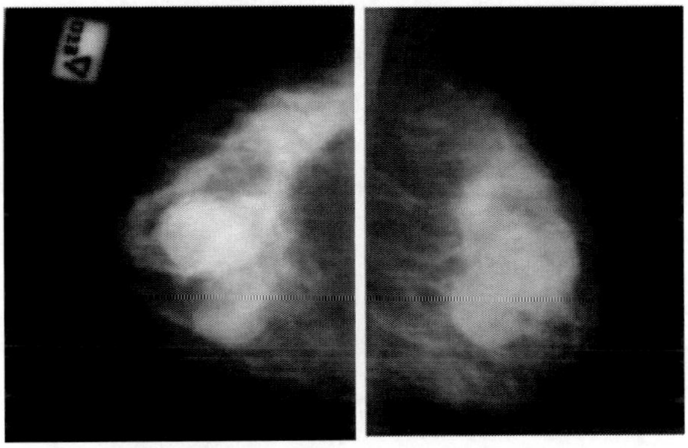

Figure 34. Mammography findings in a patient with cancer and large cysts in right breast.

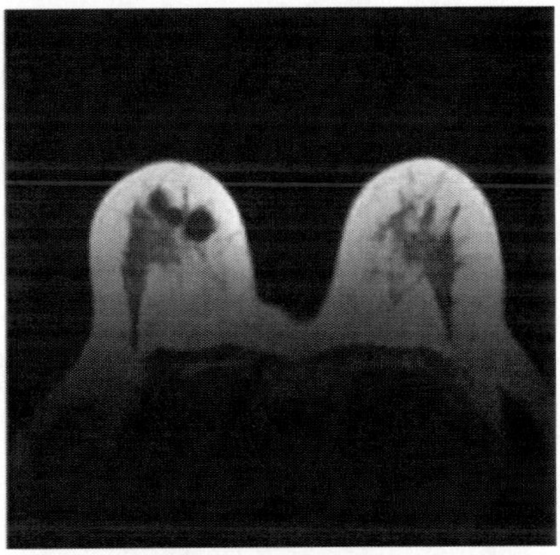

Figure 35. MRI of the same patient with breast cancer and cysts.

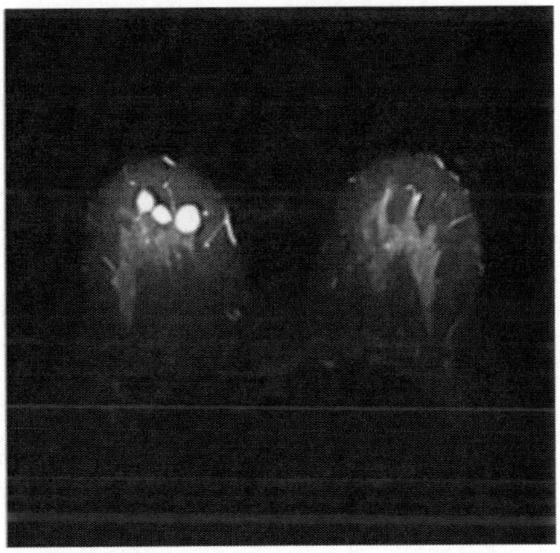

Figure 36. Abnormal enhancement on MRI.

An incomplete assessment (category 0) is used when full diagnostic imaging has not been performed and should be given only when additional imaging or clinical evaluation is recommended to establish the benignity of a finding (e.g., a possible intramammary lymph node or fat necrosis at MRI may require additional mammography and/or US examination).

7. Management

This is a description of patient management recommendations, as appropriate. If an incomplete assessment (category 0) is rendered, a specific suggestion for the next course of action should be given (physical examination, diagnostic mammography, targeted diagnostic US, etc.). Note that an incomplete assessment (category 0) should not be rendered when recommending targeted US in order to determine the feasibility of performing biopsy using sonographic guidance; such a scenario requires the use of a category 4 or 5 assessment (suspicious or highly suggestive of malignancy).

If a suspicious abnormality is detected, the report should indicate that a biopsy should be performed in the absence of clinical contraindication. This means that the radiologist has sufficient concern that a biopsy is warranted; the term "clinical contraindication" indicates that there may be reasons why the patient and her physician might wish to defer the biopsy. Concordance between BIRADS® assessment categories and management recommendations is listed in Table 7.

MRI of the breast has evolved into an important tool in breast imaging with increasing indications for its use. MRI has plenty advantages such as increased contrast of tissues, multiple views, less ionizing radiation, use of contrast enhancement time course to differentiate benign from malignant lesions, detecting lesions close to chest wall and occult breast lesions, higher sensitivity but still poor specificity. The high sensitivity of MRI but it's not so high specificity creates many false-positive results and callbacks for further evaluation, including second-look ultrasound studies and biopsies. Another disadvantage is the newly recognized but rare side effect of MRI, nephrogenic sclerosing fibrosis that is related to intravenous administration of MRI contrast agents. Special attention is needed for women with impaired renal function or renal failure [58]. The limitations of MRI include its high cost, unsuitability for some patients (those who are obese, have pacemakers, or have renal failure), the potential for unnecessary biopsies, lack of portability and the length of time required for imaging.

Table 7. Concordance between BI-RADS® Assessment Categories and Management Recommendations

Assessment	Management	Likelihood of Cancer
Category 0: Incomplete – Need additional Imaging Evaluation	Recommend additional imaging: mammogram or targeted US	N/A
Category 1: Negative	Routine breast MRI screening if cumulative lifetime risk ≥ 20%	Essentially 0% likelihood of malignancy
Category 2: Benign	Routine breast MRI screening if cumulative lifetime risk ≥ 20%	Essentially 0% likelihood of malignancy
Category 3: Probably Benign	Short-interval (6-month) follow-up)	≥ 0% but ≤ 2% likelihood of malignancy
Category 4: Suspicious	Tissue diagnosis	>2% but <95% likelihood of malignancy
Category 5: Highly Suggestive of Malignancy	Tissue diagnosis	> 95% likelihood of malignancy
Category 6: Known Biopsy-Proven Malignancy	Surgical excision when clinically appropriate	N/A

IV. COMPUTERIZED TOMOGRAPHY SCAN (CT SCAN)

A computed tomography (CT or CAT) scan is not routinely used for breast cancer screening or diagnosis, but can be useful for contrast-enhancing lesions and lesions close to chest wall (contrast enhancing lesions suggest malignancy) (Figures 37, 38, 39). CT scan is routinely used to assess for chest, liver, pelvic and bony metastases and post-treatment follow-up.

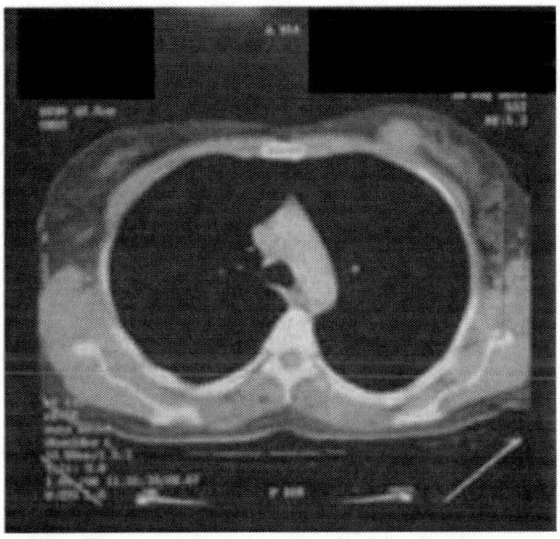

Figure 37. Breast mass in CT scan.

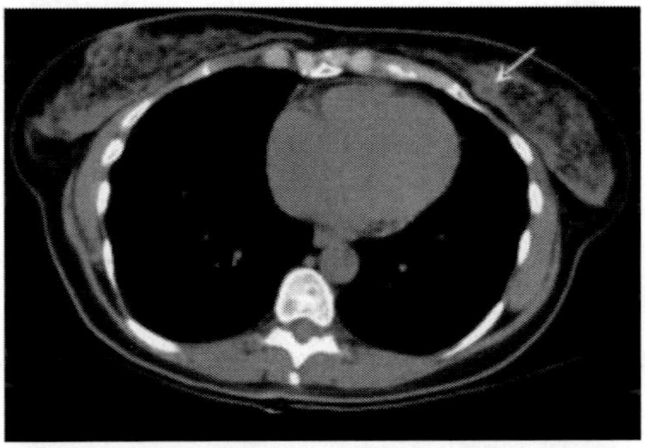

Figure 38. Breast cancer in Pre contrast CT scan.

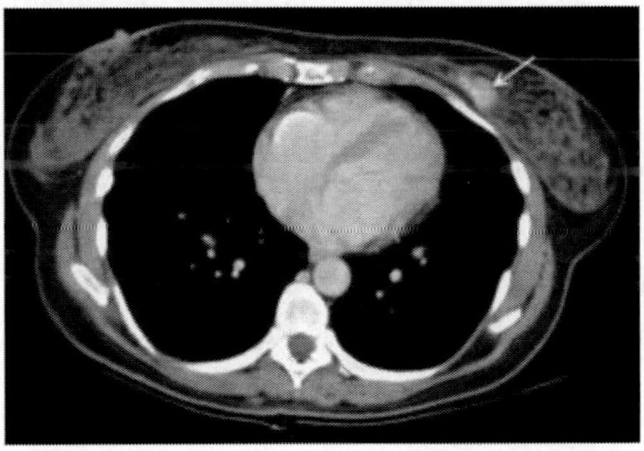

Figure 39. Post contrast CT scan enhancing lesion (yellow arrow), suggesting malignancy.

V. Positron Emission Tomography (PET) Scan

Most breast malignancies have greater metabolism than normal tissues and concentrate 18F-fluorodeoxyglucose (FDG), the agent most widely used in clinical positron emission tomography (PET) scanning [59, 60]. Whole-body PET does not have the spatial resolution needed for breast imaging. PET/computed tomography has been shown to be useful in the restaging of breast cancer, in evaluation of response to therapy, and as a problem-solving method [59, 61]. Small, dedicated PET scanners have been developed for breast imaging, which use gentle compression.

The radiopharmaceutical that is primarily used in the clinical evaluation of most cancers, including breast cancer, is FDG. FDG is widely available from commercial radiopharmacies and provides clinically important information relevant to cancer. Other radiopharmaceuticals, such as F-18 fluoroestradiol and F-18 fluoro-L-thymidine, are now being evaluated in breast cancer patients, but these radiopharmaceuticals have not assumed a clinical role at this time.

The FDG is administered intravenously in the arm opposite a known or suspected breast lesion or through a foot vein, because extravasation can result in axillary lymph node accumulation. Accumulation in an axillary lymph node could be from either metastatic disease or extravasation, so it is important not to inject in the arm on the side of the lesion. The patient should be comfortable and warm after administration of the FDG. Movement of the head and neck should be minimized to avoid accumulation in neck and shoulder girdle muscles. Furthermore, some evidence suggests that keeping the patient comfortably warm at the time of administration decreases accumulation in brown fat that may be confused with supraclavicular and internal mammary lymph node accumulation. For the evaluation of primary breast lesions, some authors have suggested the use of prone imaging and 3-hour delayed imaging.

In most studies of FDG-PET imaging in breast cancer (Figure 40), investigators have administered 10-20 mCi of FDG, and imaging is started 45-60 minutes after injection. Whole-body scans have included the external auditory meatus through the proximal thighs. Attenuation corrected scans are performed. It is unclear at this time whether 3-dimensional acquisitions will have an advantage over the 2-dimensional acquisitions that have been used until now. Furthermore, the advantages of the combined PET and computed tomography over dedicated PET scanners alone have not been demonstrated at this time.

A pilot study of positron emission mammography (PEM) by Tafra et al. evaluated 44 images. PEM demonstrated 89% of the lesions. Multifocal disease was correctly ruled out in 17 of 17 cases [62]. Berg et al. found that PEM combined with mammography and sonography yielded 47 (98%) of 48 cancers [8]. Dense breasts do not appear to negatively affect PEM as they do mammography. Lower-grade tumors are more likely to be missed, which makes sense, as the technique employed in PEM is based on FDG concentration [59].

Positron emission tomography (PET) scans are one of the tests oncologists can use to establish a baseline of whether and to what extent your cancer may have spread to other parts of your body. The problem with PET scans is that they are not very accurate, because they are not very good at finding small cancer spots. In the past, tumor needs to be at least 2cm to be seen on the scan. There are now newer scans that are a bit better and they can detect virtually all 2 cm lesions. However, they can only detect about one-third of those that are smaller than 1 cm. This means they can result in a false negative result. In addition, they often give false positive results, indicating that something might be cancer when it is really an inflammation, infection, or cells that happen to be growing rapidly.

In a prospective study that evaluated the accuracy of PET in axillary nodal staging in 360 women with newly diagnosed breast cancer, PET had a 61% sensitivity and 80% specificity [63]. Patients with small nodal metastases and with only a few lymph nodes involved have their conditions missed on PET scans. PET is not accurate enough to replace the sentinel lymph node study. In a study that evaluated the impact of the site of the primary breast cancer, patients having inner quadrant primary cancers had a much greater frequency of extra-axillary metastases than did patients having outer quadrant primaries and were twice as likely to have progression of their disease.

Several studies have evaluated the accuracy of FDG-PET in detecting primary breast cancer. A meta-analysis of the PET literature that included 606 patients demonstrated that PET had a sensitivity of 88% and a specificity of 79% [64]. The mean tumor size included in these studies ranged from 2-4 cm in diameter. Most false-negative results relate to small lesions (<1 cm), low-grade malignancy, and noninvasive cancers. False-positive results occur primarily from infectious or inflammatory lesions, such as mastitis and hemorrhagic inflammation after biopsy or surgery.

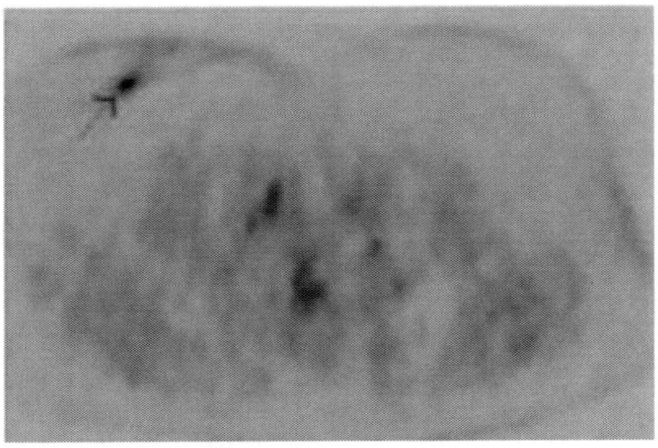

Figure 40. Invasive ductal carcinoma in PET scan (arrow).

PET in Lymph Node Staging

The evaluation of the axillary lymph nodes is important for determining prognosis (Figure 41). The 10-year survival of patients with negative axillary lymph nodes is 65% to 80% and is significantly greater than in patients with 1-3 nodes, who have a 38% to 63% 10-year survival, and in those patients with more than 3 axillary nodes, who have a 13% to 27% 10-year survival [65]. Axillary lymph node involvement influences the selection of treatment. Clinical evaluation, including conventional imaging, is not accurate in detecting axillary nodal disease. Sentinel lymph node localization is performed using Tc 99m-labeled colloids and/or blue dye in patients with invasive cancers that are 2 cm or less in diameter. Most of these patients (>80%) have negative axillary lymph nodes at surgery. Axillary nodal surgery has well-known risks, including lymphedema and diminished upper extremity motility and functioning. Metastases to the internal mammary lymph nodes have similar prognostic significance and occasionally are the only site of metastatic disease. The internal mammary lymph nodes are typically not assessed pathologically because of the extensive surgery required to sample these nodes. FDG-PET imaging has been used to evaluate whether it can replace or supplement the information available for lymphoscintigraphy and axillary lymph node staging. Several studies have evaluated FDG-PET for the detection of axillary metastatic disease. These studies have generally shown sensitivity between 50% and 100% and specificities between 67% and 100%. PET has minimal impact on patients with palpable axillary lymph nodes, because these patients will undergo axillary dissection. Thus, it is important to consider the patients with nonpalpable lymph nodes. A meta-analysis of FDG-PET has demonstrated that it has a 95% sensitivity and an 88% specificity for palpable axillary lymph nodes compared with the 90% sensitivity and 94% specificity in patients having nonpalpable lymph nodes [64].

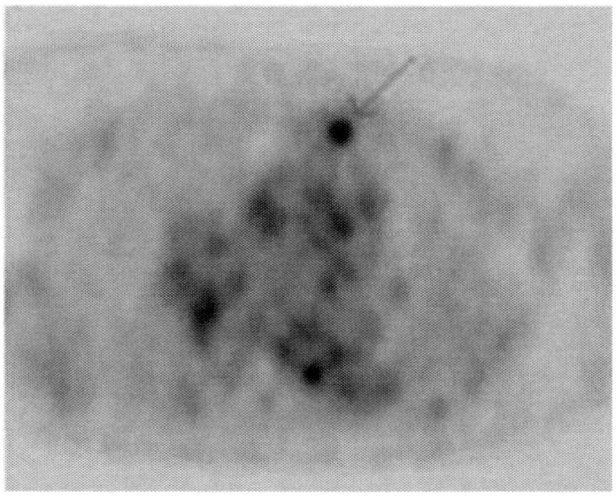

Figure 41. Breast cancer metastasis in internal mammary lymph node in PET scan (arrow).

Wahl et al., [66] performed a prospective study of axillary nodal staging. This study included 360 women with newly diagnosed breast cancer. The FDG-PET images of the draining nodal regions were interpreted qualitatively and qualitatively in a blinded manner by 3 experienced readers. The results from 308 assessable axillae were compared with axillary node pathology to determine the accuracy of the PET findings. The prevalence of axillary nodal metastases was 35%. The mean estimated area under the receiver operating characteristic curve for the 3 readers was 0.74. When at least 1 abnormal axillary focus was identified, the sensitivity was 61%, specificity was 80%, positive predictive value was 62%, and negative predictive value was 79%. False-negative results were obtained in patients who had smaller and fewer lymph nodes. The use of the standardized uptake value (SUV) normalized to lean body mass showed a positive predictive value of 90% and a sensitivity of 32% at an SUV of 1.8 or greater. If two or more foci of abnormal accumulation were noted, the predictive accuracy was 78% to 83%, but at a sensitivity of only 27%. The authors conclude that PET is not recommended for routine staging of the axilla in most patients with newly diagnosed breast cancer.

PET in Distant Metastatic Disease

In addition to detecting the primary breast cancer and loco-regional metastases, whole-body FDG-PET can detect distant metastatic disease to the soft tissues, viscera, and bone.

FDG-PET imaging has been shown to be accurate for the detection of distant metastatic disease. In a study by Dehdashti and colleagues, [67] PET had a sensitivity of 89% and specificity of 100% for differentiating benign from malignant lesions. PET has been shown to identify metastatic disease that is not detected by conventional imaging. A study by Schirrmeister and colleagues [68] evaluated 89 patients with breast cancer undergoing initial staging. FDG-PET detected distant metastatic disease in 7 patients, 3 of whom had negative conventional imaging study results. Four patients had false-positive bone scintigraphy and true-negative PET scan results.

Tran and colleagues [69] evaluated the frequency of extra-axillary metastases in the absence of axillary involvement in breast cancer patients with outer quadrant primary lesions and compared this frequency with that of inner quadrant breast cancers. Their study included 141 breast cancer patients, with 42 having inner quadrant lesions and 99 having outer quadrant lesions. The patients underwent a 3-year postscan and clinical follow-up. The patients with inner quadrant cancers had a 6-fold greater frequency of PET findings of extra-axillary metastasis compared with patients who had outer quadrant cancer. The patients with inner quadrant disease were twice as likely to experience progression of their disease as were patients with outer quadrant lesions.

Bone metastases are major contributors to the morbidity of breast cancer. The median survival of patients with metastatic disease to bone is 24 months [70]. Bone scintigraphy, the primary modality used for evaluating skeletal metastatic disease in breast cancer, has a low specificity and sensitivity for detecting osteolytic lesions. FDG-PET has been demonstrated to be more sensitive than bone scintigraphy. The FDG-PET scan is more accurate in detecting osteolytic lesions than osteoblastic lesions [71].

PET in Monitoring Therapeutic Response

The only cancer that Medicare has approved coverage for therapeutic monitoring is breast cancer. The assessment of response to therapy in patients with advanced breast cancer is important because preoperative therapy predicts outcome. Patients who respond to the chemotherapy or hormonal therapy have a better prognosis than patients who do not respond. Schelling and colleagues, [72] in a study of 22 patients with locally advanced breast cancer, demonstrated that PET correctly identified responders from nonresponders with a sensitivity of 100% and specificity of 85%. Response was defined as a decrease in the tumor SUV to less than 55% of the baseline value.

SPECT-CT Scan

SPECT-CT is where two different types of scans are taken and the images or pictures from each are fused or merged together. The fused scan can provide more precise information about how different parts of the body function and more clearly identify problems such as breast tumours. Single photon emission computed tomography (SPECT): SPECT images are obtained following an injection of a radiopharmaceutical that is used for nuclear medicine scans. The injected medication sticks to specific areas in the body, depending on what radiopharmaceutical is used and the type of scan being performed.

The radiopharmaceutical is detected by a nuclear medicine gamma camera. The camera or cameras rotate over a 360 degree arc around the patient, allowing for reconstruction of an image in three dimensions. CT scanner rotates much faster than the gamma camera, so the CT part of the study takes less time than the SPECT study.

The similarity between SPECT and CT in the method of image processing allows the images to be combined.

Preoperative imaging technologies such as scintigraphy or, recently, SPECT/CT may contribute to the precise localization of the SLN(s) and support surgical planning [74, 75]. Fluorescence imaging systems, mini gamma cameras and freehand SPECT (FhSPECT) have been suggested as alternatives that allow image-guided resection of the SLN. The first two technologies provide 2-D images of either fluorescent or radioactively labelled SLNs, [76-78] but none of the technologies has yet found its way into clinical routine. The FhSPECT technology was developed by a joint research group of the Faculty of Computer Science and the Faculty of Medicine at Technische Universität München and utilizes 3-D images, thus providing additional depth information and the possibility of image fusion with a live video of the operation sites (Figure 42) [79].

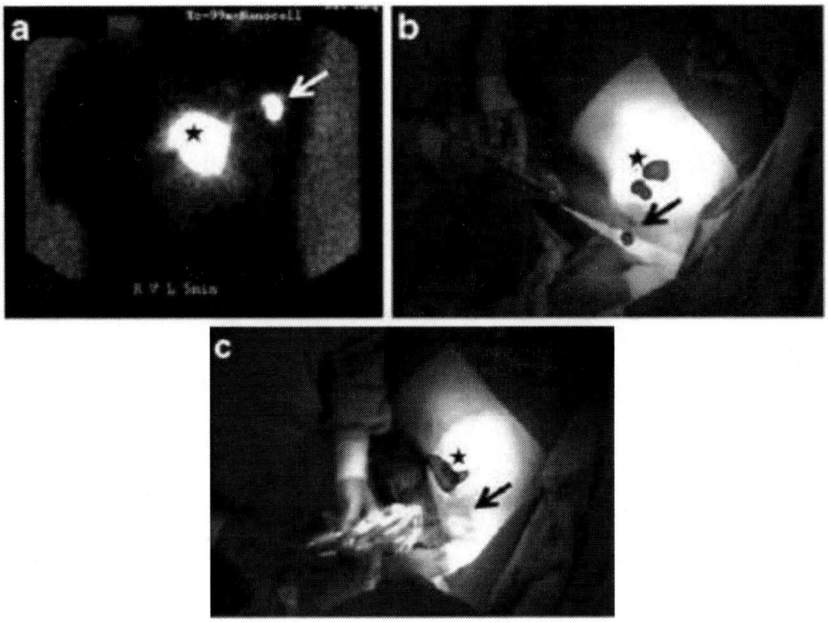

Figure 42. Patient with SLN (arrows) in the left axilla: a. preoperative scintigram; b. pre-incision FhSPECT image; c. postoperative FhSPECT image with no remaining activity (stars injection site).

FDG-PET plays an important role in the evaluation of patients with breast cancer. Its role in the detection of primary breast cancer is still under evaluation. FDG-PET is useful in the initial staging and restaging of patients with locally advanced breast cancer. FDG-PET scanning is not accurate enough to replace sentinel lymph node studies for the evaluation of axillary nodal involvement. FDG-PET scanning is rapidly becoming a critical method for monitoring response to therapy in patients with locally advanced breast cancer [73].

VI. SCINTIMAMMOGRAPHY

Another form of breast imaging that involves the functional uptake of radiotracers is scintimammography. It uses 99Tcsestamibi, which is taken up by breast cancers. A dual-head machine was tested at the Mayo Clinic, which studied more than 900 patients in 6 years [59]. The machine functions independent of breast density. Heavy compression of the breast is not required. They found a 97% concordance with mammography. Medicare charges are estimated at $1,029.69 for MRI and $292.12 for scintimammography. The final sensitivity is over 90%, making this a useful adjunct to mammography [80]. As these are emerging technologies that are not yet widely used, clinical data are still scarce.

Guidelines for Breast Cancer Screening

The American Cancer Society (ACS) guidelines for breast cancer screening currently recommend that for average-risk women mammographic screening begin at age 40 years and continuing for as long as a woman is in good health. Breast self-exam (BSE) is an option for women starting in their 20s. Women in their 20s and 30s should have a clinical breast exam every 3 years. Women over 40 years of age should have a clinical breast examination yearly. Women should be told about the benefits and limitations of breast self-examination and the importance of prompt reporting of any new breast symptoms. As long as a woman is in reasonably good health and would be a candidate for treatment, she should continue to be screened with mammography.

For women at high risk, earlier initiation of screening, shorter screening intervals, or the addition of other modalities may provide benefit. It recommended annual MRI screening in addition to mammography for BRCA mutation carriers; first-degree relatives of BRCA carriers who are untested and those patients with a calculated lifetime risk of 20% to 25% or greater as defined by BRCAPRO or other models that are largely dependent on family history. MRI is also recommended for patients who received radiation to their chest between age 10 and 30 years, patients with Li-Fraumeni syndrome and their first-degree relatives, and patients with Cowden and Bannayan-Riley-Ruvalcaba syndromes and their first-degree relatives.

Life expectancy continues to increase, and in developed countries women aged 75 years and older represent an increasing percentage of the population. Evidence-based guidelines for the regular screening of older women are lacking. Patients with life expectancies less than 5 years are not likely to derive any survival benefit from cancer screening. However, age in itself should not be a reason to stop screening but rather the patients overall health and ability to receive treatment and benefit from the screening.

REFERENCES

[1] Makariou E, Sayah A. Imaging of the surgically altered breast. In "Surgery of the breast – Principles and Art," 3rd ed, S. Spear et al, Lippincott 2011; 16-34.

[2] Berg WA. Rationale for a trial of screening breast ultrasound: American College of Radiology Imaging Network (ACRIN). *AJR Am. J. Roentgenol.* 2003;180:1225–1228.

[3] Mandelblatt JS, Cronin KA, Bailey S, et al. Effects of mammography screening under different screening schedules: model estimates of potential benefits and harms. *Ann. Intern. Med.* 2009;151(10):738–47.

[4] Hunt KK, Robertson JFR, Bland KI. The Breast. In Schwartz's Principles of Surgery, Editor-in-Chief F. Charles Brunicardi, by McGraw-Hill Education, 2015; 523-529.

[5] Crystal P, Strano SD, Shcharynski S, et al. Using sonography to screen women with mammographically dense breasts. *AJR Am. J. Roentgenol.* 2003;181:177–182.

[6] Skandalakis JE, Colburn GL, Weidman TA, Foster RS Jr, Kingsworth AN, Skandalakis LJ, Skandalakis PN, Mirilas PS. The breast. In Skandalakis' Surgical Anatomy, 2004; 185-203.

[7] Mustonen P, Farin P, Kosunen O. Ultrasonographic detection of metastatic axillary lymph nodes in breast cancer. *Ann. Chir. Gynaecol.* 1990;79:15–8.

[8] Berg WA, Gutierrez L, Ness Aiver MS, et al. Diagnostic accuracy of mammography, clinical examination, US, and MR imaging in preoperative assessment of breast cancer. *Radiology* 2004;233:830–849.

[9] Park SH, Kim MJ, Park BW, et al. Impact of Preoperative Ultrasonography and Fine-Needle Aspiration of Axillary Lymph Nodes on Surgical Management of Primary Breast Cancer. *Ann. Surg. Oncol.* 2011;18:738–744.

[10] Moore A, Hester M, Nam MW, et al. Distinct lymph nodal sonographic characteristics in breast cancer patients at high risk for axillary metastases correlate with the final axillary stage. *Br. J. Radiol.* 2008;81:630–6.

[11] Veronesi U, Paganelli G, Galimberti V, Viale G, Zurrida S, Bedoni M, et al. Sentinel-node biopsy to avoid axillary dissection in breast cancer with clinically negative lymph-nodes. *Lancet* 1997;349:1864–7.

[12] de Paredes, Ellen Shaw. Atlas of Mammography, 3rd Edition, Lippincott Williams & Wilkins, 2007;104-125.

[13] Krishnamurthy S, Sneige N, Bedi DG, et al. Role of ultrasound-guided fine-needle aspiration of indeterminate and suspicious axillary lymph nodes in the initial staging of breast carcinoma. *Cancer* 2002;95:982-988.

[14] Aragon R, Morgan J, Wong JH, Lum S. Potential Impact of USPSTF Recommendations on Early Diagnosis of Breast Cancer. *Ann. Surg. Oncol.* 2011; 18:3137–3142.

[15] Berry DA, Cronin KA, Plevritis SK, et al. Effect of screening and adjuvant therapy on mortality from breast cancer. *N. Engl. J. Med.* 2005;353(17):1784-92.

[16] Nystrom L, Andersson I, Bjurstam N, Frisell J, Nordenskjold B, Rutqvist LE. Long-term effects of mammography screening: updated overview of the Swedish randomised trials. *Lancet.* 2002;359(9310):909-19.

[17] Cady B, Michaelson JS, Chung MA. The ''tipping point'' for breast cancer mortality decline has resulted from size reductions due to mammographic screening. *Ann. Surg. Oncol.* 2011;18(4): 903–6.

[18] Virnig BA, Wang SY, Shamilyan T, Kane RL, Tuttle TM. Ductal carcinoma in situ: risk factors and impact of screening. *J Natl Cancer Inst Monogr.* 2010;(41):113-116.

[19] Ciatto S, Houssami N, Bernardi D, et al. Integration of 3D digital mammography with tomosynthesis for population breast cancer screening (STORM): a prospective comparison study. *Lancet Oncol.* 2013; 14:70134-70137.

[20] Jackson VP, Dines KA, Bassett LW, et al. Diagnostic importance of the radiographic density of noncalcified breast masses: analysis of 91 lesions. *AJR Am. J. Roentgenol.* 1991;157:25-28.

[21] Swann CA, Kopans DB, Koerner FC, et al. The halo sign and malignant breast tissues. *AJR Am. J. Roentgenol.* 1978;149: 1145-1147.

[22] Fournier DV, Weber W, Hoeffken M, et al. Growth rate of 147 mammary carcinomas. *Cancer* 1980;45:2198-2207.

[23] Heuser L, Spratt J, Polk H. Growth rates of primary breast cancer. *Cancer* 1979;43:1888-1894.

[24] Meyer JE, Kopans DB. Stability of a mammographic mass: a false sense of security. *AJR Am. J. Roentgenol.* 1981;137:595-598.

[25] Allen SD, Nerurkar A, Querci Della Rovere GU. The breast lesion excision system (BLES): a novel technique in the diagnostic and therapeutic management of small indeterminate breast lesions? *Eur. Radiol.* 2011;77(3):377-52.

[26] Kass R, Kumar G, Klimberg VS, et al. Clip migration in stereotactic biopsy. *Am. J. Surg.* 2002;184:325–331.

[27] Lamm RL, Jackman RJ. Mammographic abnormalities caused by percutaneous stereotactic biopsy of histologically benign lesions evident on follow-up mammograms. *AJR Am. J. Roentgenol.* 2000;174:753–756.

[28] Liberman L, Hann LE, Dershaw DD, et al. Mammographic findings after stereotactic 14-gauge vacuum biopsy. *Radiology* 1997;203:343–347.

[29] Kaye MD, Vicinanza-Adami CA, Sullivan ML. Mammographic findings after stereotaxic biopsy of the breast performed with large-core needles. *Radiology* 1994;192:149–151.

[30] Brenner RJ, Pfaff JM. Mammographic changes after excisional breast biopsy for benign disease. *AJR Am. J. Roentgenol.* 1996;167:1047–1052.

[31] Sickles EA, Herzog KA. Mammography of the postsurgical breast. *AJR Am. J. Roentgenol.* 1981;136:585–588.

[32] Orel SG, Schnall MD. MR imaging of the breast for the detection, diagnosis, and staging of breast cancer. *Radiology* 2001;220:13–30.

[33] Lehman CD. Role of MRI in screening women at high risk for breast cancer. *J. Magn. Reson. Imaging* 2006;24:964–970.

[34] Lee CH. Problem solving MR imaging of the breast. *Radiol. Clin. N. Am.* 2004;42:919–934.

[35] Rim A, Chellman-Jeffers M. Trends in breast cancer screening and diagnosis. *Cleve. Clin. J. Med.* 2008;75(suppl 1):S2–S9.

[36] Berman CG. Recent advances in breast-specific imaging. *Cancer Control* 2007;14(4):338–349.

[37] Buadu LD, Murakami J, Murayama S, et al. Breast lesions: correlation of contrast medium enhancement patterns on MR images with histopathologic findings and tumor angiogenesis. *Radiology* 1996;200(3):639–649.

[38] Nunes LW. Architectural-based interpretations of breast MR imaging. *Magn Reson Imaging Clin. N. Am.* 2001;9(2):303–320.

[39] Harms SE, Flamig DP, Hesley KL, et al. MR imaging of the breast with rotating delivery of excitation off resonance: clinical experience with pathologic correlation. *Radiology* 1993;187:493–501.

[40] Orel SG, Schnall MD, Powell CM, et al. Staging of suspected breast cancer: effect of MR imaging and MR-guided biopsy. *Radiology* 1995;196:115–122.

[41] Turnbull L, Brown S, Harvey I, et al. Comparative effectiveness of MRI in breast cancer (COMICE) trial: a randomized controlled trial. *Lancet.* 2010;375:563-571.

[42] Houssami N, Turner R, Morrow M. Preoperative magnetic resonance imaging in breast cancer: meta-analysis of surgical outcomes. *Ann. Surg..* 2013; 257:249-255.

[43] Jackson B, Scott-Conner C, Moulder J. Axillary metastasis from occult breast carcinoma: diagnosis and management. *Am. J. Surg.* 1995;61:431-434.

[44] Ko EY, Han B-K, Shin JH, Kang SS. Breast MRI for Evaluating Patients with Metastatic Axillary Lymph Node and Initially Negative Mammography and Sonography. *Korean J. Radiol.* 2007;8:382-389.

[45] Harvey JA, Fajardo LL, Innis CA. Previous mammograms in patients with impalpable breast carcinoma: retrospective vs blinded interpretation. 1993 ARRS President's Award. *AJR Am. J. Roentgenol.* 1993;161:1167-1172.

[46] Majid AS, de Paredes ES, Doherty RD, Sharma NR, Salvador X. Missed breast carcinoma: pitfalls and pearls. *Radiographics* 2003;23:881-895

[47] Dershaw DD. Magnetic resonance imaging as a clinical tool. In: Morris EA, Liberman L, eds. Breast MRI; Diagnosis and intervention. New York, NY: Springer, 2004:256-264.

[48] Obdeijn IM, Brouwers-Kuyper EM, Tilanus-Linthorst MM, Wiggers T, Oudkerk M. MR imaging-guided sonography followed by fine-needle aspiration cytology in occult carcinoma of the breast. *AJR Am. J. Roentgenol.* 2000;174:1079-1084.

[49] Morris EA, Schwartz LH, Dershaw DD, van Zee KJ, Abramson AF, Liberman L. MR imaging of the breast in patients with occult primary breast carcinoma. *Radiology* 1997;205:437-440.

[50] Schorn C, Fischer U, Luftner-Nagel S, Westerhof JP, Grabbe E. MRI of the breast in patients with metastatic disease of unknown primary. *Eur. Radiol.* 1999;9:470-473.

[51] Kuhl CK, Morakkabati N, Leutner CC, Schmiedel A, Wardelmann E, Schild HH. MR imaging—guided large-core (14-gauge) needle biopsy of small lesions visible at breast MR imaging alone. *Radiology* 2001;220:31-39.

[52] Zujewski J, Eng-Wong J. Sentinel lymph node biopsy in the management of ductal carcinoma in situ. *Clin. Breast Cancer* 2005;6:216-222.

[53] Sakr R, Barranger E, Antoine M, Prugnolle H, Darai E, Uzan S. Ductal carcinoma in situ: value of sentinel lymph node biopsy. *J. Surg. Oncol.* 2006;94:426-430.

[54] Lara JF, Young SM, Velilla RE, Santoro EJ, Templeton SF. The relevance of occult axillary micrometastasis in ductal carcinoma in situ: a clinicopathologic study with long-term follow-up. *Cancer* 2003;98:2105-2113.

[55] Harms SE, Flamig DP, Hesley KL, Meiches MD, Jensen RA, Evans WP, et al. MR imaging of the breast with rotating delivery of excitation off resonance: clinical experience with pathologic correlation. *Radiology* 1993;187:493-501.

[56] Friedman P, Sanders L, Russo J, Sharo R, Swaminathan S, Smith R. Detection and localization of occult lesions using breast magnetic resonance imaging: initial experience in a community hospital. *Acad. Radiol.* 2005;12:728-738.

[57] American College of Radiology. BI-RADS: Breast Imaging Reporting and Data System Atlas(BI-RADS) atlas, 5th ed. *American College of Radiology,* 2013.
[58] Deo A, Fogel M, Cowper SE. Nephrogenic systemic fibrosis: a population study examining the relationship of disease development to gadolinium exposure. *Clin. J. Am. Soc. Nephrol.* 2007;2:264–267.
[59] Cocilovo C. Breast Cancer Screening and Diagnosis. In "Surgery of the breast – Principles and Art," 3rd ed, S. Spear et al, Lippincott 2011; 13.
[60] Ringash J. Preventive health care, 2001 update: screening mammography among women aged 40–49 years at average risk of breast cancer. *Can. Med. Assoc. J.* 2001;164(4):469–476.
[61] Rosen EL, Eubank WB, Mankoff DA, et al. FDG PET, PET/CT, and breast cancer imaging. *Radiographics* 2007;27(suppl 1):S215–S229.
[62] Tafra L, Cheng Z, Uddo J, et al. Pilot clinical trial of 18 F-fluorodeoxyglucose positronemission mammography in the surgical management of breast cancer. *Am. J. Surg.* 2005;190(4):628–632.
[63] Wahl RL, Siegel BA, Coleman RE, Gatsonis CG. Prospective multicenter study of axillary nodal staging by positron emission tomography in breast cancer: a report of the staging breast cancer with PET Study Group. *J. Clin. Oncol.* 2004: 15;22(2):277-85.
[64] Samson D, Flamm CR, Aronson N. FDG Positron Emission Tomography for Evaluation of Breast Cancer. Chicago, Illinois: Blue Shield and Blue Cross Association; 2001:1-93.
[65] Hellman S, Harris JR. Natural history of breast cancer. In: Harris JR, Lippman ME, Marrow M, Osborne CK, eds. Diseases of the Breast. 2nd ed. Philadelphia, Pa: Lippincott Williams & Wilkins; 2000:407-423.
[66] Wahl RL, Siegel BA, Coleman RE, Gatsonis CG. Prospective multi-center study of axillary nodal staging with FDG positron emission tomography in breast cancer. *J. Nucl. Med.* 2003;5(suppl):77P.
[67] Dehdashti F, Mortimer JE, Siegel BA, et al. Positron tomographic assessment of estrogen receptors in breast cancer: comparison with FDG-PET and in vitro receptor assays. *J. Nucl. Med.* 1995;36:1766-1774.
[68] Schirrmeister H, Kuhn T, Guhlmann A, et al. Fluorine-18 2-deoxy-2-fluoro-D-glucose PET in the preoperative staging of breast cancer: comparison with the standard staging procedures. *Eur. J. Nucl. Med.* 2001;28:351-358.
[69] Tran A, Khatibi B, Czernis J, Phelps ME, Silvermen DH. Prognostic value of FDG-PET in staging breast cancer patients with inner quadrant primary tumors: comparison with long-term outcomes. *J. Nucl. Med.* 2003;5(suppl):77P.
[70] Mundy GR, Guise TA, Yoneda T. Biology of bone metastases. In: Harris JR, Lippman ME, Marrow M, Osborne CK, eds. Diseases of the Breast. 2nd ed. Philadelphia, Pa: Lippincott Williams & Wilkins; 2000:911-920.
[71] Cook GJ, Houston S, Rubens R, et al. Detection of bone metastases in breast cancer by 18FDG PET: differing metabolic activity in osteoblastic and osteolytic lesions. *J. Clin. Oncol.* 1998;16:3375-3379.
[72] Schelling M, Avril N, Nahrig J, et al. Positron emission tomography using [18F]fluorodeoxyglucose for monitoring primary chemotherapy in breast cancer. *J. Clin. Oncol.* 2000;18:1689-1695

[73] R Edward Coleman. PET Scanning of Breast Cancer: State-of-the-Art. http://www.medscape.org/viewarticle/461316 2003.

[74] Bluemel C, Schnelzer A, Okur A, et al. Freehand SPECT for image-guided sentinel lymph node biopsy in breast cancer. *Eur. J. Nucl. Med. Mol. Imaging* (2013) 40:1656–1661.

[75] Ibusuki M, Yamamoto Y, Kawasoe T, et al. Potential advantage of preoperative three dimensional mapping of sentinel nodes in breast cancer by a hybrid single photon emission CT (SPECT)/CT system. *Surg. Oncol.* 2010;19:88–94.

[76] Troyan SL, Kianzad V, Gibbs-Strauss SL, et al. The FLARE intraoperative near-infrared fluorescence imaging system: a first-in-human clinical trial in breast cancer sentinel lymph node mapping. *Ann. Surg. Oncol.* 2009;16:2943–52.

[77] Scopinaro F, Tofani A, di Santo G, et al. High-resolution, hand-held camera for sentinel node detection. *Cancer Biother Radiopharm.* 2008;23:43–52.

[78] Kerrou K, Pitre S, Coutant C, et al. The usefulness of a preoperative compact imager, a hand-held gamma-camera for breast cancer sentinel node biopsy: final results of a prospective double-blind, clinical study. *J. Nucl. Med.* 2011;52:1346–53.

[79] Wendler T, Hartl A, Lasser T, et al. Towards intra-operative 3D nuclear imaging: reconstruction of 3D radioactive distributions using tracked gamma probes. *Med. Image Comput Comput Assist. Interv.* 2007;10:909–17.

[80] Hruska CB, Boughey JC, Phillips SW, et al. Scientific Impact Recognition Award: Molecular breast imaging: a review of the Mayo Clinic experience. *Am. J. Surg.* 2008;196(4):470–476.

In: The Role of Imaging Technology …
Editor: Georgios Tsoulfas

ISBN: 978-1-63483-490-2

Chapter 4

THE ROLE OF IMAGING IN NEUROSURGERY

Savvas Grigoriadis[1*], Christine Karatziou[2], Maria Sidiropoulou[2], Athanasia Anastasiou[2], Eleni Tsatsali[3] and Georgios Giakoumettis[3]

[1]B' Neurosurgical Clinic, Aristotle University, Thessaloniki, Greece
[2]Department of Radiology, Hippokration Hospital, Thessaloniki, Greece
[3]Aristotle University, Thessaloniki, Greece

ABSTRACT

Sir Godfrey N. Hounsfield (28 August 1919 – 12 August 2004) was an electrical engineer who in 1979, together with Allan McLeod Cormack, received the Nobel Prize in Physiology or Medicine for developing the diagnostic technique of X-ray computed tomography (CT) [1]. The first CT scanners were designed exclusively for brain CT, and in 1972 a female with a suspected brain tumor was the first patient examined using CT scanning. In the next year, the first publication of brain CT imaging was true [2]. Early CT scans were of limited quality and demanded long scanning and processing times. Nevertheless, the following development of CT scanning provided neuroradiology with much better brain tumor images and revolutionized neurosurgical practice. A new era in modern neurosurgery had commenced [3]. The MRI, on the other hand, has literally transformed the status of neuroimaging by bringing most of the structural details of the brain and spinal cord in front of our eyes. The most important applications of the modern neuroimaging modalities in neurosurgical practice are presented in this chapter.

IMAGING IN NEUROSURGICAL ONCOLOGY

A. Brain Tumor Imaging

1. Computed Tomography

The decrease in number of the air studies, angiograms, and nuclear scans in detecting brain tumors is documented by an article from Mayo Clinic published in *Radiology* in 1975

* Correspondence to: grigo@auth.gr

[4]. In the next article of the same *Radiology* issue, the application of contrast media administration in brain tumor imaging depicted that more than 80% of intracranial mass lesions enhanced [5]. *Enhancement* is a phenomenon caused by the disruption of the tumor vasculature's blood-brain barrier (Figure 1). Following the administration of contrast agent, there is an increased difference in an imaging characteristic between a lesion and the surrounding normal tissue due to the passage of contrast agent within the tumor's interstitium [6]. Correlation of contrast enhancement to astrocytoma grade was documented in 1978 [7]. CT has evolved over the years, with improvement of image quality, reduction of scan times and cost.

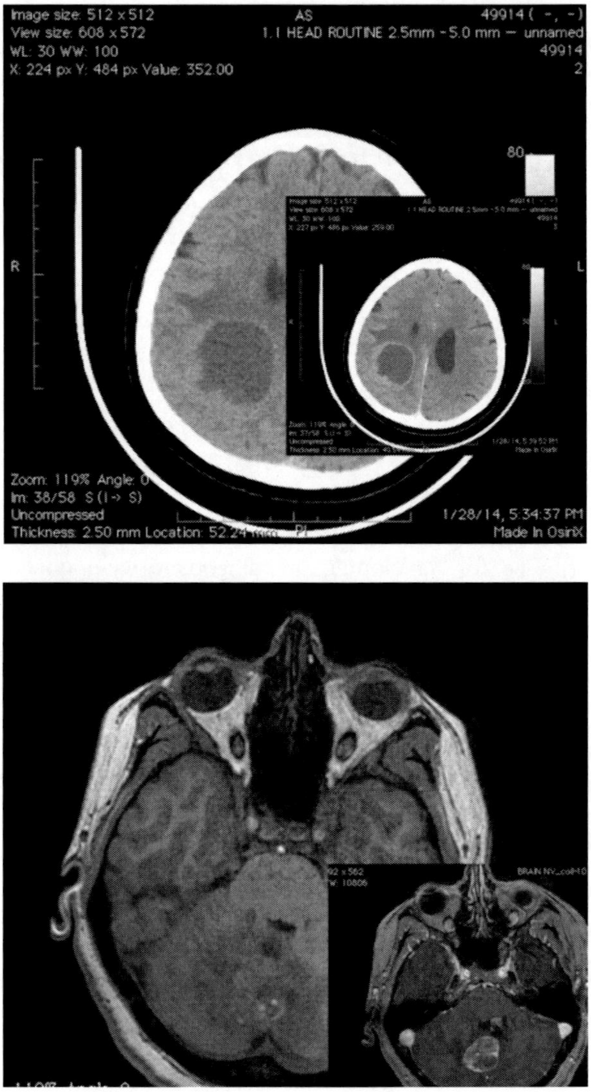

Figure 1. Enhancement of brain tumor after contrast agent administration.

Brain tumors may be *hypodense, isodense* or *hyperintense* to gray matter correlating to tumor histology and location. Small or isodense brain tumors may not be depicted on non-contrast CT scan, but they may be delineated after contrast media administration. Despite the advent of Magnetic Resonance Imaging (MRI), CT is still not only appropriate, but also necessary for emergent imaging.

CT is superior to MRI in depiction of *calcification* within brain tumors. Oligodendrogliomas, ependymomas, gangliogliomas, choroid plexus papillomas, astrocytomas, central neurocytomas and metastases are the intra-axial brain tumors that more often present calcifications. Extra-axial tumors that have calcifications are craniopharyngiomas, meningiomas, chondrosarcomas and chordomas. Additionally, CT contributes to detection of *osseous changes* secondary to brain tumor.

Hemorrhage which is characteristic of oligodendroglioma, glioblastoma multiforme, and metastases from melanoma, breast and lung cancer, is readily evaluated on CT scans.

Fat presents characteristic negative HU values on CT and is encountered in lipomas, teratomas and dermoid cysts.

Last but not least, patients suffering from claustrophobia, with metallic devices or pacemakers, critically ill or unstable benefit from CT exams [6].

Perfusion CT

Perfusion CT (PCT) is an imaging technique that is usually applied in the evaluation of patients with acute brain infarct. Additionally, PCT has been used during the previous years as an imaging biomarker with parameters such as tumor blood volume, blood flow, vascularity permeability, and size of extravascular extracellular space that are applied to patients with brain tumor [8-10]. Data obtained by PCT is used for tumor grading and prognosis, as well as for estimation of the response to antiangiogenic agents.

Perfusion CT consists of acquiring sequential CT images during the wash-in and washout of an iodinated contrast agent through the brain tissue._Following the rapid administration of a contrast medium bolus and serial image scanning at short intervals, maps of perfusion parameters are obtained:

a) Cerebral blood volume (CBV)
b) Cerebral blood flow (CBF)
c) Mean transit time (MTT), and
d) Permeability surface-area product maps [11-13]

PCT is able to differentiate low- and high-grade gliomas presenting high sensitivity and specificity [11]. Additionally, PCT can distinguish enhancing grade III from grade IV astrocytic tumors and delineate heterogeneity of gliomas [10].

PCT can be useful in differentiating gliomas from tumefactive demyelinating lesions, mass-like lesions of vasculitis or angiopathy and lymphoma, as well as in distinguishing recurrent tumor from radiation necrosis [12].

It has also been demonstrated that metastases from different primaries can be distinguished from one another using CT perfusion in the majority of cases [14].

Finally, it is worth pointing out that PCT provides absolute quantification of perfusion parameters and has no susceptibility artifacts due to hemorrhage, which may be present in post-operative patients [13].

2. MRI Techniques

MR Perfusion

Perfusion imaging permits insight into angiogenesis, a process essential for neoplastic growth [15]. Angiogenesis leads to development of tumoral neovasculature that commonly exhibits increased endothelial permeability [16]. Neoplastic vessels are abnormally structured vessels that tend to be leaky, and thus neoplasms have *increased permeability parameters* [15].

Perfusion is the process by which nutrients and oxygen are delivered to tissue and metabolic products are removed by blood flow.

Perfusion MRI provides measurement of the parameters of cerebral microvascularisation:

a) Regional blood volume (RBV)
b) Mean transit time (MTT), and
c) Regional blood flow (RBF)

Measurement of tissue perfusion depends on the ability to serially measure concentration of a tracer agent in a target-organ of interest [17].

MR perfusion is based on the use of a tracer that may be *exogenous* or *endogenous* (spin labeling).

Imaging techniques acquired with exogenous contrast agents are dynamic susceptibility contrast (DSC) MRI and dynamic contrast enhanced (DCE) MRI.

Endogenous tracer MR perfusion takes advantage of signal loss resulting from magnetically labeled water protons flowing into the imaging plane and exchanging with tissue protons. Water protons within inflowing arterial blood are magnetically labeled ("tagged") by the application of a special radiofrequency pulse [17]. Arterial spin labeling (ASL) MRI is a routine endogenous tracer MR perfusion sequence.

CBV calculated by DSC-MRI is strongly correlated to tumor grade [18-20]. Areas of malignant transformation or tumor dedifferentiation in low-grade lesions at risk before they are visible on conventional MRI can be depicted, allowing accurate targeting of biopsies, and potentially more accurate estimation of tumor grade [23].

Astrocytoma rCBV is strongly correlated to astrocytoma grading but this should be limited to fibrillary astrocytomas because other gliomas (especially oligodendrogliomas) may present high rCBV despite grade [18, 22, 23]. Oligodendrogliomas are characterized by delicate neoangiogenic vessels ("chicken-wire" vasculature) and *even low-grade oligodendrogliomas present elevated rCBV that may be as high as in glioblastoma* [23].

Lymphoma can be differentiated from primary high-grade neoplasms and high-grade glial neoplasms on MRI perfusion parameter basis [24, 25].

Metastatic brain tumors contain capillaries that resemble the organ where the systemic cancer arose and not those of the brain [26].

Discrimination between high-grade glioma and metastatic brain lesion can be provided by examining the peritumoral lesion where the differences in mechanisms underlying peritumoral edema affect microvascularity [27]. Higher CBV values are documented around high-grade gliomas as compared to around metastases [24].

Regional changes in MR perfusion parameters that occur early during treatment can be used to construct a paramagnetic response map, which can predict overall survival in high-grade glioma, and may even distinguish pseudoprogression in temozolomide-treated glioblastoma multiforme [28, 29].

MRI perfusion techniques can differentiate between tumor recurrence (high CBV) and radiation necrosis (low CBV).

Diffusion Weighted Imaging

Diffusion weighted imaging is an MRI method that is sensitized to the random motion of water molecules in all directions ('Brownian motion"). Random water motion is not possible in various pathologies and this is called "restricted diffusion." Lesions are characterized according to the presence of unrestricted or restricted diffusion. Lesions with restricted diffusion present high signal on diffusion weighted images while they are hypointense on Apparent Diffusion Coefficient (ADC) maps [30].

ADC is inversely proportional to cellular density and reflects the intensity of diffusion of water molecules in a tissue and ADC maps quantify the degree of water molecule mobility.

Although initial reports between minimum ADC and glioma grade were promising, there is a significant overlap in ADC values among different grades of glioma [31].

Metastatic cerebral neoplasms present an elevated ADC. There is an overlap of ADC values between primary and secondary brain tumors. Measuring ADC values in peritumoral regions can differentiate primary (high ADC) from secondary (low ADC) brain tumors [32].

Medulloblastoma, lymphoma and meningioma present low ADC values. A necrotic tumor presents high ADC value whereas an abscess has low ADC value.

Also, an arachnoid cyst (low ADC) can be distinguished from an epidermoid (high ADC).

MR Spectroscopy

MRS is the only noninvasive technique that measures chemicals within the body. MRS distinguishes metabolites according to their slightly different chemical shifts or resonance frequencies [33]. Proton MR spectroscopic imaging (^{1}H-MRSI) incorporates spatial localization of MRI with biochemical data of ^{1}H-MRSI [34].

Brain tumors present different spectra from normal brain tissue. Choline (Cho, 3.24ppm) signal is elevated in nearly all tumor types due to alteration of membrane metabolism. Cho is a basic component of the cell membrane and contains contributions from Cho-containing compounds involved in membrane synthesis and degradation [35]. Cho also correlates with cellular density of the tumor [36], cell proliferation, and with degree of tumor infiltration into brain tissue [37]. *N*-acetyl-aspartate (NAA, 2.02 ppm) is a marker of neuronal activity.

NAA decreases due to loss, dysfunction, or displacement of normal neuronal tissue [38]. In almost all brain tumors, NAA signal is decreased and Cho signal often increased (increase of Cho/NAA ratio).

The Cr signal is the sum of Cr and phosphocreatine. Cr is associated with short-term energy storage and is decreased when there is rapid cell proliferation [34]. Lactate (Lac) is not normally encountered in the adult brain and is a marker of anaerobic glycolysis [39]. The presence of lipids has been correlated with necrosis where cellular death results in membrane breakdown [40]. Increased levels of myo-inositol (ml) reflect increase of glial cells. The most useful parameters in MRS for the diagnosis and differential diagnosis of brain tumors are the following ratios: Cho/Cr, Cho/NAA, and NAA/Cr.

MRS, in combination with conventional MRI imaging, can aid to differentiate a tumor from a non-neoplastic lesion (Figure 2). Non-neoplastic lesions that mimic a tumor may be infectious (abscess), ischemic, or demyelinating (tumefactive demyelination) [35]. Some non-neoplastic lesions may present elevated Cho, making differential diagnosis difficult. For example, increased Cho, often increased lactate and decreased NAA can be found not only in brain tumors but also in acute demyelination lesions [41].

MRI is the most sensitive imaging modality for the detection of brain tumors. However, it lacks specificity as different lesions may share similar MR features.

Studies have suggested the correlation of tumor grade to Cho levels, implying that higher-grade tumors have greater Cho concentrations [42]. However, some high-grade tumors due to necrosis may present lower Cho levels than lower grade tumors. Heterogeneous tumors with central necrosis and proliferative rims, and invasion of surrounding brain tissue reflect metabolic heterogeneity also. ^{1}H-MRS is useful in studying changes in metabolic profile during the malignant transformation from diffuse to anaplastic astrocytoma [34].

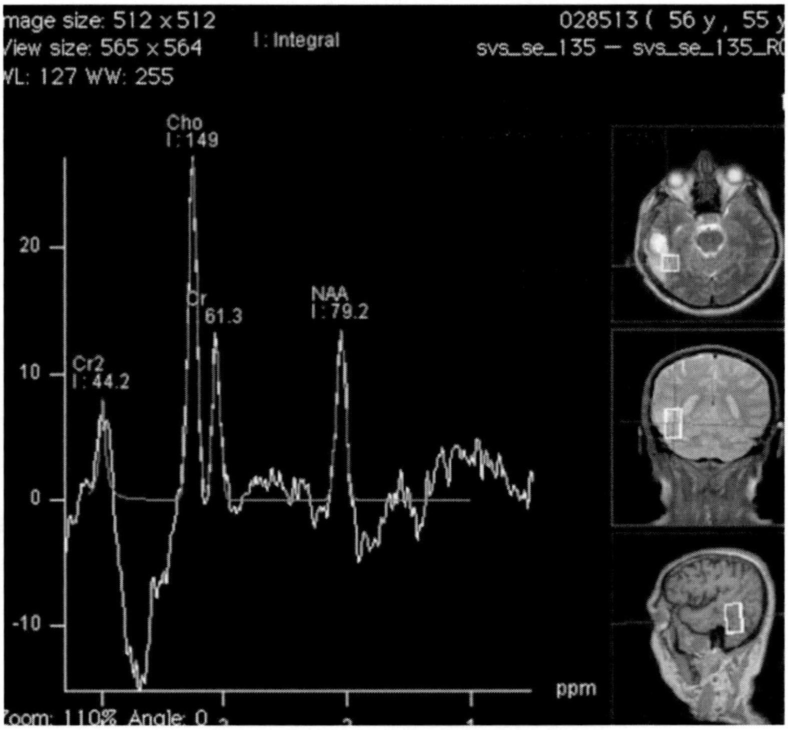

Figure 2. MR spectroscopy. The values of Cho, Cr and NAA are depicted.

MRS should be anticipated as an adjunct imaging modality that may aid to differential diagnosis rather than a modality diagnosing the exact type of a brain tumor on its own.

Investigation of peri-enhancing tumor regions can facilitate discrimination of solitary metastases from primary brain tumors. As gliomas are infiltrating lesions, Cho is elevated in surrounding tissue. On the contrary, as metastatic lesions tend to be more encapsulated, surrounding tissue does not demonstrate high Cho levels [43].

MPS can significantly aid the differential diagnosis between abscess and neoplasm. The acquisition of a single-voxel spectrum with short TE, besides the low Cho signal, will detect the presence of other minor peaks not encountered in neoplasia (e.g., succinate, acetate, leucine, alanine) [44].

In the study of Crawford et al. [45] GBM patient survival was studied in correlation to pre-surgical metabolic and physiological parameters. Survival was poor in patients with large areas of contrast enhancement, restricted diffusion, and abnormal metabolism. Survival time was also negatively associated with high lactate and lipid levels and the ADC in the enhancing area. Metabolic indices however have not always been proven to be prognostic in survival prediction in other brain tumors.

Total resection of the brain tumor is the basic goal in neuro-oncology. However, high-grade gliomas have indistinct boundaries and infiltration. MRS can aid proper tissue sampling at brain biopsy. Areas of increased angiogenesis, vascular permeability, and high metabolic activity should be sampled [46].

The dilemma between recurrent tumor and radiation necrosis, a focal reaction to radiation in patients undergoing radiation therapy, is common. Radiation necrosis demonstrates T2-hyperintense signal and enhancement after contrast medium administration, findings that are difficult to differentiate not only from tumor progression, but also from pseudo-progression (increase in edema, mass effect, and contrast enhancement that resolves over time) [47]. Increased Cho signal is indicative of recurrence whereas reduced Cho levels indicate radiation necrosis [48]. MRS cannot differentiate between tissue containing mixed tumor-radiation necrosis and either tumor or radiation necrosis, although it did achieve good separation between pure necrosis and pure tumor [49].

Functional MRI (fMRI)

The functional magnetic resonance imaging (fMRI imaging) is a non-invasive neuroimaging technique that can be used for studying the function of the human brain in vivo. The fMRI technique extends the use of classical MRI imaging beyond the anatomical information and provides information about the biological function. The study of the functional organization of the brain was the main interest of researchers since the late 19th century. In 1881 the Italian physiologist Angelo Mosso observed that the neural activity of a human is associated with the local brain cerebral blood flow (CBF). A few years later similar observations have been made by Charles Roy and Charles Sherrington in lab-animals. Unfortunately the objections of other researchers and the lack of sufficient experimental means led to a decrease in interest in this observation. It was not until half century passed that this observation came forth again, when researchers proved that the oxygenated hemoglobin is repelled, while the deoxyhemoglobin is attracted by magnetic fields. This phenomenon was used by Seiji Ogawa in order to prove that with the technique of imaging the oxygen level of blood [Blood Oxygenation Level Dependent imaging] (BOLD imaging), one can visualize the brain function. This is a standard technique used to create images in functional magnetic resonance imaging studies (fMRI) and is based on differences in cerebral blood flow in brain regions that show increased activity. The first successful attempt to elucidate the functional organization and mapping of the brain using magnetic resonance carried out in 1991 in the MRI center of the Massachusetts General Hospital in Boston. After that, identifying brain areas activated during a specific test offered a very satisfactory level of spatial resolution of 2 mm and a degree of temporal resolution of few seconds.

Blood flow to the brain is locally controlled and is in response to oxygen and carbon dioxide of the cortical tissue. When an area of the cortex increases its activity in response to a process, initially there is a fall of oxygenated hemoglobin (oxyHb) and an increase in deoxygenated hemoglobin (deoxyhemoglobin, deoxyHb). After a delay of 2-6 seconds, the cerebral blood flow (CBF) increases by providing an excess of oxygenated hemoglobin, replacing deoxyhemoglobin. This increase in local tissue oxygenation can be imaged. The reason that the fMRI is able to detect this change is due to a fundamental difference in the paramagnetic properties of oxyhemoglobin (oxyHb) and deoxyhemoglobin (deoxyHb), whereas the latter is paramagnetic, while the first is not. However, there are some limitations of BOLD imaging and other CBF imaging techniques. Therefore, i) cerebral blood flow is only an indirect indicator of activity, rather than direct visualization of cortical activation, ii) the smallest unit of the brain that is able to regulate its blood flow, it is measured in millimeters in diameter and finally iii) the increase in blood flow is in conjunction with the increase of the activity having a 2-6 seconds delay.

Statistical analysis of data obtained from BOLD technique is important and crucial for brain mapping with functional MRI. Thanks to wide range of experiments done with fMRI several statistical models and approaches can be applied in order to extract useful information. The simplest statistical model data analysis of BOLD technique is the t-test where the statistical parameter taken into consideration is the p-value, which reflects the level of confidence. The proposed p-value is $p < 0.05$ with a confidence level of 95%. Moreover, the selection of a certain threshold is equally important for the sensitivity of the signal that is to be received. The goal is not to identify the voxels that have a signal greater than the threshold, but to identify those voxels whose change of signal is much larger than expected and the level of statistical significance depends on the threshold applied according to predefined statistical parameters. Data analysis is done by software that processes the data of anatomical images and of fMRI. Before that, images of fMRI are aligned (alignment), normalized (normalization), smoothed and motion-corrected. Then statistical analysis is applied after using a threshold in signal sensitivity and the results of fMRI are displayed on high-definition three-dimensional anatomical images. The representation of functional areas is in accordance with a chromatic scale and the intensity of the signal is proportional to the threshold. The signal from brain activity is subtracted from the signal at rest. Changes in signal intensity are represented by the number Z, which is defined as:

$$Z = \frac{\text{average signal difference}}{\text{standard deviation}}$$

Low values of Z generate results of low resolution and specificity. High values of Z allow visualization of areas with high signal and have high resolution. Thus, setting this statistical parameter is depended on the signal intensity.

The idea of mapping functional areas of the brain for a safe navigation during a brain surgery is dated in the middle of 20th century. Although invasive techniques, such as transcortical stimulation, are a gold standard in functional neurosurgery, they do not allow the preoperative designing of the surgery, whilst neuropsychological tests do not offer precision. Thus, the need for an accurate preoperative technique in order to design and execute as safely as possible a brain surgery, has brought in the use of fMRI. Brain mapping is done in order to identify and surgically preserve eloquent areas such as motor speech area, sensorimotor cortex, motor cortex and other brain areas that are responsible for writing, calculating, spatial perception, memory etc. Moreover brain mapping helps individualize an operation offering maximum surgical result. Consequently, fMRI contributes not only to the preoperatively design and to a safe neuronavigation during surgery, but it is also established as a decision-making examination for surgery. Finally, fMRI is widely used in neuroscience contributing to research, studying anatomy as well as brain diseases.

Diffusion Tensor Imaging

Diffusion tensor imaging (DTI) consists a rapidly growing area of research, as well as clinical application in intracranial tumors [50]. DTI is the only non-invasive *in vivo* method for mapping white matter tract in the human brain [51]. DTI is based on the concept of *anisotropic diffusion*. Water diffusion in the white matter is not equal in all 3 dimensions but tends to move along the long axis of the fiber bundle because myelin sheath allows less water diffusion perpendicularly [50, 51]. The portion of overall diffusion that is therefore directional is referred as fractional anisotropy (FA) [52] and permits visualization of white matter fiber direction. FA maps quantify changes in FA values as loss of brightness (gray scale) and direction of white matter tracts in color: fiber orientation is represented by different colors. Diffusion-based MRI tractography is an imaging tool that generates 3-D reconstructions of white matter fiber tracts as an aid to identifying safe margins of resection [53]. DTI can evaluate the relation of a brain tumor to the adjacent white matter tracts [54, 55]. White matter involvement by a tumor can be deviated, infiltrated, edematous and destroyed. DTI contributes to planning for brain tumor surgery as it indicates white matter tracts relative to the tumor.

B. Spinal Tumor Imaging

Tumors of the spine compose a vast group of lesions that are derived from diverse tissues: neoplasms from the spinal cord, the leptomeninges, extradural soft tissues, primary and metastatic bone lesions as well as paraspinal soft tissue tumors. This long list of tumors is usually categorized according to the site of origin [56].

CT consists the method of choice for delineating osseous involvement, calcifications and the degree of bone loss [57]. CT can demonstrate tumor destruction. Multidetector CT obtains axial, sagittal, and coronal reformatted images [57].

Bone metastases are the most common neoplasms of the spine. Spinal bone metastases consist the most common site of bone metastasis. Vertebral metastases are the cause of initial presentation of symptoms in a significant group of patients with cancer. Vertebral metastases are located at the lower thoracic, lumbar and, at a lesser degree, at the cervical spine.

Vertebral metastases originate from cancer of the breast, lung, prostate, gastrointestinal system and thyroid gland.

Osteolytic metastases present low signal on T1 and high signal on T2 images (Figure 3). Contrast media should be administrated at the end of basic sequences because the enhanced bone metastasis may be impossible to differentiate from the surrounding vertebra.

Osteosclerotic metastases are depicted with low signal on both T1 and T2 images.

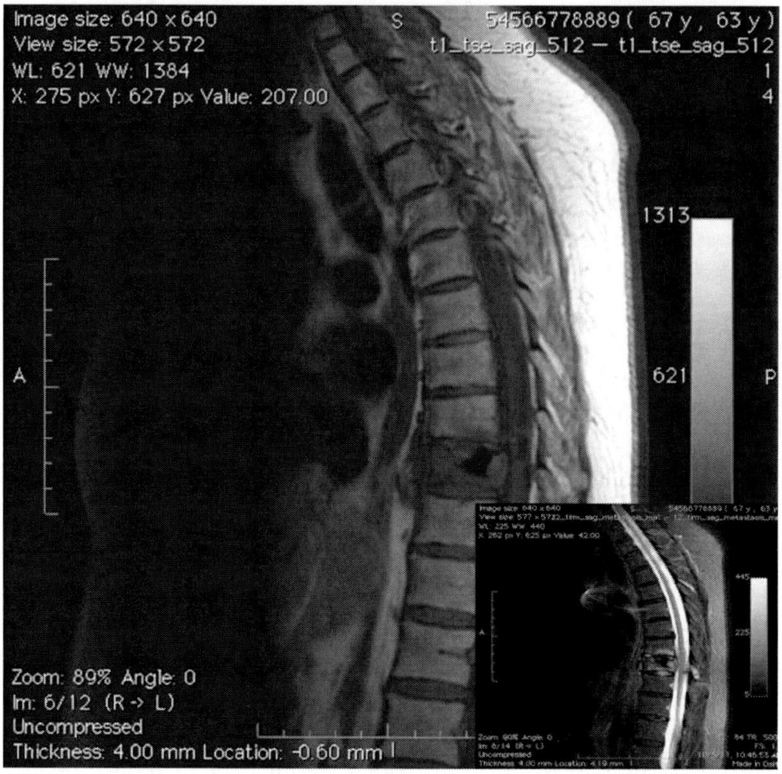

Figure 3. Metastatic spinal tumor with characteristic low signal on T1WI and high signal on T2WI.

In cases of spinal involvement in leukemia, bone marrow presents low T1 signal and intervertebral discs seem bright ("bright disk sign").

Hemangioma is the most common benign vertebral lesion. Hemangiomas are mailnly located at the lower thoracic and lumbar spine. T1 signal is high or low according to ratio of vascular to fatty component of the lesion. Hemangiomas have saturation of high signal on STIR sequences.

Osteoid osteoma is a benign lesion with characteristic CT features.

MRI is the most sensitive imaging method for evaluation of the spinal cord. Infiltration of nerve roots, thecal sac, paraspinal soft-tissues as well as vertebral bone marrow is markedly revealed [58].

Spinal tumors are classified as intradural (intra-medullary and extra-medullary) and extradural (epidural and from the vertebral column) (Figure 4).

There are 3 significant features in MRI images while evaluating patients suspected of having an intramedullary spinal lesion: cord expansion, degree of enhancement, and the presence of a cyst [58].

Ependymoma is the most common intramedullary spinal tumor in adults [60]. Myxopapillary ependymoma consists a rare, variant type of ependymoma, usually without connection with the spinal cord. Cord ependymomas occur most commonly in the cervical spine. Most spinal cord ependymomas are iso- or hypo- intense on T1 images. Rarely, they may present hyperintensity on T1 due to hemorrhage. On T2 images, ependymomas may be hyperintense or isointense.

Astrocytoma has poorly defined margins and is iso- to hypointense on T2 and hyperintense on T2 images. A degree of contrast enhancement is depicted. Cyst is a common finding. In more than half cases, astrocytoma is eccentric within the spinal cord [59].

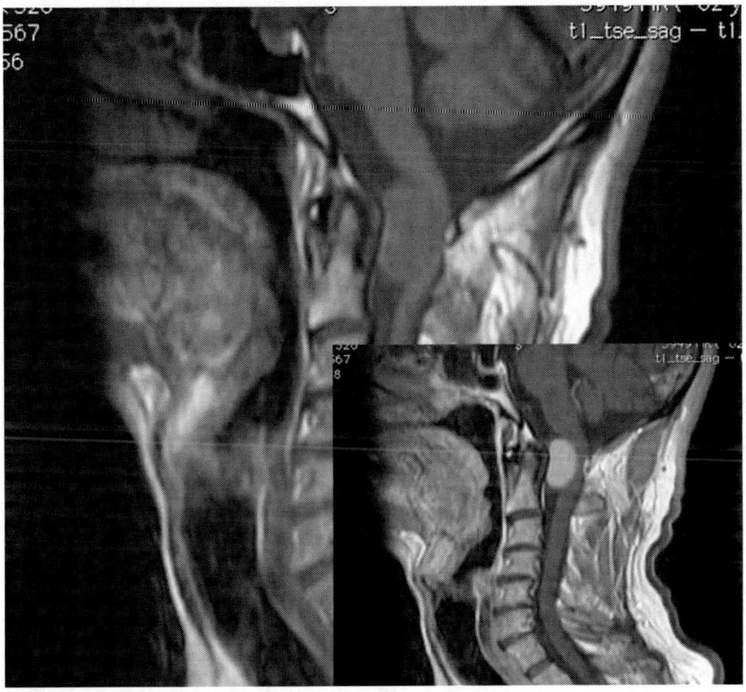

Figure 4. Cervical MRI showing an intradural extramedullary tumor (meningioma).

C. Intraoperative MRI

Ferenc Jolesz at the Brigham and Woman's Hospital in Boston in 1990 first conceived the idea of operating under real MRI guidance. Intraoperative MRI (ioMRI) can identify any residual tumor, delineate the degree of brain shift and update the neurosurgical navigation system [61].

Additionally, potential intracranial complications such as hemorrhage, hydrocephalus and cerebral edema could be depicted [62].

In the first reports of patients in which ioMRI data was used, the image quality was able to identify residual tumor in most cases [63].

Low-field ioMRI in the following years however was not able to efficiently depict residual tumor, especially low-grade glioma [64, 65].

High-field ioMRI enhances the extent of resection, even for non-enhancing gliomas [66].

In high-field ioMRI, operations are performed using conventional, non-MR compatible equipment. The disadvantage however is that more time is required to obtain a scan and real-time imaging is unavailable [61].

Other distinct advantages of ioMRI include the excellent soft tissue discrimination, the ability to view the surgical site in three dimensions, and the ability to "see" tumor beyond the surface visualization of the surgeon's eye. The enhanced ability to view the tumor being biopsied or resected allows the surgeon to choose a safe surgical corridor that avoids critical structures, maximizes the extent of the tumor resection, and confirms that an intraoperative hemorrhage has not resulted from surgery [67].

CT AND MRI IN THE EMERGENCY DEPARTMENT

A. Craniocerebral Injuries

CT is the preferred method for evaluating patients after traumatic CNS traumatic injuries. The principal tool for imaging severe acute craniocerebral trauma is the Multidetector Computed Tomography (MDCT). It is used for the detection of:

a) Intracranial hemorrhage
b) Mass effect
c) Cerebral contusions
d) Cerebral edema and herniation
e) Skull fractures (Figure 5)
f) Displaced bone fragments
g) Foreign bodies
h) Intracranial air

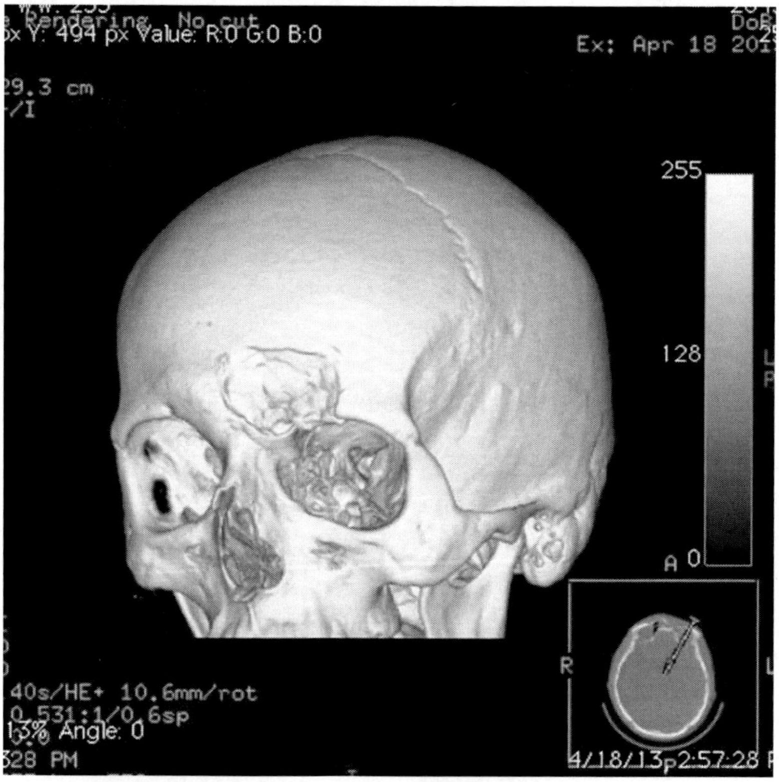

Figure 5. Cranial CT after 3-D reconstruction. Depressed skull fracture (frontal bone).

MRI is relatively insensitive for the detection of skull fractures and small bone fragments [68, 69]. However, the role of MRI is growing in the assessment of acute, subacute and chronic phase of craniocerebral trauma. MRI is more sensitive than CT to certain injuries like:

a) Diffuse axonal injury (DAI)
b) Small extra-axial fluid collections
c) Cortical contusions, and
d) Brainstem injuries [70]

In the acute or subacute phase of trauma:

FLAIR sequence presents high sensitivity for DAI, edema, subarachnoid and intraventricular hemorrhage [71].

Gradient echo T2* and SWI sequences are sensitive for detection of DAI, intracranial hemorrhage and blood degradation products with paramagnetic properties.

DWI-ADC map sequences are useful in the evaluation of DAI, cytotoxic edema and hypoxic-ischemic brain damage in cases of non-accidental head injury (e.g., child abuse) [72, 73].

Finally, MRI using a complex variety of sequences can provide data about the "age" of an intracranial hemorrhage.

As a general rule, MRI is indicated in stable patients in whom there is a significant discrepancy between the patient's clinical condition and CT findings [68, 74].

In the chronic phase of trauma:

MRI is superior to CT for the detection of chronic subdural hematomas (CSH), which are often isodense to CSF on non-contrast CT scans.

FLAIR and Gradient echo T2* sequences are superior to T2 sequence in the detection of small subdural hematomas, with different signals due to varying phases of the blood-breakdown process.

Gradient echo T2* and SWI sequences demonstrate hypointense hemosiderin deposits after DAI.

Post-traumatic encephalomalacia and gliosis are much better appreciated with FLAIR sequence. On FLAIR, the area of tissue loss is isointense to CSF and is surrounded by a rim of gliosis that is hyperintense.

B. Spine Injuries

MR imaging has supplanted CT as the modality of choice for the majority of CNS conditions including neoplasms and vascular lesions. However, in some instances, CT provides a diagnostic advantage for the evaluation of spinal pathology especially in evaluating spine-trauma patient. CT with multiplanar reformatted images and 3D-display remains the method of choice for the detection of fractures and their patterns, displacement or retro-pulsed bony fragments and narrowing of the spinal canal, information that is critical for the appropriate management of trauma victims (Figure 6).

The size, shape, integrity, as well as the degree of canal compromise are best assessed with CT. It is often the only modality to demonstrate subtle lesions especially small cortical fractures, pars interarticularis defects, widening of the apophyseal joints, locked facets, occult fractures of the posterior elements and fractures of the occipital condyles [75, 76]. Evaluation also includes assessment of the disc, nerve root and paraspinous soft tissue including ligaments and evaluation of stability. When further evaluation of the cord and roots or an expanding extramedulary hematoma is indicated, MRI is preferable to CT, to reproduce the internal architecture of the spinal cord and the injured cord parenchyma.

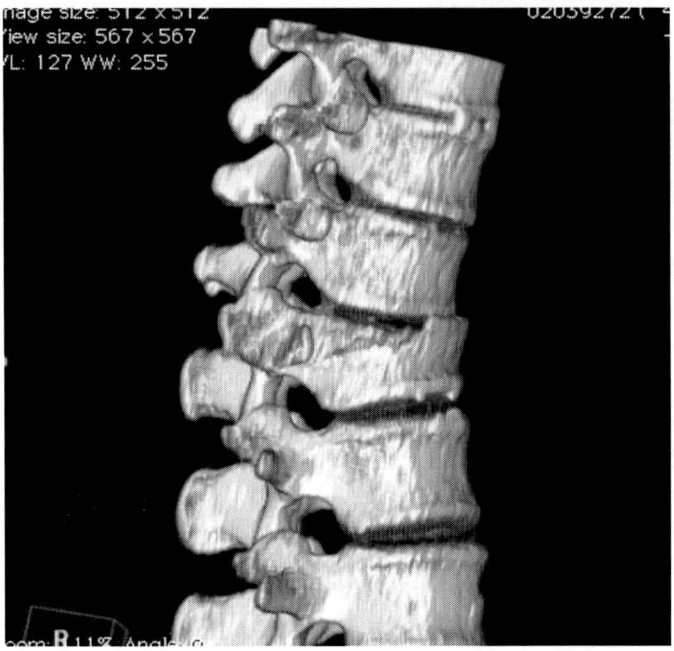

Figure 6. Spine CT after 3-D reconstruction shows a traumatic vertebral fracture.

Except from the comprehensive display of spinal anatomy and pathology, CT can be performed with the same settings as CT for the other traumatic injuries of the body areas [77, 78]. In addition CT angiography is an accurate, rapid, noninvasive diagnostic alternative in the initial evaluation of patients who present to the emergency department with possible carotid and vertebral arterial injuries [79, 80].

Imaging of Stroke

Stroke can be defined as a sudden or rapid onset of a neurologic deficit due to a cerebrovascular lesion, lasting longer than 24 hours. If the neurologic deficit lasts <24 hours, it is called *transient ischemic attack* (TIA). There are four main etiologies for stroke:

a) Cerebral infarction (80%)
b) Intraparenchymal hemorrhage (ICH) (15%),
c) Non-traumatic subarachnoid hemorrhage (SAH) (5%)
d) Venous infarction (1%) [89]

Acute *ischemia* constitutes approximately 80% of all strokes and is an important cause of morbidity and mortality in the United States [81]. Stroke is the third leading cause of death in the USA, and cerebral infarction is the most common cause of disability among adult Americans [88].

Until recently, before effective therapies were introduced for acute ischemic stroke, imaging was used primarily to exclude "stroke mimickers." There is a long list of conditions that mimic the symptoms of acute ischemic stroke, such as intracranial hemorrhage, neoplasms, infection, migraine, seizures, functional and metabolic disorders and vasogenic edema syndromes [88]. It is therefore very important to confirm that the cause is an ischemic lesion, before therapy is started, as these non-ischemic stroke mimickers should not be treated with thrombolysis.

The development of new treatment options, such as intra-arterial and intravenous thrombolysis, have led to the evolution of imaging technology in order to decide which stroke victim will benefit from the new therapeutic modalities [81]. The new aggressive therapies are aimed to re-establish the blood flow in the infarcted area, to reduce the size of the infarcted tissue and to protect the surrounding brain at risk, which is called the *penumbra*. Brain tissue is exquisitely sensitive to ischemia. In the complete absence of blood flow, the available energy can maintain neuronal viability for approximately 2-3 minutes. However, in acute stroke, ischemia is more often incomplete, because uninjured arterial and leptomeningeal vessels supply blood to the injured area of the brain [81]. Therefore, acute cerebral ischemia may result in an infracted core, which is the ischemic region that is irreversibly injured, and the penumbra, which is defined as the brain tissue that is hypoperfused and is in danger of infarcting. Penumbra is the region that is potentially salvageable with early recanalization. Neuroimaging can provide excellent estimates of the core and penumbra in individual patients and help the clinicians to decide which stroke victim will benefit from thrombolysis.

The goals of neuroimaging in acute stroke ischemia are:

a) To assess brain parenchyma
b) To rule out hemorrhage and other stroke mimickers
c) To assess the intra- and extracranial circulation in order to depict endovascular thrombi
d) To assess the perfusion of the brain tissue, the size of the infarcted core, and the surrounding penumbra [81]

1. Non Contrast CT (NCCT)

The speed, widespread availability, low cost, and accuracy in detecting subarachnoid and intracranial hemorrhage have led conventional unenhanced computed tomography (NCCT) scanning to become the first-line diagnostic tool for the emergency evaluation of acute stroke.

CT findings that are useful in the detection of acute ischemia are focal parenchymal hypodensity, obscuration of the lenticular nuclei and the insular cortex, sulcal effacement due to brain edema, loss of gray-white matter differentiation, and the hyperdence MCA sign due to an acute thrombus in an intracranial vessel which has typically high attenuation [81, 87] (Figure 7).

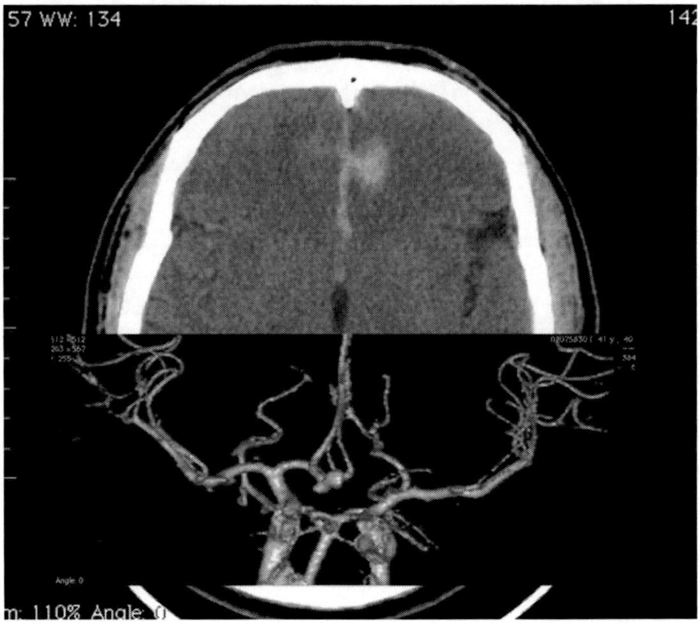

Figure 7. Non-contrast CT of the brain with evidence of subarachnoid hemorrhage and interhemispheric hematoma.

2. CT Angiography (CTA)

CT angiography is the next step in assessing intracranial and extracranial circulation. It is a widely available, fast and simple technique that is capable of detecting endovascular thrombi. CT angiography is performed after intravenous injection of contrast agent and it visualises vessels from the aortic arch to the circle of Willis. Multiplanar reformatted images and maximum intensity projection images are produced at a three-dimensional display workstation [81] (Figure 8).

CTA can detect endovascular thrombi and can define the level of intracranial vascular occlusion in patients presenting within 6 hours of embolic stroke onset [87]. It can detect large vessel occlusion but it can also provide information about collateral flow and lesion extent. Plaque burden at the origins of internal carotid arteries and arterial dissection can also be detected by CTA [87]. CTA plays a major role in the exclusion of unnecessary thrombolysis in patients presenting with acute embolic stroke, but who don't have large vessel occlusions amenable to thrombolysis [87]. CT angiographic demonstration of a significant thrombus burden, can guide appropriate therapy in the form of intra-arterial or mechanical thrombolysis, as it is known that intra-arterial thrombolysis may be more efficacious than intravenous therapy in patients with acute stroke and a significant thrombus burden [81]. Unlike MRA, CTA is an anatomic imaging technique and therefore it is not likely to yield false-positive results for occlusion due to slow flow or artefact [87].

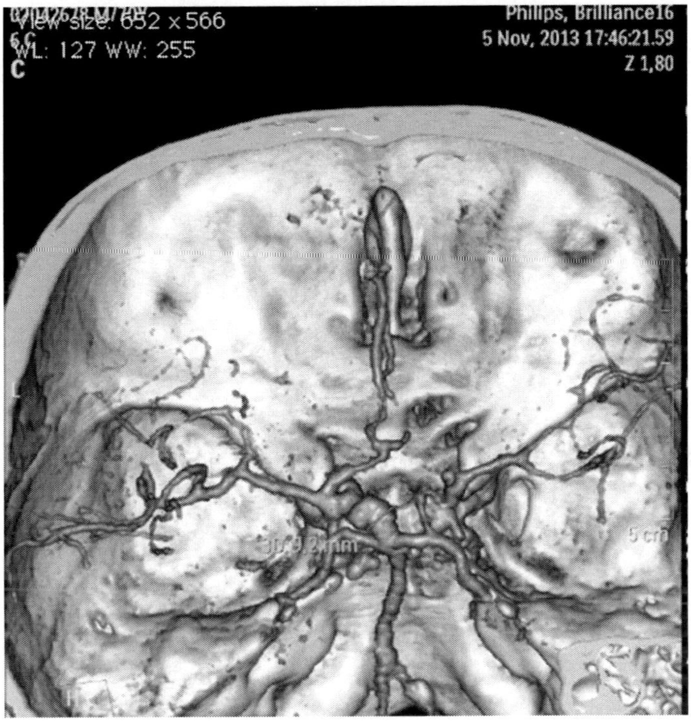

Figure 8. CT Angiography: a saccular aneurysm of the basilar tip is depicted.

3. CT Perfusion Imaging

CT perfusion imaging (CTP) in addition to CTA is fast, available and safe and adds no more than 10 minutes to the time required to perform a standard NCCT. CTP is based on dynamic i.v. administration of a contrast agent, which is tracked with serial imaging during its first pass circulation through the brain tissue capillary beds. Depending on the assumptions regarding the arterial inflow and venous outflow of the tracer, perfusion parameters can be estimated mathematically. CT perfusion maps then can be generated in a short time at an appropriate workstation.

CT perfusion imaging is used to estimate the following perfusion parameters:

- Cerebral blood volume (CBV), which is the volume of blood per unit of brain tissue (normal range, 4–5 mL/100g)
- Cerebral blood flow (CBF) defined as the volume of blood flow per unit of brain tissue per minute (normal range in gray matter, 50–60 mL/100 g/min)
- Mean transit time (MTT), defined as the time difference between the arterial inflow and venous outflow (MTT= CBV/CBF)
- Time to peak enhancement (TTP), which represents the time from the beginning of contrast material injection to the maximum concentration of contrast material within a region of interest (ROI) [81].

As mentioned before, the infarcted core is a region of brain tissue which is severely hypoperfused and irreversibly infarcted or is destined to infarct regardless of therapy. It is defined as an area with prolonged MTT, markedly decreased CBF and markedly reduced CBV.

The ischaemic penumbra, which in most cases surrounds the infarct core, also has prolonged MTT but in contrast has only moderately reduced CBF and importantly near normal or even increased CBV (due to autoregulatory vasodilatation) [83]. Hence, functional images can help differentiate between:

- A favourable pattern of ischemic stroke which consists of a small infarcted core and a large penumbra
- An unfavourable pattern with a large core and a small penumbra
- An intermediate pattern with relatively equal size of core and penumbra, and
- Malignant pattern with a very large core and small penumbra

This way the clinicians are guided in their decision-making process on weather to attempt revascularization or not [84].

4. MRI Imaging

Conventional MRI used in the evaluation of acute stroke, typically includes T1-weighted spin-echo, T2-weighted fast spin-echo, fluid-attenuated inversion recovery, T2*-weighted gradient-echo, and gadolinium-enhanced T1-weighted spin-echo sequences [81].

MRI can diagnose infarcts of all stages of evolution but it is most sensitive after the hyperacute stage. The basic findings during the hyperacute stage are loss of flow voids on T2-weighted images, FLAIR hyperintensity in the affected vessels and stasis of contrast material in the vessels of the affected territory [87]. Typical MR imaging findings in the acute phase include hyperintense signal in white matter on T2- weighted images and FLAIR images, with a resultant loss of grey-white matter differentiation. Sulcal effacement and mass effect can also be demonstrated. In the subacute phase, parenchymal swelling and enhancement after contrast administration may be seen [87].

T2*-weighted gradient-echo images and susceptibility-weighted imaging (SWI) depict an acute intracranial hemorrhage as an area of abnormal blooming. Compared with CT and other MR imaging methods, these techniques are superior in detecting very small cerebral hemorrhages in patients with acute stroke. However the impact of depicting these small hemorrhages in the infarcted area in deciding thrombolytic therapy is not strongly established yet [81, 92].

MR angiography (MRA) is divided into non-contrast (TOF MRA and Phase-contrast MRA) and contrast-enhanced techniques (Figure 9). TOF MRA is a gradient echo sequence that depicts vascular flow. Phase-contrast MRA is a gradient echo sequence that depicts blood flow by quantifying differences in the transverse magnetization between stationary and moving tissue. Contrast-enhanced MRA is usually obtained from the arch to the scull base. Three-dimensional TOF MRA is quite sensitive and specific for the evaluation of intracranial proximal stenoses and occlusions. Phase-contrast MRA can evaluate collateral flow patterns in the circle of Willis. MR angiography is useful for detecting intravascular occlusion due to a thrombus and for evaluating the carotid bifurcation in patients with acute stroke. However MRA is relatively insensitive in depicting stenoses in distal intracranial vessels [87].

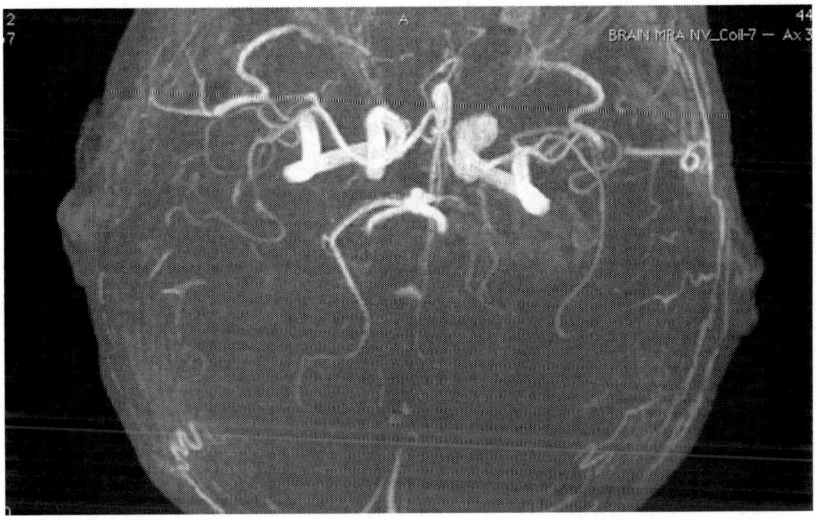

Figure 9. MR Angiography.

5. Diffusion Weighted Imaging

Diffusion weighted imaging (DWI) was introduced in the clinical setting in the mid-1990s and today is the most reliable method for detecting acute ischemia and it can be accomplished in less than 2 minutes [81]. The abnormal finding of infarction is an area of hyperintensity on DWI. This is likely caused by the cessation of ATP production and the dysfunction of Na^+-K^+ pump, which is unable to remove excess water from the cells, resulting in cytotoxic edema [88]. The actual diffusion coefficient cannot be measured by using diffusion-weighted MR imaging, for a number of reasons. Hence, the diffusion coefficient obtained from orthogonal diffusion-weighted MR images in all three planes is called the apparent diffusion coefficient (ADC) [81]. The ADC map is used to confirm that the signal abnormality on DWI is caused by restricted diffusion. Acute infarction is demonstrated as a hyperintence area on DWI and as an area of low signal intensity on ADC map and it corresponds to the irreversibly infarcted brain tissue. Diffusion restriction with reduced signal on ADC map has been observed as early as 30 minutes after the onset of ischemia. This information is critical as thrombolytic therapy can be started within the "golden period" of *3 hours from the onset of symptoms* resulting in early reperfusion of the hypoperfused tissue. In the hyperacute stage of infarction (<6 hours) the DW signal intensity is increased with a corresponding low ADC. In the acute phase (6 hours to 3 days) there is a further increase of the DW signal of the infarcted tissue and also a lower ADC. In the subacute phase (3 days to 3 weeks), there is a pseudonormalisation of the ADC. This is likely due to the development of vasogenic edema along with the persistence of cytotoxic edema. In the chronic stage (3 weeks to 3 months) there is an increase in ADC with a bright signal on ADC map [88]. In contrast to unenhanced CT or conventional MR imaging, which have low sensitivities (50%) for acute ischemia detection within the first 6 hours after onset of symptoms, diffusion-weighted imaging was reported to have had high sensitivity and specificity, of 88%-100% and 86%-100%, respectively, in various studies [81].

6. Perfusion-Weighted MR Imaging (PWI)

While diffusion-weighted MR imaging is most useful for detecting irreversibly infarcted tissue, perfusion-weighted imaging may be used to identify areas of reversible ischemia as well. Perfusion-weighted MR Imaging describes techniques that study perfusion by visually depicting hemodynamic conditions at the microvascular level. Perfusion-weighted imaging techniques rely on measurement of the concentration within each voxel of a contrast agent that is dissolved in the blood. Multiple echo-planar images are made with a high temporal resolution.

Various post-processing algorithms are used to convert the sequence of dynamically acquired images into synthetic maps that depict any of perfusion parameters for each brain voxel [87].

What is the clinical role of PWI in conjunction with DWI? In the acute stroke setting, a region that shows both diffusion and perfusion abnormalities is thought to represent irreversibly infarcted tissue, while a region that shows only perfusion abnormalities and has normal diffusion likely represents viable ischemic tissue, or a penumbra. These are very helpful information in order to decide thrombolytic therapy [81, 85].

7. CT versus MR Imaging in Acute Stroke Evaluation

CT is widely available, and a stroke imaging protocol that consists of unenhanced CT, CT angiography, and CT perfusion imaging can be executed in 5 minutes for the comprehensive evaluation of the extra- and intracranial circulation, the amount of infarcted brain tissue, and the penumbra. The MR imaging protocol for evaluation of stroke, which includes conventional MR imaging, diffusion-weighted imaging, MR angiography, and perfusion-weighted imaging, may take a little longer (15 minutes) [81]. NCCT is a widely available tool and a very reliable one in detecting acute hemorrhage. Until recently, it is considered to be superior than MRI in depicting hemorrhage, however recent studies have shown that MRI, including T2*-weighted gradient-echo images or susceptibility-weighted imaging, can also depict hyperacute haemorrhage [91-93]. These new techniques, as mentioned before, are superior to CT in depicting old hemorrhages and hemorrhagic transformation in the infarcted area [92]. DWI is definitely superior to CT in evaluating the irreversibly infarcted tissue even in the hyperacute phase [87, 88]. CTA may be superior to MRA in depicting vessel occlusion because MRA is vulnerable to motion artifacts. The two modalities including CTP and PWI are equally useful for evaluating acute stroke and provide equivalent depiction of the penumbra. Some authors have pointed out that whereas CT is simple to perform, MR findings are simple to interpret [81]. Disadvantages of CT are ionizing radiation and higher risk for anaphylaxis and toxic effects on kidneys because of the administration of iodinated contrast material. On the other hand MRI is not so widely available as CT, it cannot be performed in patients with pacemakers, aneurysm clips, or other ferromagnetic materials in their bodies and it may not be easy to perform in patients who need life support equipment [82]. Acute stroke imaging protocols vary among institutions, depending on the availability of imaging time, software, and expertise.

8. Intracranial Hemorrhage (ICH)

All hemorrhages, according to WHO classification are divided into cerebral, subarachnoid, subdural and intraventricular [90].

a. Etiologies of Intracranial Hemorrhage

Hypertension, hemorrhagic transformation of a previous cerebral infarction and cerebral amyloid angiopathy, are the most frequent causes of intraparenchymal hemorrhage in patients older than 60 years. In younger patients, we have to consider as possible causes of intraparenchymal hemorrhage, underlying cerebrovascular malformations such as arteriovenous malformations and cavernous angiomas, vasculopathy and venous infarctions due to venous thrombosis. Cerebral hemorrhage can also occur at any age in the case of an underlying tumor. Hemorrhage may be the first manifestation of a previously unknown tumor. Bleeding diathesis, coagulopathy due to anticoagulants and thrombolytic drugs administration should also be taken into account. Usage of illicit drugs and alcohol, endocarditis, congenital heart defects and long operations on heart should also be considered as possible causes of cerebral hemorrhage. Other more rare causes include eclampsia, encephalitis and brain abscess, Moyamoya disease, vasculitis, and hereditary hemorrhagic telangiectasia [86, 90, 94].

Non-traumatic subarachnoid hemorrhage (SAH) is usually related to an aneurysmal rupture (in 75% of cases) or a vascular malformation [89].

Subdural and epidural hematomas are most frequently caused by trauma. When there is no history of previous trauma we have to think of AVM rupture, dural arteriovenous fistulas, or coagulopathy [90].

The most frequent non-traumatic reasons for intraventricular hemorrhage are hypertonic hemorrhage in the basal ganglia, AVM rupture and deep cavernoma.

Dural sinus and cerebral vein thrombosis can lead to venous infarctions. Common causes of venous thrombosis are dehydration, pregnancy, infection, oral contraceptives, coagulopathies, malignancies, collagen vascular diseases and trauma [86, 90]. Detection of hemorrhage and identification of the etiology of non-traumatic intracranial hemorrhage is the major task of every neuroimaging method and it is crucial for the patient's therapeutic management.

b. What Are the Imaging Recommendations for Detecting a Spontaneous Nontraumatic Intracranial Hemorrhage?

Radiologists and clinicians should always take into consideration the patient's clinical history and physical examination's findings in order to decide which imaging modalities are suitable for each patient.

Non-contrast computed tomography (NCCT) is, in most hospitals, the first imaging modality used to investigate primary intraparechymal hemorrhage. CT scan is an excellent tool for depicting acute hemorrhage. It can demonstrate the location and size of hemorrhage as well as the possible complications of it such as intraventricular hemorrhage, hydrocephalus, edema and herniations [82]. If the patient is old and suffers from hypertension and NCCT reveals an hematoma in the region of basal ganglia, which is typical for hypertensive intraparenchymal hemorrhage, there is no need for further radiological investigation. If there is no clear cause of hemorrhage or an atypical appearance on NCCT, MRI (including Diffusion-weighted imaging and T2*-weighted imaging or susceptibility-weighted imaging) should be performed [89].

T2*-weighted imaging or susceptibility-weighted imaging, are able to detect intracranial hemorrhage in the hyperacute stage and in chronic stage as well [91-93]. Multifocal black dots demonstrated on T2*-weighted imaging or susceptibility-weighted imaging, guide us to hypertensive or amyloid angiopathy [86, 90].

MRI with gadolinium administration contributes to investigate an underlying pathology such as tumors or vascular anomalies. CT angiography (CTA) and MR angiography (MRA) are the methods of choice for investigation of vascular anomalies such as aneurysms or AVMs, while CT venography (CTV) and MR venography (MRV) can reveal dural sinus and cerebral vein thrombosis. If the cause of intracerebral hemorrhage remains unclear we have to proceed to DSA. MRI can be used for the follow up [89].

c. What Is the Best Imaging Modality in Order to Investigate Spontaneous Intracranial Hemorrhage. CT or MRI?

Non-contrast computed tomography (NCCT) is in most hospitals the first imaging modality used to detect ICH. It is widely available, fast and can be performed in patients who are unable to tolerate an MRI examination or who have contraindications to MRI such as pacemakers, aneurysm clips, or other ferromagnetic materials in their bodies [82]. In addition, CT scan is more accessible to patients who need special equipment for life support. CT scan, as mentioned before, is an excellent tool for depicting acute hemorrhage and its potential complications. Contrast-enhanced CT scanning can be used easily for patients at risk for hematoma expansion [82]. NCCT in combination with contrast enhanced CT (CECT), CTA and CTV can reveal underlying abnormalities such as aneurysms, arteriovenous malformations, pre-existing tumors. However NCCT is less sensitive than MRI in depicting and visualizing ischemic changes in a very early stage, or small infarcts especially situated in the brainstem or posterior cranial fossa. Patient's exposure to ionizing radiation and possible allergic reactions to the iodinated contrast medium are also disadvantages of CT [81].

On the other hand, MRI is much more sensitive than CT in depicting ischemic changes in a very early stage. Diffusion-weighted imaging (DWI) is able to detect ischemic changes 30 minutes after vessel occlusion [81]. The usage of DWI and perfusion weighted imaging (PWI) can also detect the extent of the infarcted core and the penumbra. These are very significant elements for the decision of management and use of thrombolysis. In the past, MRI has been considered unable to detect hemorrhage in the hyperacute stage. In recent years there have been studies that support that MRI, including T2*-weighted imaging or susceptibility-weighted imaging, can be very sensitive in the detection of hyperacute cerebral hemorrhage [91, 93].

Some authors also noticed that MRI was more sensitive than CT in depicting hemorrhagic transformation of an ischemic infarction, which may play a role in deciding thrombolytic therapy [81, 92]. MRI is also much more sensitive than CT in detecting hemorrhages in chronic phases and old microbleeds, which also contributes to the diagnosis and therapeutic management [92]. However, MRI is less sensitive than CT to differentiate small acute hemorrhages from chronic ones, because small acute hemorrhages, with minimal or no edema, may have similar characteristics to calcifications or endovascular clot [92]. MRI with gadolinium administration, MRA and MRV can help visualize the possible cause of cerebral hemorrhage. Some authors support that routine multimodal MRI adds diagnostic yield to NCCT and helps changing the therapeutic management [94]. Others have decided to examine patients with suspected cerebral ischemia only with MRI in order to save time and if there is no hemorrhage demonstrated on MRI, thrombolysis may be started [96]. However MRI is not so widely available as CT, some hospitals are supplied with low field strength equipment, with which the modern sequences cannot be performed and MRI is sometimes difficult to perform in critically ill patients who need life support equipment.

d. Radiological Findings of ICH on CT and MRI

Based on time, all hemorrhages can be divided in 5 stages, the huperacute (the first 24 hours), the acute (1-3 days), the early subacute (3-7 days), the late subacute (7-14 days), and the chronic stage (later than 14 days) [95].

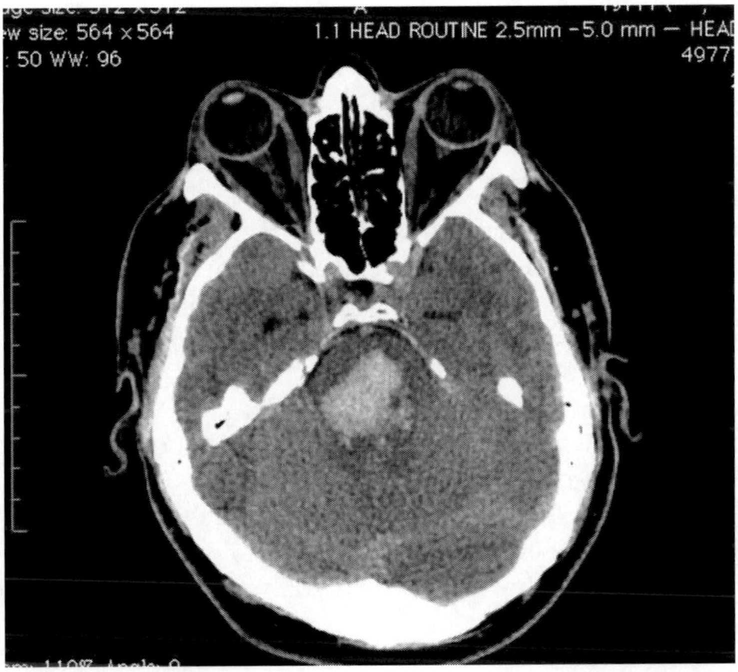

Figure 10. Brain CT showing a mesencephalic hematoma.

The acute extravasated blood is hyperdense on CT scans. The hematoma's density in the first few hours can reach 60-80 HU [90]. On MRI, hyperacute hemorrhage containing oxyhemoglobin, appears to be made of three parts: a center, a periphery and a surrounding rim. The center is slightly hypointense or isointense relative to the brain on T1-weighted images. On T2-weighted images the center is heterogeneous and slightly hyperintense relative to the brain. The periphery of the hematoma appears hypointense and the surrounding rim, which corresponds to perilesional edema, appears hyperintense. On T2*-weighted imaging or susceptibility-weighted imaging, the center appears heterogeneous iso- or hyperintense, but the peripherya appears hypointense. As time passes there is progressive enlargement of the periphery of the lesion towards the center [93]. Such lesions do not enhance after the administration of a gadolinium-based contrast agent.

During the acute stage, hematoma continues to appear hyperdense on CT (Figure 10). On MRI, the hematoma appears iso- to hypointense on T1 weighted images, markedly hypointense on T2 weighted images due to the formation of deoxyhemoglobin [89, 95]. In this phase perilesional edema increases [90].

In the subacute phase there is a progressive decrease in hematoma's density on CT. In the early subacute stage, hematoma appears hyperintense on T1 weighted images and hypointense on T2 weighted images due to the existence of intracellular methemoglobin [89, 90]. In the late subacute stage, the hematoma appears hyperintense on both T1 and T2 weighted images due to exracellular methemoglobin [89, 90].

In the chronic stage, at last, hematoma appears as a hypodense area on CT with density close to CSF. It may also appear as a slit-like lesion or calcinated areas [89, 90]. On MRI hematoma appears hypointense on both T1 and T2 weighted images because of the existence of hemosiderin and extracellular ferritin. In the subacute and chronic stage peripheral rim enhancement may be noticed after contrast administration either on CT and MRI [89, 95].

e. Radiological Appearances of Specific Causes of ICH

Hypertensive Hemorrhage

Hypertensive hemorrhage is the most common cause of intracranial hemorrhage and it most commonly involves the lenticulostriate arterial branches of the middle cerebral artery, leading to putaminal or caudate hemorrhage. It may also result from rupture of the small perforating branches, in which case it leads to pontine or thalamic bleeds. Large hematomas often dissect into the ventricles, causing intraventricular extension [95].

Hemorrhagic Transformation of Cerebral Infarction

Infarcted brain tissue has a propensity to bleed, particularly when reperfused in the acute phase. Infarcted brain tissue can be recognized on MRI and especially Diffusion -weighted images. Hemorrhagic transformation in the infracted area can be demonstrated on T2*-weighted imaging or susceptibility-weighted imaging. However, early massive bleeding may obscure the underlying infarct. The risk of bleeding in venous infarction is higher than arterial infarction [95].

Amyloid Angiopathy

Cerebral amyloid angiopathy (CAA), is caused by the deposition of beta-amyloid in the arterial media and/or adventitia of small arteries and arterioles in the meninges, cortex, and cerebellum [95]. Unlike the hemorrhages due to hypertension, which are usually located in the basal ganglia, the presense of multiple and small hemorrhages in the cortex and subcortical white matter of cerebral hemispheres, and rarely in the cerebellum, is typical for amyloid angiopathy [90]. MRI is the best imaging tool to depict old bleeds on T2*-weighted imaging or susceptibility-weighted imaging [92].

Intratumoral Hemorrhage

There is an increased risk for hemorrhage in brain tumors with significant neovascularity. High-grade tumors, such as glioblastoma multiforme, and certain metastases (eg, melanoma, renal cell carcinoma, thyroid carcinoma, choriocarcinoma, lung cancer) are more likely to bleed than others. In the case of an intratumoral hemorrhage, blood of different ages may be present and admixed with abnormal neoplastic tissue. That explains why MRI appearances are often atypical and complex. There is usually delay of the evolution of changes in MRI signal intensity of hemorrhage inside the tumor. Vasogenic edema is greater with brain tumors than with primary ICH. The edema surrounding a primary ICH usually resolves after 4-8 weeks, while edema due to intratumoral hemorrhage persists even into the chronic phase of hematoma. Administration of contrast medium may reveal tumor enhancement [95].

Cerebrovascular Malformations (CVMs)

Cerebrovascular malformations are a heterogeneous group of disorders that represent lesions affecting arteries, veins, capillaries or various types of vessels. Arteriovenous malformations (AVMs) and cavernous malformations, may hemorrhage abruptly without any warning sign. Developmental venous anomalies and capillary telangiectasias are generally benign lesions and clinically silent [89]. MRI with gadolinium administration, including T2*-weighted imaging or susceptibility-weighted imaging and MRA, can reveal cerebrovascular malformations.

Catheter angiography is often needed to further evaluate AVMs and arteriovenous dural fistulaes. On MRI, AVM appears as a tightly packed honeycomb of flow voids like a "bag of worms" caused by high-velocity signal loss. Areas of hemorrhages in different stages can be seen [89].

Arteriovenous dural fistulaes are a network of tiny vessels in the wall of a thrombosed dural venous sinus [89].

Cavernous hemangiomas have a typical popcorn-like appearance with locules of variable size containing blood products of different ages [89]. Multiple lesions at different locations are seen in 50% of patients with cavernous hemangiomas [95].

Developmental venous anomalies, formerly known as venous angiomas, appear like an umbrella collection of enlarged medullary veins (Medusa head) [89].

Non-Traumatic Subarachnoid Hemorrhage (SAH)

Nontraumatic subarachnoid hemorrhage (SAH) accounts for 5% of all acute strokes. As mentioned before, the most common cause of SAH is a ruptured intracranial saccular (berry) aneurysm (aSAH). Saccular aneyrusms are focal sac or berry like arterial dilatations. They are most commonly located on the circle of Willis and the middle cerebral artery bi- or trifurcation. That is the reason why most aSAHs are located in the suprasellar cistern and the sylvian fissure. Other types of aneurysms are pseudoaneurysms, blood blister-like aneurysms and fusiform aneurysms [89]. The imaging modality recommended for investigating SAH is NCCT, which can demonstrate blood as hyperdense material in the sulci and cisterns. CTA with multiplanar reformation can be the next step as it can depict an aneurysm in 90-95% of cases, if the aneurysm is larger than 2mm [89]. If CTA is negative, we can proceed to DSA

(Figure 11). On MRI, SAH may be demonstrated as high signal intensity material in sulci, compared with normally hypointense CSF spaces on Fluid-Attenuated Inversion Recovery (FLAIR) images. FLAIR MRI is similar to CT in terms of its findings in SAH [95]. It can be more sensitive than CT in detection of small SAH but it is less specific as infectious material in the CSF spaces can present with the same signal intensity [89]. T2*-weighted images can potentially demonstrate SAH as an area of low signal intensity in normally hyperintense subarachnoid spaces. On T1-weighted images, acute SAH may appear as intermediate or high signal intensity in the subarachnoid space [95] and subacute SAH may appear as high signal intensity in CSF spaces [90]. Magnetic resonance angiography (MRA) may be useful in the evaluation of aneurysms and other vascular lesions that cause SAH. Factors that limit the utility of MRA in the diagnosis of acute SAH are its low sensitivity for aneurysms less than 5 mm, its inability to depict small aneurysm contour irregularities, and its difficulty in providing high-quality images in patients who are agitated or confused [95].

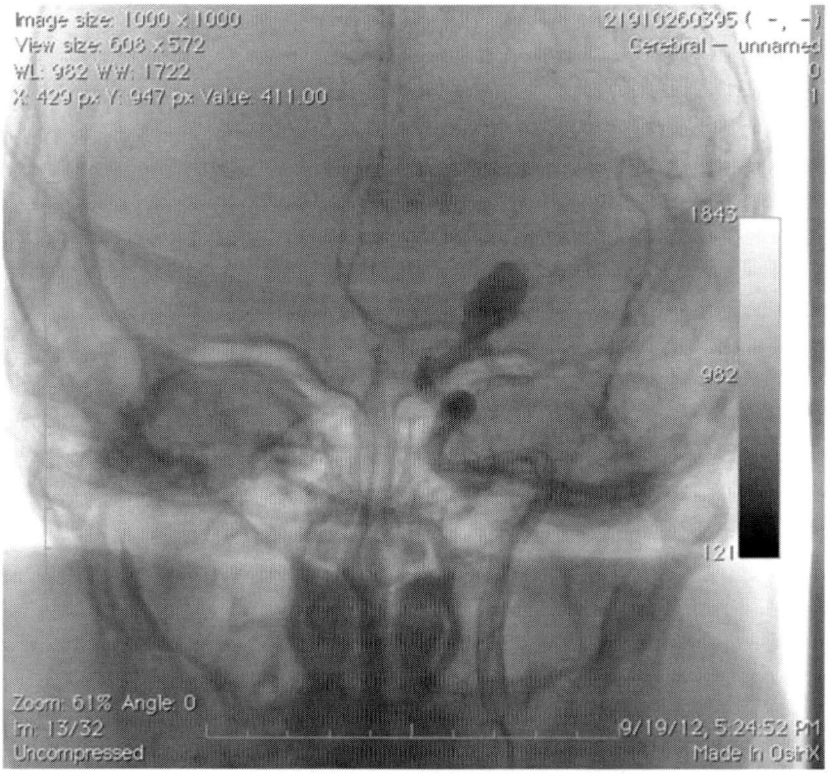

Figure 11. Digital Subtraction Angiography (DSA). A large saccular aneurysm of the left ICA bifurcation is shown.

Venous Infarction

Venous infarction can be a challenging diagnosis and it is caused by cerebral venous thrombosis, complicating both dural sinus thrombosis and deep cerebral vein thrombosis. Several conditions can lead to venous thrombosis, as mentioned before, like acute dehydration, hypercoaguable states, infection and malignancy [86]. The imaging modalities recommended are NCCT where thrombosed sinuses and cortical veins appear hyperdense and cortical/subcortical hemorrhages and edema can be demonstrated. The next step can be

CECT. Empty delta sign is produced by enhancing the dura that surrounds the non-enhancing thrombus in a thrombosed sinus. CTV can demonstrate the thrombus as a filling defect in the sinus. If the CT exams are negative and there is a high clinical suspicion of venous thrombosis we can proceed to MRI including T2*-weighted imaging or susceptibility-weighted imaging and MRV (Figure 12) with gadolinium administration, in order to visualise the thrombus [89]. MRI is superior to CT in detecting the complications of sinus thrombosis. Edema is easier to be detected on T2-weighted images and FLAIR images, while infarcted areas are best demonstrated on DWI. Hemorrhage may be detected on CT and MRI as well.

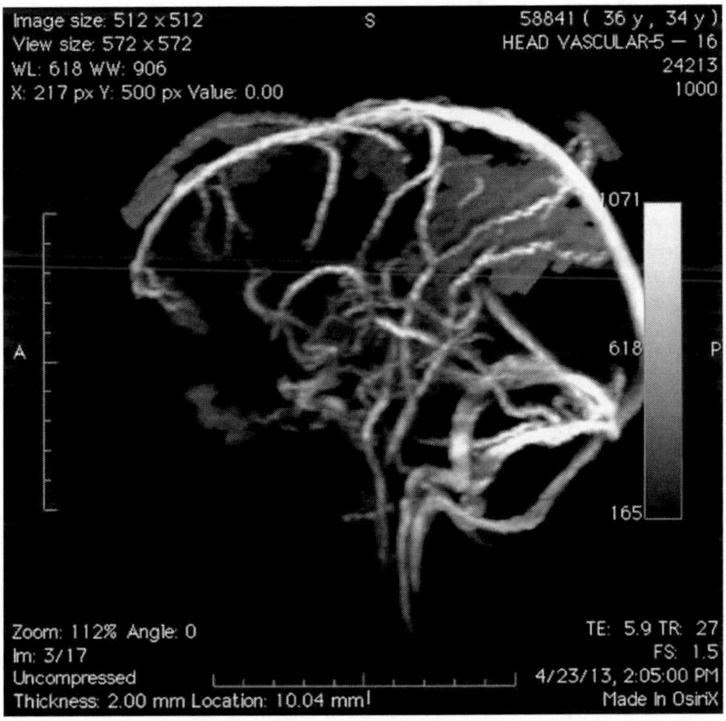

Figure 12. MR Venography with normal findings.

REFERENCES

[1] Castillo M. History and evolution of brain tumor imaging: insights through Radiology. *Radiology*: Volume 273: Number 2 (Suppl)-November 2014; S111-S125.

[2] Ambrose J, Hounsfield C. Computerized transverse axial tomography. *Br. J. Radiol* 1973; 46Q 148-9.

[3] Kirkman MA. The role of imaging in the development of neurosurgery. *Journal of Clinical Neuroscience* 2015; 22: 55-61.

[4] Baker HL Jr. The impact of computed tomography on neuroradiographic practice. *Radiology* 1975; 116(3): 637-640.

[5] Kramer RA, Janetos GP, Peristein G. An approach to contrast enhancement in computed tomography of the brain. *Radiology* 1975; 116(3): 641-647.

[6] Drevelegas A and Papanikolaou N. Imaging Modalities in brain tumors. In: A. Drevelegas (eds). Imaging Brain Tumors with Histological Correlations. Berlin Heidelberg, Germany: Springer-Verlag 2011.

[7] Burler AR, Horii SC, Kricheff II, Shammon MB, Budzilovich GN. Computed Tomography in astrocytomas. A statistical analysis of the parameters of malignancy and the positive contrast-enhanced CT scan. *Radiology* 1978; 129(2): 433-439.

[8] Law M, Young RJ, Babb JS, et al. Gliomas: predicting time to progression or survival with cerebral blood volume measurements at dynamic susceptibility- weighted contrast-enhanced perfusion MR imaging. *Radiology* 2008; 247: 490–98.

[9] Law M, Yang S, Babb JS, et al. Comparison of cerebral blood volume and vascular permeability from dynamic susceptibility contrast- enhanced perfusion MR imaging with glioma grade. *AJNR Am. J. Neuroradiol.* 2004; 25: 746–55.

[10] Jain R, Ellika SK, Scarpace L, et al. Quantitative estimation of permeability surface-area product in astroglial brain tumors using perfusion CT and correlation with histopathologic grade. *AJNR Am. J. Neuroradiol.* 2008; 29: 694–700.

[11] Ellika SK, Jain R, Patel SC, Scarpace L, Schultz LR, Rock JP, et al. Role of perfusion CT in glioma grading and comparison with conventional MR features. *AJNR Am. J. Neuroradiol.* 2007; 28: 1981-1987.

[12] Jain R. Perfusion CT imaging of brain tumors: an overview. *AJNR Am. J. Neuroradiol.* 2011; 32: 1570-1577.

[13] Huang APH, Tsai JC, Kuo LT, Lee CW, Lai HS, Tsai LK, et al. Clinical application of perfusion computed tomography in neurosurgery. Clinical article. *J. Neurosurg.* 2014; 120: 473-488.

[14] Dolgushin MB, Pronin IN, Holodny EA, Fadeeva LM, Holodny AI, Kornienko VN. Use of CT perfusion to discriminate between brain metastases from different primaries. *Clin. Imaging* 2015; 39: 9-14.

[15] Al-Okaili RN, Krejza J, Wang S, Woo JH, Melhem ER. Advanced MR Imaging techniques in the diagnosis of intraaxial tumors in adults. *RadioGraphics* 2006; 26: S173-S189.

[16] Jayson GC, Zweit J, Jackson A, et al. Molecular imaging and biological evaluation of HuMV833 anti-VEGF antibody: implications for trial design of antiangiogenic antibodies. *J. Natl. Cancer Inst.* 2002; 94(19): 1484-93.

[17] Patella JR and Provenzale JM. MR perfusion imaging of the brain: techniques and applications. *AJR* 2000; 175: 207-219.

[18] Aronen HJ, Gazit IE, Louis DN, et al. Cerebral blood volume maps of gliomas: comparison with tumor grade and histologic findings. *Radiology* 1994; 191(1): 41-51.

[19] Law M, Yang S, Wang H, et al. Glioma grading: sensitivity, specificity, and predictive values of perfusion MR imaging and proton MR spectroscopic imaging compared with conventional MR imaging. *AJNR Am. J. Neuroradiol.* 2003; 24(10): 1989-98.

[20] Ludemann L, Grieger W, Wurm R, et al. Comparison of dynamic contrast-enhanced MRI with WHO tumor grading for gliomas. *Eur. Radiol.* 2001; 11(7): 1231-41.

[21] Di Costanzo A, Scarabino T, Trojsi F, et al. Multiparametric 3T MR approach to the assessment of cerebral gliomas: tumor extent and malignancy. *Neuriradiology* 2006; 48(9): 622-31.

[22] Lev MH, Ozsunar Y, Henson JW, et al. Glial tumor grading and outcome prediction using dynamic spin-echo MR susceptibility mapping compared with conventional

contrast-enhanced MR: confounding effect of elevated rCBV of oligodendrogliomas. *AJNR Am. J. Neuroradiol.* 2004; 25: 214-21.

[23] Cha S. Update on brain tumor imaging: from anatomy to physiology. *AJNR Am. J. Neuroradiol.* 2006; 27: 475-87.

[24] Cha S, Knopp EA, Johnson G, Wetzal SG, Litt AW, Zagzag D. Intracranial mass lesions: dynamic contrast-enhanced susceptibility-weighted echo-planar perfusion MR imaging. *Radiology* 2002; 223(1): 11-29.

[25] Hartmann M, Heiland S, Harting I, et al. Distinguishing of primary cerebral lymphomas from high-grade glioma with perfusion-weighted magnetic resonance imaging. *Neurosci.* 2003; 338(2): 119-122.

[26] Long DM. Capillary ultrastructure in human metastatic brain tumors. *J. Neurosurg.* 1979; 51:53-58.

[27] Thompson G, Mills SJ, Stivaros SM, Jackson A. Imaging of Brain Tumors: Perfusion/Permeability. In: State of the Art Brain Tumor Diagnostic, Imaging, and Therapeutics. Neuroimaging Clinics of North America. *SK Mukherji* (ed). August 2010; 20(3): 293-310.

[28] Galban CJ, Chenevert TL, Mayer CR, et al. The parametric response map is an imaging biomarker for early cancer treatment outcome. *Nat. Med.* 2009; 15(5): 572-6.

[29] Tsien C, Galban CJ, Chenevert TL, et al. Parametric response map as an imaging biomarker to distinguish progression from pseudoprogression in high-grade glioma. *J. Clin. Oncol.* 2010; 28(13): 2293-9.

[30] Sanghvi DA. Recent advances in imaging of brain tumors. *Indian Journal of Cancer* 2009; 46(2): 82-87.

[31] Cha S. Update on brain tumor imaging: from anatomy to physiology. *AJNR Am. J. Neuroradiol.* 2006; 27: 475-87.

[32] Al-Okaili RN, Krejza J, Wang S, Woo JH, Melhem ER. Advanced MR Imaging techniques in the diagnosis of intraaxial tumors in adults. *RadioGraphics* 2006; 26: S173-S189.

[33] Sanghvi DA. Recent advances in imaging of brain tumors. *Indian Journal of Cancer* 2009; 46(2): 82-87.

[34] Chapter 5. MRS in brain tumors. In: Barker PB, Bizzi A, De Stefano N, Gullapalli RP, Lin DDM. Clinical MR Spectroscopy: Techniques and Applications. New York, United States of America: Cambridge University Press 2011.

[35] Horská A, Barker PB. Imaging of Brain Tumors: MR Spectroscopy and Metabolic Imaging. In: State of the Art Brain Tumor Diagnostic, Imaging, and Therapeutics. Neuroimaging Clinics of North America. SK Mukherji (ed). August 2010; 20(3): 293-310.

[36] Gupta RK, Cloughesy TF, Sinha U, et al. Relationships between choline magnetic resonance spectroscopy, apparent diffusion coefficient and quantitive histopathology in human glioma. *J. Neurooncol.* 2000; 50(3): 215-226.

[37] Croteau D, Scarpace L, Hearshen D, et al. Correlation between magnetic resonance spectroscopy imaging and image-guided biopsies: semi-quantitative and qualitative histopathological analyses of patients with untreated glioma. *Neurosurgery* 2001; 49(4): 823-9.

[38] Barker PB. N- acetyl-aspartate-a neuronal marker? *Ann. Neurol.* 2001; 49(4): 423-4.

[39] Miller JC. Magnetic Resonance Spectroscopy in the brain. Radiology Rounds. *Massachusetts General Hospital Imaging*. July 2012; 10(7): 1-6.

[40] Remy C, Fouilhe N, Barba I, et al. Evidence that mobile lipids detected in rat brain glioma by 1H nuclear magnetic resonance correspond to lipid droplets. *Cancer Res.* 1997; 57: 407-414.

[41] Saindane AM, Cha S, Law M, et al. Proton MR spectroscopy of tumefactive demyelinating lesions. *AJNR Am. J. Neuroradiol.* 2002; 23(8) : 1378-1386.

[42] Hourani R, Horska A, Albayram S, et al. Proton magnetic resonance spectroscopic imaging to differentiate between nonneoplastic lesions and brain tumors in children. *J. Magn Reson Imaging* 2006; 23(2): 99-107.

[43] Fan G, Sun B, Wu Z, et al. In vivo single-voxel proton MR spectroscopy in the differentiation of high-grade gliomas and solitary metastases. *Clin. Radiol.* 2004; 59(1): 77-85.

[44] Law M, Hamburger M, Johnson G, et al. Differentiating surgical from non-surgical lesions using perfusion MR imaging and proton MR spectroscopy imaging. *Technol. Cancer Res. Treat* 2004; 3(6): 557-65.

[45] Crawford FW, Khayal IS, McGue C, et al. Relationship of pre-surgery metabolic and physiological MR imaging parameters to survival for patients with untreated GBM. *J. Neurooncol.* 2009; 91(3): 337-51.

[46] Klingebiel R, Bohner G. Neuroimaging. Recent results. Cancer Res 2009; 171: 175-190.

[47] Yang I, Aghi MK. New advances that enable identification of glioblastoma recurrence. *Nat. Rev. Clin. Oncol.* 2009; 6(11): 648-57.

[48] Taylor JS, Langston JW, Reddick WE, et al. Clinical value of proton magnetic resonance spectroscopy for differentiating recurrent or residual brain tumor from delayed cerebral necrosis. *Int. J. Radiat. Oncol. Biol. Phys.* 1996; 36(5): 1251-61.

[49] Rock JP, Hearshen D, Scarpace L, et al. Correlations between magnetic resonance spectroscopy and image-guided histopathology, with special attention to radiation necrosis. *Neurosurgery* 2002; 51(4): 912-9.

[50] Cha S. Update on brain tumor imaging: from anatomy to physiology. *AJNR Am. J. Neuroradiol.* 2006; 27: 475-87.

[51] Field AS, Wu YC, Alexander AL. Principal diffusion direction in peritumoral fiber tracts: Color map patterns and directional statistics. *Ann N Y Acad Sci* 2005; 1064: 193-201.

[52] Young RJ, Brennan N, Fraser JF, Brennan C. Advanced Imaging in Brain Tumor Surgery. In: State of the Art Brain Tumor Diagnostic, Imaging, and Therapeutics. Neuroimaging Clinics of North America. SK Mukherji (ed). August 2010; 20(3): 293-310.

[53] Farquharson S, Tournier JD, Calamante F, Fabinyi G, Schneider-Kolsky M, Jackson GD, Connelly A. White matter fiber tractography: why we need to move beyond DTI. *J. Neurosurg.* 2013; 118(6): 1367-77.

[54] Goebell E, Fiehler J, Ding XQ, Paustenbach S, Nietz S, Heese O, et al. Disarrangement of fiber tracts and decline of neuronal density correlate in glioma patients: A combined diffusion tensor imaging and ^{1}-H-MR Spectroscopy study. *AJNR Am. J. Neuroradiol.* 2006; 27: 1426-31.

[55] Field AS, Alexander AL, Wu YC, Hasan KM, Witwer B, Badie B. Diffusion Tensor Eigenvector Directional color imaging patterns in the evaluation of cerebral white matter tracts altered by tumor. *J. Magn Reson Imaging* 2004; 20: 555-562.

[56] Neoplastic disease of the spine. Maravilla KR, Cohen WA. In MRI Atlas of the Spine. Martin Dunitz London UK 1991.

[57] Rodallec MH, Feydy A, Larosserie F, Anract P, Campagna R, Babinet A, Zins M, Drape JL. Diagnostic imaging of solitary tumors of the spine: what to do and say. *Radiographics* 2008; 28: 1019-1041.

[58] Fuchs B, Boos N. Primary Tumors of the Spine. In: Spinal Disorders: Fundamentals of diagnosis and treatment. Boos N, Aebi M(eds). Springer-Verlag 2008; 951-976.

[59] Koeller KK, Rosenblum RS, Morrison AL. Neoplasms of the spinal cord and filum terminale. *Radiographics* 2000; 20: 1721-1749.

[60] Terrance L, Mastronardi L, Celli P, Lunardi P, Acqui M, Fortunately A. Intramedullary spinal cord ependymomas: a study of 45 cases with long-term follow-up. *Act Neurochir.* 1992; 119: 74-79.

[61] Young RJ, Brennan N, Fraser JF, Brennan C. Advanced Imaging in Brain Tumor Surgery. In: State of the Art Brain Tumor Diagnostic, Imaging, and Therapeutics. Neuroimaging Clinics of North America. SK Mukherji (ed). August 2010; 20(3): 293-310.

[62] Foroglou N and Black PM. Mid-Field Suite Design. In: Intraoperative MRI-Guided Neurosurgery. Hall WA, Nimsky C, Truwit CL (eds). First edition. Thieme 2010.

[63] Black PM, Moriarty T, Alexander E 3rd, et al. Development and implementation of intraoperative magnetic resonance imaging and its neurosurgical applications. *Neurosurgery.* 1997 Oct; 41(4): 831-42; discussion 842-5.

[64] Zimmermann M, Seifert V, Trantakis C, Raabe A. Open MRI-guided microsurgery of intracranial tumours in or near eloquent brain areas. *Acta Neurochir* (Wien). 2001; 143(4): 327-37.

[65] Nimsky C, Ganslandt O, Tomandl B, Buchfelder M, Fahlbusch R. Low-field magnetic resonance imaging for intraoperative use in neurosurgery: a 5-year experience. *Eur. Radiol.* 2002 Nov; 12(11): 2690-703.

[66] Mohammadi AM, Sullivan TB, Barnett GH, Recinos V, Angelov L, Kamian K, Vogelbaum MA. Use of high-field intraoperative magnetic resonance imaging to enhance the extent of resection of enhancing and nonenhancing gliomas. *Neurosurgery.* 2014 Apr; 74(4): 339-48; discussion 349; quiz 349-50.

[67] Hall WA, Truwit CL. Intraoperative magnetic resonance imaging. *Acta Neurochir. Suppl.* 2011; 109: 119-29.

[68] Lee B, Newborg A. Neuroimaging in Traumatic Brain Imaging. *Neuro* RX 2005 Apr;2(2): 372-383

[69] Haydel MJ, Preston CA, Mills TJ, Luber S, Blaudeau E, DeBlieux PM. Indications for Computed Tomography in patients with minor head injury. *N. Engl. J. Med.* 2000; 343: 100-105.

[70] Coles JP. Imaging after brain injury. *Br. J. Anaesth*, 2007;99(1):49-60.

[71] Ashikaga R, Araki Y, Ishida O. MRI of head injury using FLAIR. *Neuroradiology* 1997; 39: 239-242.

[72] Medana IM, Esiri MM. Axonal damage: a key predictor of outcome in human CNS diseases. *Brain.* 2003; 126(pt): 513-530.

[73] Dans PC. Head trauma. *AJNR Am. J. Neuroradiol.* 2007;28(8): 1619-1621
[74] Mittl RL, Grossman RI, Hiehle JE etal. Prevalence of MR evidence of diffuse axonal injury in patients with mild head injury and normal head CT findings. *AJNR Am. J. Neuroradiol.* 1994; 15(8): 1583-1589.
[75] Klanders AE, Croul SE. Spinal Trauma. In: Atlas S., ed. Magnetic Resonance Imaging of the brain and spine. Lippincott Williams and Wilkins, 2002 pp1769-1823.
[76] Olsen WL, Chakeres DW, Berry I, Richard J. Spine and Spinal Cord Trauma. In: Munelfe C., ed. Imaging of the Spine and Spinal Cord. Raven Press, New York, 1992 pp407-444.
[77] Munera F, Rivas LA, Nunez DB, Cluncer RM. Imaging evaluation of adult spinal injuries: Emphasis on Multidetector CT in Cervical Spine Trauma. *Radiology* 2012; 263(3): 645-660.
[78] Larson DB, Johnson LW, Schnell BM, Salisburg SR, Forman HP. National trends in CT use in the emergency department: 1995-2007. *Radiology* 2011: 258(1): 164-173.
[79] Chokshi FH, Munera F, Rivas LA, Henry RP, Cluencer PM. 64MDCT angiography of blunt vascular injuries of the neck. *AJR Am. J. Roentgenol.* 2011; 1966(3): w309-W315.
[80] Sliker CW, Shanmuganathan K, Mirvis SE. Diagnosis of blunt cerebrovascular injuries with 16-MDCT: accuracy of whole-body MDCT compared with neck MDCT angiography. *AJR Am. J. Roentgenol.* 2008; 190(3): 790-799.
[81] Ashok Srinivasan, Mayank Goyal, Faisal Al Azri, and Cheemun Lum. State-of-the-Art Imaging of Acute Stroke. *RadioGraphics* 2006 26: suppl_1, S75-S95.
[82] David S Liebeskind, J Stephen Huff, Howard S Kirshner, Richard S Krause, Helmi L Lutsep, Denise Nassisi, Jeffrey L Saver, Francisco Talavera, Chief Editor: Robert E O'Connor. Hemorrhagic Stroke Workup. Medscape Reference.
[83] Dr Tim Luijkx and Dr Frank Gaillard et al. CT perfusion in ischaemic stroke Radiopaedia.org.
[84] Josef Tacke. *Acute Stroke Imaging*. ECR Live 2014 (Video)
[85] Girish M. Fatterpekar, Thomas P. Naidich, Peter M. Som. The Teaching Files: Brain and Spine. Elsevier Health Sciences 2011.
[86] David M. Yousem, Robert I. Grossman. Neuroradiology: The Requisites, Third Edition. Elsevier Health Sciences, 2010.
[87] R. Gilberto González, Joshua A. Hirsch, Michael H. Lev, Pamela W. Schaefer, Lee H. Schwamm. Acute Ischemic Stroke: Imaging and Intervention. Springer Science & Business Media, 2010.
[88] Toshio Moritani, Sven Ekholm, Per-Lennart A. Westesson. Diffusion-Weighted MR Imaging of the Brain. Springer Science & Business Media, 2009.
[89] Anne G. Osborn, Karen L. Salzman, A. James Barkovich. Diagnostic Imaging: Brain. Amirsys, 2010.
[90] Valery N. Kornienko. Diagnostic Neuroradiology. Springer Science & Business Media, 2008.
[91] Montserrat Alemany Ripoll. MRI Diagnosis of Intracranial Hemorrhage: Experimental and Clinical Studies. *Department of Oncology, Radiology and Clinical Immunology*, 2003.
[92] Kidwell CS, Chalela JA, Saver JL, et al. Comparison of MRI and CT for Detection of Acute Intracerebral Hemorrhage. *JAMA*. 2004; 292(15): 1823-1830.

[93] Italo Linfante, MD; Rafael H. Llinas, MD; Louis R. Caplan, MD; Steven Warach, MD, PhD. MRI Features of Intracerebral Hemorrhage Within 2 Hours From Symptom Onset. *Stroke.* 1999 Nov; 30(11): 2263-7.

[94] Christine AC Wijman, Ryan Snider, Chitra Venkatasubramanian, Anna Finley-Caulfield, Marion Buckwalter, Irina Eyngorn, Nancy Fischbein, Alisa Gean, Daniel F Hanley, Carlos S Kase, Jonathan T Kleinman, Neil ESchwartz, Maarten G Lansberg, Gregory W Albers, Michael Mlynash, Stephanie Kemp, Demi Thai, Rashmi Narayana, Michael Marks, Roland Bammer, and Mike Moseley. Diagnostic Accuracy of MRI in Spontaneous intra-cerebral Hemorrhage. The DASH study – Final Results. Stanford Neurocritical Care Program, Stanford Stroke Center Stanford University Medical Center.

[95] Jitendra L Ashtekar, Tufail Ahmed Patankar, David S Levey, C Douglas Phillips, Robert M Krasny, Chief Editor: L Gill Naul. Intracranial Hemorrhage Evaluation with MRI. Medscape Reference.

[96] Fiebach JB, Schellinger PD, Gass A, Kucinski T, Siebler M, Villringer A, Olkers P, Hirsch JG, Heiland S, Wilde P, Jansen O, Röther J, Hacke W, Sartor K; Kompetenznetzwerk Schlaganfall B5. Stroke magnetic resonance imaging is accurate in hyperacute intracerebral hemorrhage: a multicenter study on the validity of stroke imaging. *Stroke.* 2004 Feb; 35(2): 502-6.

In: The Role of Imaging Technology ...
Editor: Georgios Tsoulfas

ISBN: 978-1-63483-490-2

Chapter 5

THE ROLE OF IMAGING IN PARATHYROID SURGERY

I. Koutelidakis*, A. Doundis, A. Ananiadis, S. Kalaitzis, T. Kaltsikis and V. Papaziogas

2nd Department of Surgery, Medical School,
Aristoteleio University of Thessaloniki, Greece

ABSTRACT

Primary hyperthyroidism (PHPT) is mainly caused by a parathyroid adenoma. The localization of this parathyroid lesion is essential for the surgical treatment of the disease. Various invasive and non-invasive localizing tests are available for evaluating PHPT. The traditional non-invasive imaging modalities include ultrasonography, scintigraphy, computed tomography and magnetic resonance imaging. In the era of minimally invasive parathyroidectomy (MIP), the utilization of SPECT and SPECT/CT in radioimaging, the 4D CT and various combinations of individual visualization techniques have established parathyroid imaging as an essential supplement to parathyroid surgery.

INTRODUCTION

There are typically two superior and two inferior parathyroid glands (PG) in humans. The superior PG develops from the dorsal wing of the third pharyngeal pouch and the inferior of the fourth. PG are composed mainly of chief cells, oxyphil cells and adipose tissue. The normal weight of each PG is about 40 to 50mg and measuring about 5 × 3 × 1 mm. The inferior thyroid artery is the predominant vascular supply to both superior and inferior PG in the majority of the cases [1].

The PG are located in the posterior surface, adjacent to the poles of the lobes of the thyroid gland. A nomenclature of possible locations of the PG is shown in figure 1 [2]. It should be mentioned that the inferior PG are consistently anterior (ventral) to the recurrent laryngeal nerve (RLN) and the superior PG posterior (dorsal) to the RLN [3].

* Corresponding Author: I. Koutelidakis, Email: iokoutel@gmail.com

In approximately 10% of patients supernumerary glands and less than four glands have been reported. When the PG are situated above or below the level of the thyroid gland or they are distant from its posterior aspect, they are considered ectopic. Ectopic PG are usually intrathyroidal, in the carotid sheath, the trachealesophageal groove or in the thymus or the superior mediastinum [4].

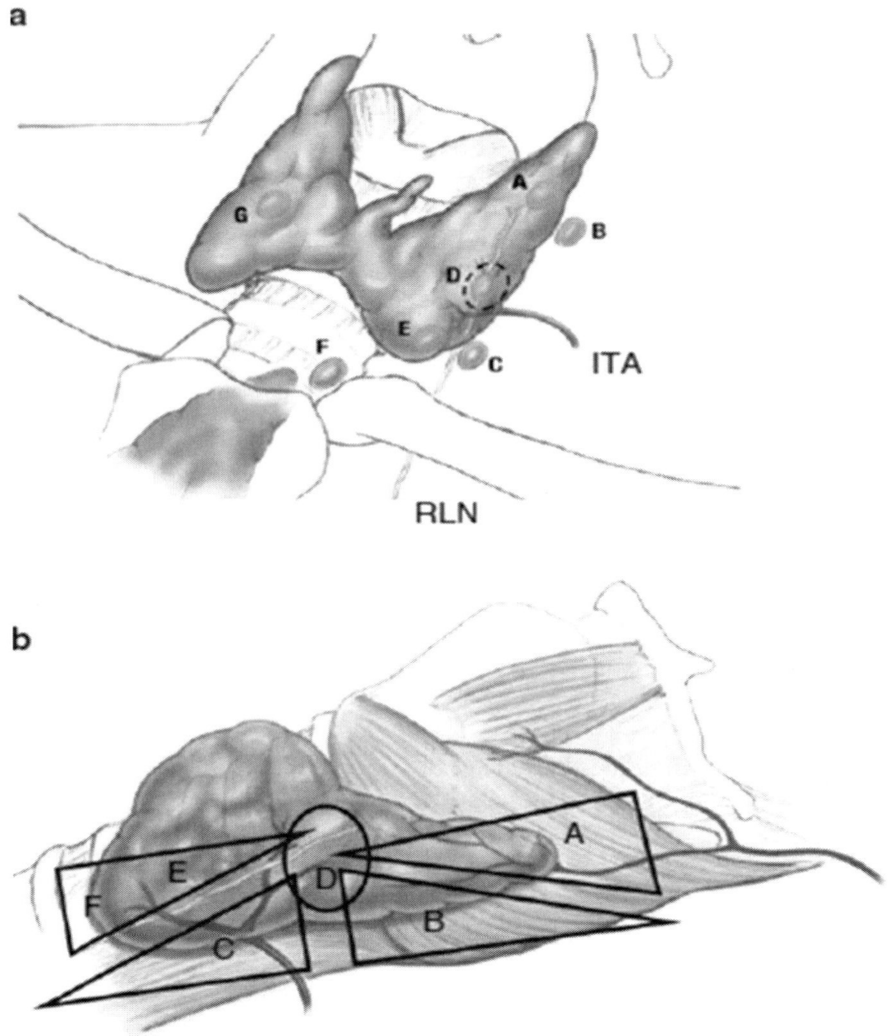

Figure 1. (a) Anterior view displaying nomenclature of possible locations of parathyroid adenomas. A: Superior gland, in proximity of posterior surface of thyroid parenchyma, may be intracapsular/ compressed. B : Superior gland, fallen posteriorly into tracheoesphageal groove, no contact with posterior surface of thyroid tissue in the cranio-caudal confines of thyroid lobe. C : Superior gland, fallen posteriorly into tracheoesphageal groove, no contact with posterior surface of thyroid tissue and is caudal/inferior to cranio-caudal confines of thyroid lobe. D : Superior or inferior gland, in mid region of posterior surface of thyroid parenchyma near junction of RLN and inferior thyroidal artery. E : Inferior gland, in region inferior to thyroid parenchyma, anterior to trachea. F : Inferior gland, descended into thyrothymic ligament or superior thymus and may appear in mediastinum. G : Intrathyroidal parathyroid. (b) Lateral view [2].

PG secrete parathyroid hormone (PTH) which is the key regulator of calcium homeostasis. Hyperfunction of the PG is leading to a condition known as primary hyperparathyroidism (PHPT). Secondary hyperparathyroidism is commonly due to chronic kidney disease, in which low serum calcium concentrations stimulate diffuse gland hyperplasia, In those patients PT glands may continue to grow and become overactive, resulting in typical asymmetric hypertrophy because of autonomous function (tertiary hyperparathyroidism) [5]. Most cases of PHPT are caused by a single parathyroid adenoma (90%). Other causes include hyperplasia of all four glands (5%), double adenomas (5%), and, rarely, parathyroid carcinoma. There is an increased incidence of parathyroid hyperplasia in multiple endocrine neoplasia type I. Another rare cause of PHPT is familial hypocalciuric hypercalcemia [6].

PHPT is a common disease occurring in about 1% of the adults. It is 2-3 times more common in women than men and peaks around the fifth decade of life. Diagnosis of PHPT is accomplished by biochemical findings. The most common presenting symptoms of PHPT include fatigue, hypertension, bone pain, muscle weakness, and psychiatric illness. All symptomatic patients and asymptomatic patients younger than 50 years, as well as patients meeting specific criteria are candidates for surgical therapy [7].

The traditional approach to parathyroid surgery consists of bilateral neck exploration in order to identify and visually inspect all four parathyroid glands. The success of this approach exceeds to 90-95%. However, cervical exploration requires a larger incision, longer operating time and can have higher morbidity [1].

With the progress in parathyroid imaging a minimally invasive approach can be accomplished. The minimally invasive parathyroidectomy (MIP) includes small incision, out-patient parathyroidectomy, endoscopic or video assisted surgery and operation under local anesthesia. MIP is associated with significant reductions in operative time and hospital stay, provides a better cosmetic result while decreasing the potential complications of bilateral exploration [8].

Various invasive and non-invasive localizing tests are available for evaluating PHPT. The traditional non-invasive imaging modalities include ultrasonography, scintigraphy, computed tomography and magnetic resonance imaging.

In the era of MIP, the utilization of SPECT and SPECT/CT in radioimaging, the 4D CT and various combinations of individual visualization techniques have established parathyroid imaging as an essential supplement to parathyroid surgery.

ULTRASONOGRAPHY

Ultrasonography of the neck (US) is the most generally available and cheap examination in parathyroid imaging.

With the use of high-frequency 12- or 15-MHz transducers and the patient in supine position with his or her neck hyperextended, the neck is examined from the carotid bifurcation superiorly to the sternal notch inferiorly and the carotid artery/internal jugular vein laterally [9].

Normal PG are rarely visualized by US, because of their small size and insufficient acoustic difference compared to adjacent thyroid tissue. However, parathyroid adenomas, hyperplasia, and carcinomas exhibit a relatively hypoechogenic pattern, due to their compact cellularity relative to thyroid tissue [10].

Parathyroid adenomas are usually well-circumscribed ovoid, longitudinal in shape and tend to be solid and homogenously hypoechoic relative to echogenic thyroid tissue. An echogenic line that separates the thyroid gland from the enlarged parathyroid gland can usually be seen. Larger adenomas are more likely to have cystic change, lobulations, increased echogenicity due to fatty deposition, and occasional calcifications [11]. (Figure 2).

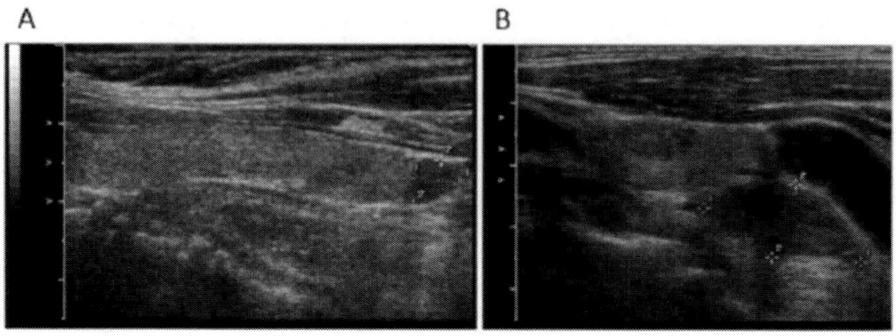

Figure 2. Hypoechoic left lower pole (A) and behind the left lower pole (B) parathyroid adenomas identified by ultrasound [1].

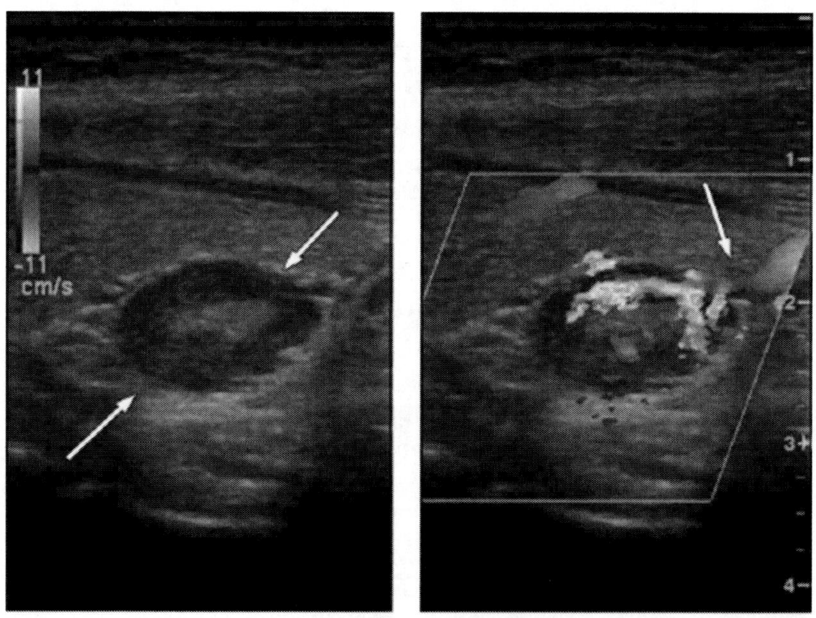

Figure 3. 44-year-old woman with hyperparathyroidism due to right inferior parathyroid adenoma. Resected gland weighed 629 mg, nearly 15 times weight of a normal gland (40–50 mg). A, Sonogram shows typical hypoechoic adenoma (arrows) deep in relation to lower pole of thyroid. B, Color Doppler sonogram shows peripheral feeding vessel (arrow) characteristic of parathyroid adenomas. Also note typical arc or rim vascularity [21].

Color Doppler US (CDUS) has also been used to localize enlarged parathyroid glands, while Contrast-Enhanced US (CEUS) has not yet shown a potential benefit. In CDUS, parathyroid adenomas tend to be hypervascular lesions. An extrathyroidal artery may lead to a parathyroid adenoma in the majority of patients. An extrathyroidal feeding vessel may provide a roadmap to an otherwise inconspicuous gland. Characteristically, the extrathyroidal artery enters at one pole of the gland (polar artery). However, color Doppler sonograms of parathyroid adenomas may not show increased vascularity until the lesions are 1 cm in size [12]. (Figure 3).

Thc scnsitivity of US for detecting enlarged parathyroid glands ranges from 70% to 100% as it is, to a great degree, depended to the experience of the examiner, the size of the PG lesion and the pathology of the adjacent thyroid tissue. An advantage of US is the fact that the identified concurrent thyroid disease can be addressed by fine needle aspiration (FNA) preoperatively or intraoperatively.

Additionally, even when US findings are atypical, US can be helpful leading to further investigation [10, 13-14].

False positive or negative sonographic diagnosis may be due to thyroid nodules, prominent blood vessels, cervical lymph nodes, esophagus and longus colli muscle and poor visualization of neck structures due to previous surgery . It must be stressed that US does not enable localisation of parathyroid glands placed in the mediastinum or in retrotracheal or retrooesophageal regions due to acoustic shadows from bones or air spaces [15].

RADIOIMAGING

The use of radionucleotid agents (radioimaging) is the most widely adopted method in parathyroid imaging.

Among several radiotracers that have been used in the past or are still in use, Hexakis-2-methoxy-isobutyl-isonitrile labeled with technetium- 99m (99mTc-sestamibi) holds a predominant place.

99mTc-sestamibi consists of monovalent cationic lipophilic molecules which after intravenous (i.v.) injection distribute according to blood flow. These molecules cross the cell membranes according to the electrochemical gradient and intracellularly accumulate in the mitochondria of the oxyphil cells. 99mTc-sestamibi is also taken up by the thyroid gland, but it washes out more rapidly from normal thyroid tissue than out of PT glands.99mTc-sestamibi is sequestered also in the myocardium, the salivary glands and in brown fat, which often is noted as a mild supraclavicular shade [16].

Two different protocols can be used in 99mTc sintigraphy.

The dual-phase protocol uses 99mTc-sestamibi alone. Early (10–30 min after injection) and delayed (1.5–2.5 h after injection) high-count images are obtained of the neck and chest. The concept of this technique is based on the different washout of the radiofactor between the thyroid and the abnormal parathyroid gland. Dual-phase imaging with 99mTc-tetrofosmin appears not to be useful because of rapid washout from parathyroid tissue. It should be mentioned that it is mainly a functional technique as it visualizes the difference in the wash out of the radiofactor between the thyroid and the parathyroid gland [17]. (Figure 4).

The dual-tracer protocol uses the coadministration of 99mTc-sestamibi as a substitute to Tl-201, 123I- or 99mTc pertechnetate. The thyroid images generated are then digitally subtracted from the 99mTc-sestamibi image and the residual signal after subtraction of the thyroid image is indicative of parathyroid uptake [17]. (Figure 5).

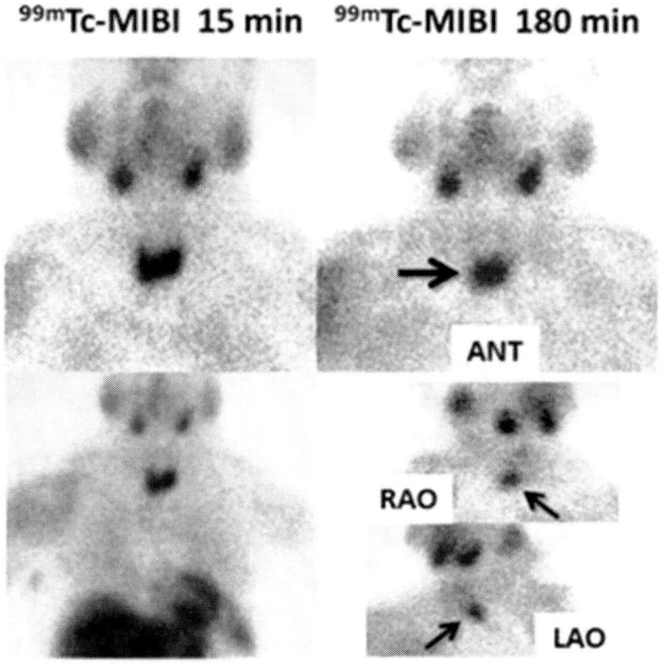

Figure 4. Double phase 99mTc-sestamibi (99mTc-MIBI) parathyroid scintigraphy. In delayed imaging focal tracer retention is seen in the lower part of the thyroid gland (arrow). In the right and left anterior oblique views (RAO and LAO, respectively) the abnormal focus "changes its position significantly" relative to the submandibular salivary glands, indicating that it is located in the thyroid area and not deep in the neck [16].

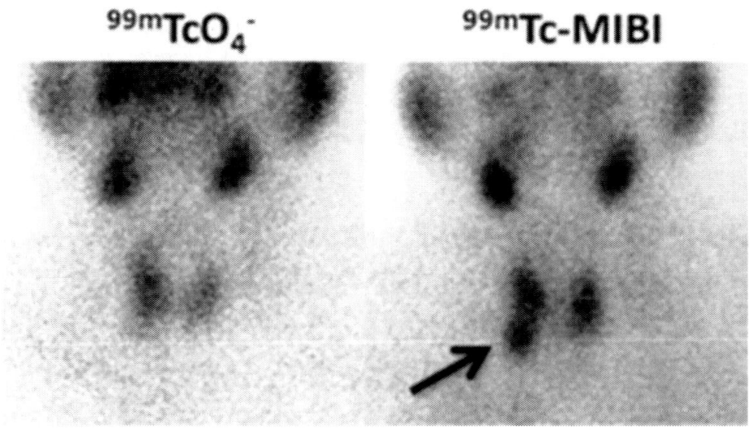

Figure 5. In a patient with primary hyperthyroidism double tracer parathyroid scintigraphy shows a solitary focus adjacent to the lower pole of the right thyroid lobe which takes up 99mTc-sestamibi but not 99mTcO4 -. It is very likely that this patient suffers from a single adenoma and he is suitable for a targeted surgical treatment [16].

Two-dimensional planar PG scanning has been the standard technique for many years, the three-dimensional single photon emission tomography (SPET) was added later on and more recently the latter is combined with computed tomography (SPET/CT) leading to higher sensitivity rates [16]. (Figure 6).

If a dual-phase study is performed, then a high-resolution parallel-hole collimator or a pinhole or converging collimator can be used. Pinhole collimators are preferred if SPECT or SPECT/CT is not part of the imaging protocol. The range of intravenously administered radioactivity in adults is 740–1,110 MBq (20–30 mCi) [17].

In the double tracer subtraction technique the patient should remain immobile between the two successive scans and images should be carefully subtracted to avoid artifacts. In scanning in secondary HPT it is advised to withhold drugs refraining PG hyperfunction, namely calcimimetics for 2 weeks and vitamin D supplements for 1-4 weeks. If a subtraction technique is used, iodine-containing preparations should be avoided for >4 weeks and thyroxine for 3 weeks. If 123I is used for thyroid scanning, thyrostatic drugs should be stopped for 1 week [18].

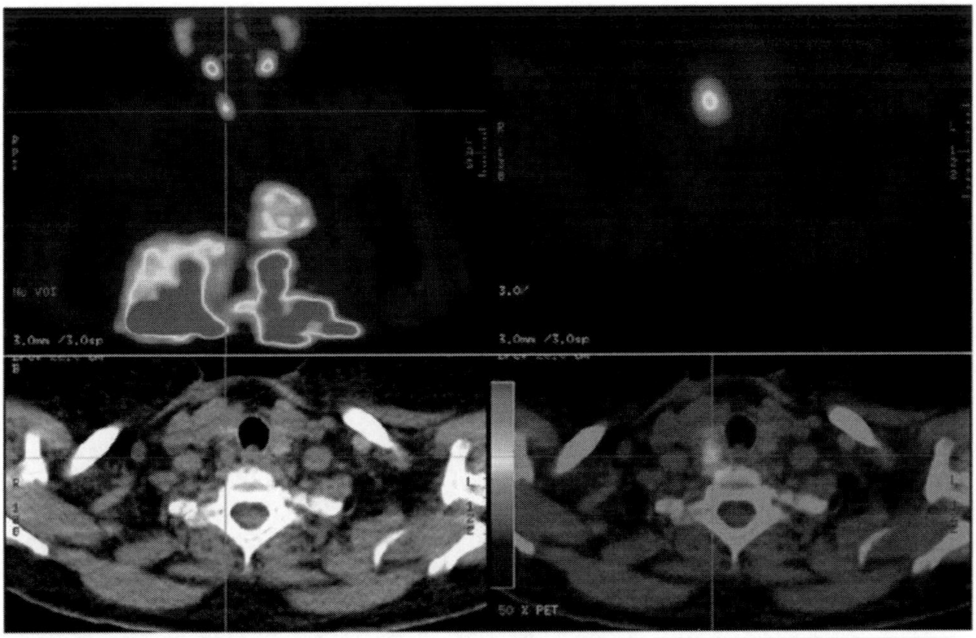

Figure 6. SPECT/CT demonstrating a right side parathyroid adenoma [1].

Sensitivity of 99mTc-sestamibi sintigraphy is reported to be about 80-100%.

Regional perfusion, gland size and functional activity, cell cycle phase, and prevalence of mitochondria-rich cells are some of the factors affecting the diagnostic accuracy of the method [19].

One further advantage of radioimaging is that the use of gamma probe intraoperatively can assist to the localization of the PG lesion and navigate the surgeon through challenging anatomies, especially in cases of ectopic PG [20].

Computed Tomography

Computed tomography (CT) scanning was considered to be an effective adjunct to the conventional first line imaging techniques (US and radioimaging), reserved for cases of reccurent PHPT or cases of altered anatomy [21].

With the induction of 4D CT , therefore the addition of changes in the perfusion of contrast over time to the three dimensional anatomic CT images allowed for further functional information to the anatomic images due to the rapid uptake and washout of the contrast from the hyperfunctioning gland to the anatomic data and improved the sensitivity of the method [22, 23].

Furthermore, 4D CT can be combined with US and this combination technique appears to be an excellent and cost effective preoperative localizing method for hyper-functioning parathyroid glands [24].

CT acquisition involves intravenous administration of nonionic iodinated contrast at a dose of 2 mL per kg patient weight. This technique relies on the vascularity of the parathyroid glands and their relative enhancement with contrast compared to the surrounding structures. A prominent feeding artery at the margin of a parathyroid adenoma (polar vessel), first described on ultrasound, may be seen in up to two thirds of parathyroid adenomas on high-quality 4D-CT studies. This finding can increase diagnostic confidence that a suspicious lesion is a parathyroid adenoma instead of a lymph node or thyroid nodule [25]. (Figure 7 and 8).

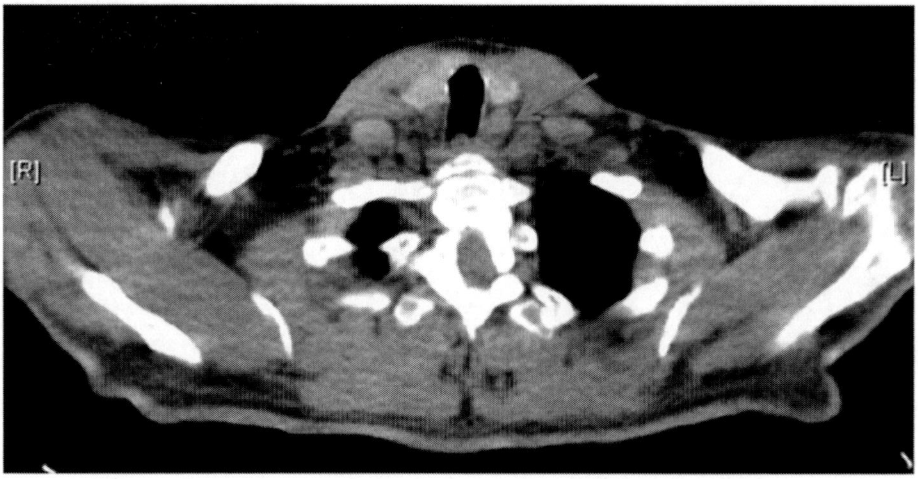

Figure 7. Computed tomography demonstrating a left sided parathyroid adenoma [1].

A 3-phase 4D-CT protocol with helical acquisition at 1.25-mm slice thickness from the bottom of the mandibular teeth down to the carina with noncontrast, early postcontrast, and delayed postcontrast imaging. The first noncontrast images can be helpful to distinguish adenomas from the intrinsically dense iodine-rich thyroid gland, while the early and delayed postcontrast imaging highlight the hypervascular nature of adenomas and their characteristic early washout [26].

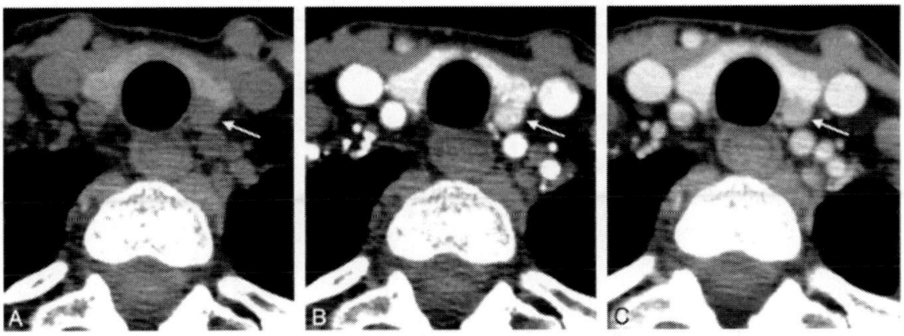

Figure 8. Axial noncontrast (A), axial early phase postcontrast (B), and axial delayed phase postcontrast (C) images show a hypoattenuated hypodense nodule contiguous with the left posterior thyroid gland, which demonstrates avid early contrast enhancement and washout. Pathology revealed a 600-mg parathyroid adenoma [23].

Most modern multiphase 4D-CT techniques report a sensitivity and specificity exceeding 90%. In a CT picture, a parathyroid adenoma can be difficult to differentiate from lymph nodes, normal vessel structures or an exophytic thyroid tuberculum, particularly in patients who have previously undergone an operation within the neck. PG can be difficult to identify by CT at the area of the sternal notch and mediastinum due to streak artifact or being mistaken with lymph nodes. CT is also not particularly useful in identifying the parathyroid glands in patients who are not able to receive IV contrast [22].

MAGNETIC RESONANCE IMAGING

Magnetic Resonance Imaging (MRI) is an expensive and not always available technique; therefore, like CT scanning, MRI is reserved for cases of recurrent PHPT and ectopic PG lesions, despite the advantage of lack of ionizing radiation.

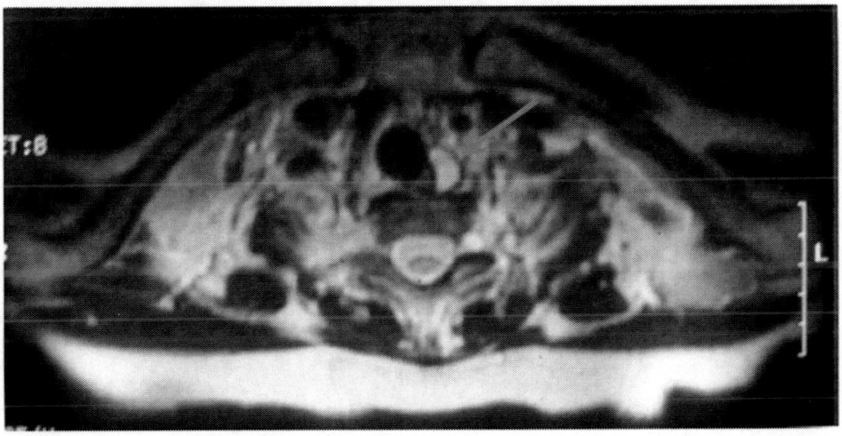

Figure 9. MRI demonstrating a left parathyroid adenoma [1].

Normal parathyroid glands usually are not seen on MRI. Parathyroid adenomas are isointense relative to the surrounding muscle and have low intensity on T1 weighted images.

They are generally hyper intense on T2 weighted images; however, hyper-functioning parathyroid glands show intense contrast enhancement on T1 weighted images [27]. (Figure 9).

The sensitivity of MRI in detecting abnormal parathyroid glands is reported from 70% to 90%. Factors resulting in false positive disease are concomitant thyroid disease and enlarged cervical lymph nodes that may mimic parathyroid adenomas. MRI is less sensitive and specific in identifying hyperplastic glands compared to parathyroid adenomas [28].

POSITRON EMISSION TOMOGRAPHY

Positron Emission Tomography/ Computed Tomography (PET/CT) with 18F-Fluorodeoxyglucose (18F-FDG) as an imaging tool in parathyroid cancer is not clearly reported in the literature, although there is a potential role of PET/CT in assessing the extent of disease and response to treatment which are the general principles used to correctly evaluate disease status. It has been proposed that FDG-PET can provided additional information related to the location and extent of parathyroid carcinoma, compared to CT, MRI and 99mTc-sestamibi [29,30]. (Figure 10).

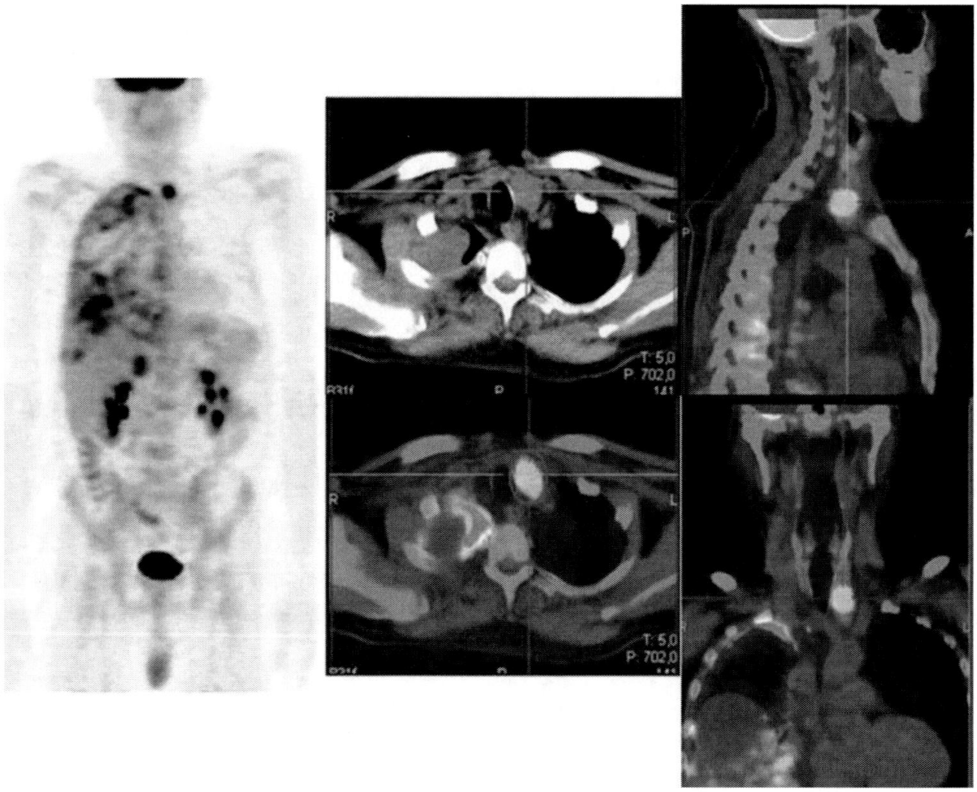

Figure 10. Staging. Right: At Maximum intensity projection the parathyroid and pleural involvements are visible; Central and left: High 18F-Fluorodeoxyglucose-uptake is clearly displayed corresponding to the left parathyroid gland and right pleura in coronal, transverse and sagittal planes [30].

Invasive Methods

The invasive methods used for diagnosing primary hyperparathyroidism are quite sensitive. Selective angiography shows 60% sensitivity, and intra-operative determination of parathormone in venous blood 80%. If both examinations are used, the sensitivity will increase to as much as 91–95%. These examinations help to accurately localize an adenoma (angiography) and to identify further adenomas or hyperplasia (PTH in venous blood). Unfortunately, the methods may involve dangerous complications, including neurological disorders, embolism or renal failure [31].

Conclusion

The role of imaging in parathyroid surgery is more than crucial as it is the factor that can alter the operative strategy and offer to the surgeon the ability for more precise, focused and minimally invasive techniques.

With US and 99mTc sestamibi sintigraphy SPECT or SPECT/CT as first line examinations and the implication of 4D CT and MRI for selected cases, the majority of PG lesions can be precisely visualized and surgically removed.

The combination of different methods has been showed to increase the sensitivity of parathyroid imaging and the intraoperative measurement of PTH can provide confidence to the surgeon and lead to safer parathyroid surgery for the patient.

References

[1] Mohebati A, Shaha AR. Imaging techniques in parathyroid surgery for primary hyperparathyroidism. *Am. J. Otolaryngol.* 2012 Jul-Aug;33(4):457-68. doi: 10.1016/j.amjoto.2011.10.010. Epub 2011 Dec 7.

[2] Elizabeth G. Grubbs , Beth S. Edeiken , Maria K. Gule , Brett J. Monroe, Edmund Kim, Thinh Vu, and Nancy D. Perrier Chapter 2 Preoperative Parathyroid Imaging for the Endocrine Surgeon Handbook of parathyroid diseases A case-based practical guide Khan, MD ,AA; Clark O.H. (Eds.) 2012

[3] Wang C. The anatomic basis of parathyroid surgery. *Ann. Surg.* 1976;183(3):271–5.

[4] Thompson NW, Eckhauser FE, Haven JG. The anatomy of primary, *hyperparathyroldism Surgery* 1982:92:814-821.

[5] Gopinath P, Mihai R. Hyperparathyroidism. *Surgery* (Oxford) 2011; 29: 451-8.

[6] Ruda JM, Hollenbeak CS, Stack BC Jr. A systematic review of the diagnosis and treatment of primary hyperparathyroidism from 1995 to 2003. *Otolaryngol. Head Neck Surg* 2005; 132:359–372

[7] Eigelberger MS, Cheah WK, Ituarte PH, Streja L, Duh QY, Clark OH. The NIH criteria for parathyroidectomy in asymptomatic primary hyperparathyroidism: are they too limited?. *Ann. Surg. Apr* 2004;239(4):528-35.

[8] Norman J, Chheda H, Farrell C. Minimally invasive parathyroidectomy for primary hyperparathyroidism: decreasing operative time and potential complications while improving cosmetic results. *Am. Surg.* 1998 May;64(5):391-5; discussion 395-6.

[9] Leupe PK, Delaere PR, Vander Poorten VL, Debruyne F. Pre-operative imaging in primary hyperparathyroidism with ultrasonography and sestamibi scintigraphy. *B-ENT.* 2011;7(3):173-80.

[10] Gilat H, et al. Minimally invasive procedure for resection of a parathyroid adenoma: the role of preoperative high-resolution ultrasonography. *J. Clin. Ultrasound.* 2005; 33(6):283–7. [PubMed: 16134156]

[11] Solbiati L, et al. Ultrasound of thyroid, parathyroid glands and neck lymph nodes. Eur Radiol. 2001; 11(12):2411–24. [PubMed: 11734934]

[12] Lane MJ, Desser TS, Weigel RJ, Jeffrey RB Jr. Use of color and power Doppler sonography to identify feeding arteries associated with parathyroid adenomas. *AJR Am. J. Roentgenol.* Sep 1998;171(3):819-23.

[13] Boi F, Lombardo C, Cocco MC, Piga M, Serra A, Lai ML, Calò PG, Nicolosi A, Mariotti S. Thyroid diseases cause mismatch between MIBI scan and neck ultrasound in the diagnosis of hyperfunctioning parathyroids: usefulness of FNA-PTH assay. *Eur. J. Endocrinol.* 2012 Dec 10;168(1):49-58. doi: 10.1530/EJE-12-0742. Print 2013 Jan.

[14] Chandramohan A, Sathyakumar K, John RA, Manipadam MT, Abraham D, Paul TV, Thomas N, Paul MJ. Atypical ultrasound features of parathyroid tumours may bear a relationship to their clinical and biochemical presentation. *Insights Imaging.* 2014 Feb;5(1):103-11. doi: 10.1007/s13244-013-0297-x. Epub 2013 Nov 29.

[15] Barbaros U, et al. The characteristics of concomitant thyroid nodules cause false-positive ultrasonography results in primary hyperparathyroidism. *Am. J. Otolaryngol.* 2009; 30(4):239–43. [PubMed: 19563934]

[16] Moralidis E. Radionuclide parathyroid imaging: a concise, updated review. *Hell J. Nucl. Med.* 2013 May-Aug;16(2):125-33. doi: 10.1967/s002449910083. Epub 2013 May 20. Review. PMID: 23687643

[17] Greenspan BS, Dillehay G, Intenzo C, Lavely WC, O'Doherty M, Palestro CJ, Scheve W, Stabin MG, Sylvestros D, Tulchinsky M. SNM practice guideline for parathyroid scintigraphy 4.0. *J. Nucl. Med. Technol.* 2012 Jun;40(2):111-8. doi: 10.2967/jnmt.112.105122. Epub 2012 Mar 27.

[18] Hindié E, Ugur Ö, Fuster D et al. 2009 EANM parathyroid guidelines. *Eur. J. Nucl. Med. Mol. Imaging* 2009; 36: 1201-16.

[19] Torregrosa JV, et al. (99m)Tc-sestamibi scintigraphy and cell cycle in parathyroid glands of secondary hyperparathyroidism. *World J. Surg.* 2000; 24(11):1386–90. [PubMed: 11038211]

[20] Daliakopoulos SI, Chatzoulis G, Lampridis S, Pantelidou V, Zografos O, Ioannidis K, Sapranidis M, Ploumis A. Gamma probe-assisted excision of an ectopic parathyroid adenoma located within the thymus: case report and review of the literature. *Cardiothorac Surg.* 2014 Mar 31;9:62. doi: 10.1186/1749-8090-9-62.

[21] Johnson NA, Tublin ME, Ogilvie JB Parathyroid imaging: technique and role in the preoperative evaluation of primary hyperparathyroidism. *AJR Am. J. Roentgenol.* 2007 Jun;188(6):1706-15. Review.

[22] Rodgers SE, et al. Improved preoperative planning for directed parathyroidectomy with 4- dimensional computed tomography. *Surgery.* 2006; 140(6):932–40. discussion 940-1. [PubMed: 17188140].

[23] Chazen JL, Gupta A, Dunning A, Phillips CD. Diagnostic accuracy of 4D-CT for parathyroid adenomas and hyperplasia. *AJNR Am. J. Neuroradiol.* 2012 Mar;33(3):429-33. doi: 10.3174/ajnr.A2805. Epub 2011 Dec 1.

[24] Kutler DI, et al. Parathyroid localization with modified 4D-computed tomography and ultrasonography for patients with primary hyperparathyroidism. *Laryngoscope*. 2011.

[25] Bahl M, Muzaffar M, Vij G, Sosa JA, Choudhury KR, Hoang JK. Prevalence of the Polar Vessel Sign in Parathyroid Adenomas on the Arterial Phase of 4D CT. *AJNR Am. J. Neuroradiol.* Aug 14 2013.

[26] Chazen JL, Gupta A, Dunning A, Phillips CD. Diagnostic accuracy of 4D-CT for parathyroid adenomas and hyperplasia. *AJNR Am. J. Neuroradiol.* Mar 2012;33(3):429-33.

[27] Abikhzer G, Levental M, Rush C. High resolution MRI in the detection of an intrathymic parathyroid adenoma. *Br. J. Radiol.* 2006; 79(945):e78–80. [PubMed: 16940365].

[28] McDermott VG, et al. Preoperative MR imaging in hyperparathyroidism: results and factors affecting parathyroid detection. *AJR Am. J. Roentgenol.* 1996; 166(3):705–10. [PubMed: 8623655].

[29] Neumann DR, Esselstyn CB, Kim EY. Recurrent postoperative parathyroid carcinoma: FDG-PET and sestamibi-SPECT findings. *J. Nucl. Med* 1996; 37: 2000-2001.

[30] Evangelista L, Sorgato N, Torresan F, Boschin IM, Pennelli G, Saladini G, Piotto A, Rubello D, Pelizzo MR. FDG-PET/CT and parathyroid carcinoma: Review of literature and illustrative case series. *World J. Clin. Oncol.* 2011 Oct 10;2(10):348-54. doi: 10.5306/wjco.v2.i10.348.

[31] Gawrychowski J, Buła G. Imaging diagnostics for primary hyperparathyroidism. *Endokrynol. Pol.* 2013;64(5):404-8. doi: 10.5603/EP.2013.0024. PMID: 24186598.

In: The Role of Imaging Technology …
Editor: Georgios Tsoulfas
ISBN: 978-1-63483-490-2

Chapter 6

THE ROLE OF IMAGING IN ADRENAL SURGERY

K. Sapalidis[1,*], I. Anastasiadis[2], E. Kotidis[3], M. G. Pramateftakis[4] and I. Chrysogonidis[5]

[1]Assistant Professor of Surgery, 3rd Surgery Department, AHEPA University Hospital, Thessaloniki, Greece
[2]General Surgery Chief Resident, 3rd Surgery Department, AHEPA University Hospital, Thessaloniki, Greece
[3]Lecturer of Surgery, 3rd Surgery Department, AHEPA University Hospital, Thessaloniki, Greece
[4]Senior Colorectal Fellow, Guy's and St Thomas' NHS Foundation Trust
[5]Assistant Professor of Radiology, Department of Radiology, AHEPA University Hospital, Thessaloniki, Greece

ABSTRACT

The adrenal glands constitute an indispensable part of human physiology and the diseases affecting them, ranging from benign to malignant ones, are often a challenge for the medical and surgical team. As a result, knowledge of the latest imaging technology is critical for the diagnosis and management of these diseases, in order to provide our patients with the best possible care. This chapter will present the various imaging modalities used for the adrenal glands, as well as discuss the advantages and disadvantages of each, in order to provide our readers with a practical decision-making guide.

INTRODUCTION

The adrenal glands constitute indispensable components of normal physiology. In terms of fundamental anatomy, the adrenal is divided in an outer layer, known as the cortex and in an inner layer, the medulla [1-2]. Each gland weighs approximately 2-4 grams [1-2]. Being of

* Corresponding author: Sapalidis Konstantinos, E- mail: sapalidis@med.auth.gr

significant interest in surgical practice, their blood supply can arise from several different vessels including the aorta, the celiac trunk, the inferior phrenic or the renal arteries [1-2]. The adrenal cortex secretes glucocorticoids, mineralocorticoids and sex hormones, while the adrenal medulla secretes catecholamines (epinephrine and norepinephrine and dopamine) [3]. From an embryology perspective, the adrenal cortex tissue stems from the intermediate mesoderm, whilst the medulla is derived from neural crest cells through a complex migration process [4-5]. Indeed, understanding the basis of embryonic adrenal development is a key aspect of deciphering certain pathology of this gland.

To begin with, lesions affecting the adrenal cortex have a higher prevalence than lesions located in the gland's medulla [6]. Further classification is focused on determining whether the lesion is primary or metastatic. Notably, primary adrenal lesions are metabolically functional in several cases leading to the clinical manifestations of hormone excess (e.g., Cushing syndrome, Conn syndrome, pheochromocytoma etc.). This is rare with metastatic adrenal tumors [7]. In respect with lege artis medicine, Radiologic Imaging proves to be indispensable in diagnosis and staging. Predominantly, adrenal imaging can be accomplished with Computed Tomography (CT), Magnetic Resonance Imaging (MRI), Ultrasonography (US), nuclear imaging and angiography which are implemented with regard to current guidelines and the surgical team's judgment [8].

METHODOLOGY

This chapter was composed after consulting with the PRISMA Statement (2009) [9]. A review of literature was conducted using PubMed (Medline). Inclusion criteria were: papers published in English which reported on humans. Both primary research (case reports, case series, clinical trials etc.) and secondary research (reviews and meta-analyses) were deemed eligible. Exclusion criteria were: papers published in a language other than English, experimental studies on animals, Editorials and commentaries or letters to the editor. Pre-decided keywords were applied to search the database and include the following: *adrenal lesion imaging, adrenal lesion CT, adrenal lesion MRI, adrenal lesion US, adrenal lesion nuclear imaging, adrenal lesion angiography, laparoscopic adrenalectomy, robotic adrenalectomy.*

MINIMALLY INVASIVE ADRENALECTOMY: NOVEL DIRECTIONS AND LIMITATIONS

I. The Role of Laparoscopy in Adrenal Surgery

Gagner introduced laparoscopy in the field of adrenal surgery in 1992 [10]. Indisputably, in the 21st century, laparoscopic adrenalectomy has prevailed over conventional open surgery as the gold standard of care, mainly due to diminished ICU and hospital stay, fewer post-operative complications and higher cosmetic satisfaction expressed by patients. The fact that the adrenals are located in the retroperitoneal space ignited the genesis of several approaches such as: the lateral retroperitoneal, the transperitoneal, the posterior retroperitoneal and even the transthoracic technique [11].

Lateral Retroperitoneal Approach

The patient is subjected to general anaesthesia and placed in the lateral decubitus position. The ipsilateral, to the affected side, arm is suspended approximately 60°, whilst the contralateral arm safely rests on a special board protected with padding. Moreover, under the contralateral axilla a soft cushion is applied [11-12]. Left adrenalectomies usually require four trocar portals. On the other hand, it is typical to utilize 5 portals when performing right adrenalectomies [11-12]. Trocars are inserted transversally along the posterior auxiliary and mid-clavicular line (just below the rib cage). During left adrenalectomy special care must be given out to the splenic flexure, the spleen and the tail of the pancreas. When working in close approximation to the right colonic flexure, the surgeon must be cautious in order to avoid inflicting injury to right lobe of the liver. Indeed, identification and clipping of the adrenal vein constitute priorities of paramount significance.

Transperitoneal Approach

This technique bears a most distinctive advantage. The surgeon has optimal visualization of the abdomen, which effectively decreases technical difficulties and leads to improved post-operative outcomes [13]. The transperitoneal approach constitutes a wise choice for pheochromocytomas and malignant tumours.

Posterior Retroperitoneal Approach

Walz et al. introduced this approach in which the adrenal is resected from the superior pole of the kidney prior to adrenal vessel ligation [14-15]. Even though this technique has been questioned [11], Cleveland clinic series [16] and systematic reviews have revealed that the posterior retroperitoneal is similar in outcomes with the lateral retroperitoneal approach if not superior [17]. Limitations exist though, as these results can only be regenerated when the procedure is performed by experienced surgeons in carefully selected groups of patients.

Transthoracic Approach

This technique was initially described in 2001. Four ports were utilized without pneumo-insufflation. The diaphragm was incised under ultrasound guidance and the adrenal was visualized in the retroperitoneal space. Ultimately vessel ligation and specimen resection was successful. Gill et al. conclude that this approach is oriented towards patients with significant abdominal and retroperitoneal fibrosis from previous surgeries [18].

Indications and Contraindications to Laparoscopic Adrenalectomy

The usual scenario involves a benign, solitary, adrenal lesion with either cortical or medullary location. Specifically, non-secreting cortical adenomas represent the vast majority of cases, with secreting adenomas (e.g aldosteronomas, glucorticoid secreting tumors), pheochromocytomas and metastases accounting for just a minor percentage of the total number of adrenal lesions. Other rare lesions regard neuroblastomas, myelolipomas, sex-hormone secreting tumors, ganglioneuromas and adrenal cysts [19]. As far as contraindications are concerned there is no widely-accepted consensus amongst Endocrine

Surgeons. However, open adrenalectomy is preferable to the laparoscopic procedure in cases involving lesions larger than 8cm or malignant adrenal tumours; especially in the event of infiltration of adjacent structures [11, 17].

Chai et al. highlight that size criteria were less restrictive with laparoscopic lateral transperitoneal adrenalectomy [17]. Notably, a solitary metastatic adrenal lesion does not constitute an absolute contraindication for laparoscopic adrenalectomy [11].

II. The Role of Robotics in Adrenal Surgery

The first series of robotic adrenalectomy were described in 1999 by Piazza et al. and Hubbens et al. [20-21] The Da Vinci ® system is superior to its predecessor (AESOP 2000 ®) on account of the EndoWrist technique and the three-dimensional vision [23]. A 2014 meta-analysis comparing robotic to laparoscopic adrenalectomy confirmed that the transperitoneal approach is the most widely implemented method with both techniques (72.5% of robotic adrenalectomies, 75.5% of laparoscopic adrenalectomies, p = 0.27). Conversion rates, OR time and incidence of post-operative complications did not differ statistically for the two techniques. However, laparoscopically treated patients did experience heavier intraoperative bleeding and required longer hospitalization than patients who underwent robotic adrenalectomy [24].

APPLICATIONS OF IMAGING IN ADRENAL SURGERY

Differential diagnosis between benign and malignant lesions is accomplished with the contribution of Radiology. With the progress of technology, current imaging equipment can offer highly detailed anatomical information and clues about a lesion's physiological behaviour. All of the above assist the Surgeon in implementing the most appropriate procedure for the patient.

I. Adrenal Cortical Adenoma

Adrenal cortical adenoma is usually a benign mass and in most cases nonfunctional. If the lesion is active it produces symptoms related to hypersecretion of cortisol or aldosterone, while its potential malignancy is increased with size (>3cm). Sex-hormone secreting tumors have commonly malignant behavior.

They produce androgens, estrogens or both. For androgen secreting tumors, high blood concentration of testosterone and DHEA-s levels combined with urine 17-ketosteroids forge the diagnosis. For estrogen secreting tumors, high blood concentration of estrogens and urine 17-ketosteroids serve the same cause.

Imaging is crucial in the evaluation of incidentalomas. It's also valuable to correlate current and previous imaging, as malignant lesions tend to change over time, unlike non-malignant ones. Adrenal lesions can be divided to typical and atypical according to their appearance [25].

Typical adenomas: small: < 3 cm, homogeneous and with low density.

Atypical adenomas:

> 3 cm, may present: hemorrhage, calcification, necrosis, absence of adipose tissue

> 4 cm: 70% malignant (excluding adrenal myelolipomas which are easily recognized due to adipose tissue presence, and pheochromocytomas which are usually recognized with biochemical markers.

> 6 cm: 85% malignant potency [25]

Radiographic Approach

Computed Tomography (CT): Adrenal masses are usually first identified by CT scan. Most of adrenal adenomas (about 70%) contain significant intracellular fat and therefore CT presents with high sensitivity and specificity in their identification. Calculating the mean Hounsfield units (HU) of an adrenal lesion first at non-enhancing CT (between -10 Hounsfield units and 10 HU) and early and delayed enhanced CT using the region of interest. A washout rate, usually of 15-min-delayed CT, is most useful in the diagnosis of adrenal adenomas. CT is the most reliable test to differentiate between benign and malignant adrenal lesions. However, the diagnosis of lipid-poor adenomas is quite harder [26].

Magnetic Resonance Imaging (MRI): MRI is mainly utilized when CT results are inconclusive. Chemical shift imaging demonstrates a high diagnostic reliability, as it is highly sensitive to little amounts of intracellular fat and therefore a signal intensity drop can be measured in the majority of adenomas. The adenoma can also be compared in and out of phase, using other adjacent tissues as reference (apart from the liver). Restricted diffusion is usually detected in malignant lesions [27] (Figures 3, 4).

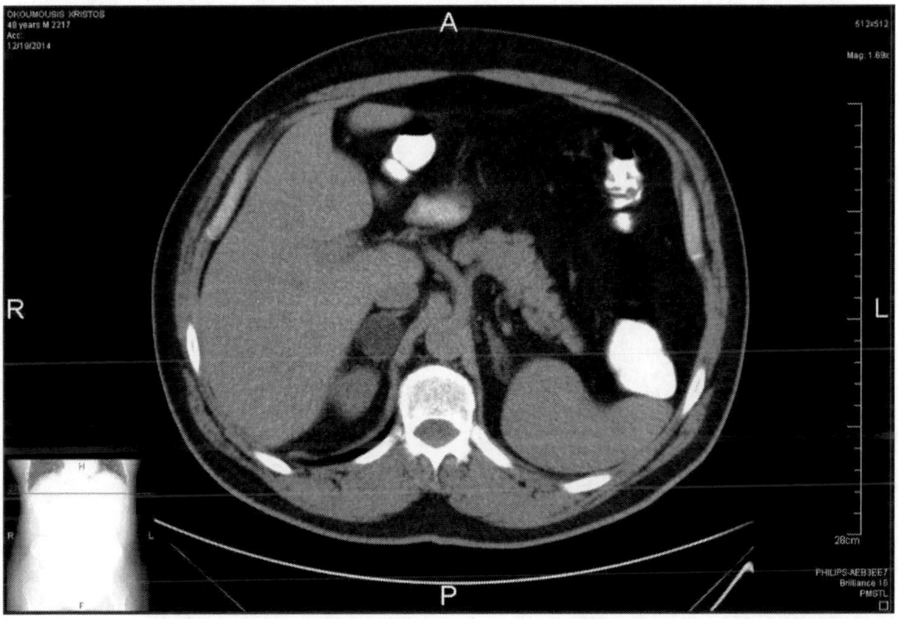

Figure 1. Right adrenal mass. Thin-section non-enhanced CT image, attenuation levels are at 15 HU, because of abundant intracytoplasmatic lipid in the cortex.

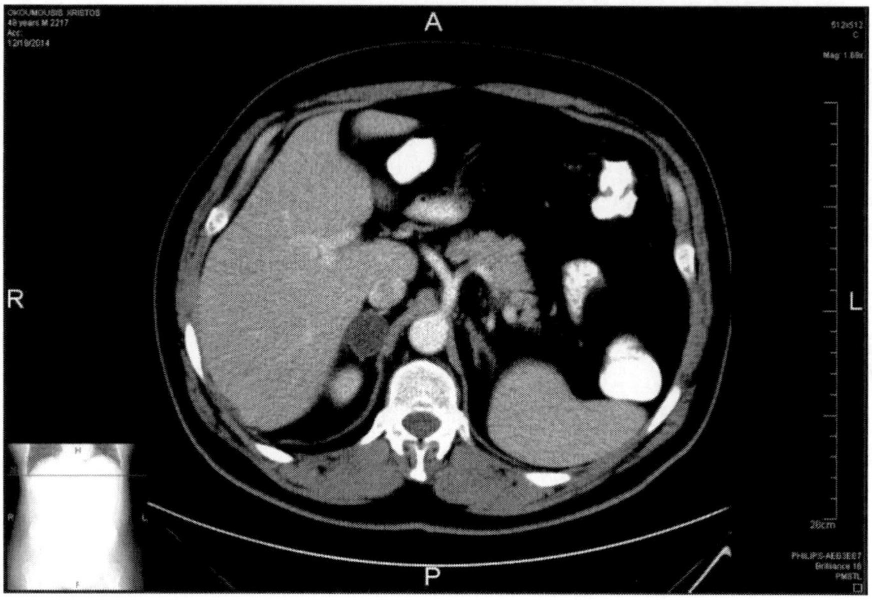

Figure 2. Right adrenal mass. Thin-section enhanced CT image. During the arterial phase of enhancement, density measurements reach 122 HU, dropping to 72 HU during the portal phase of enhancement.

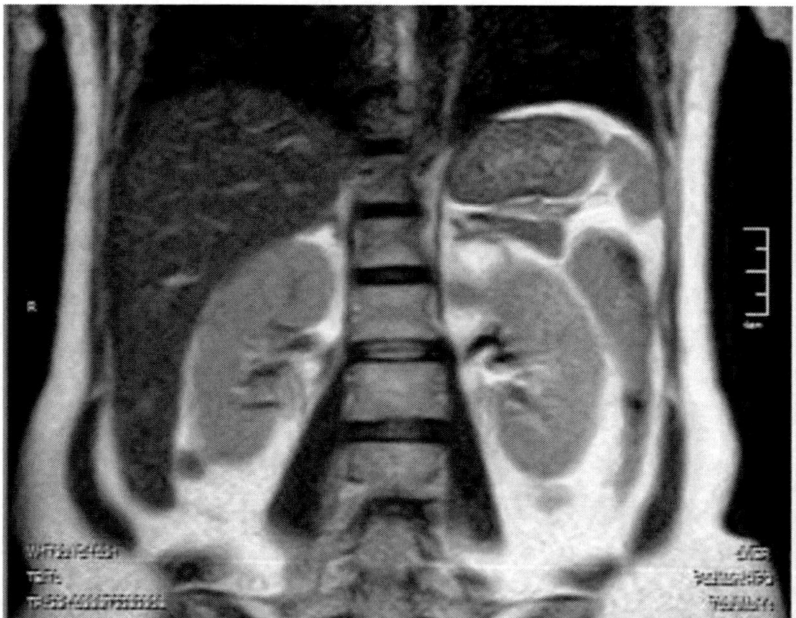

Figure 3. Adrenal adenoma. A coronal T1-weighted out-of-phase MR image shows relative signal loss within the lesion, when compared with the signal loss of the spleen and paraspinal muscle. The signal loss on opposed-phase images related to intracellular lipid is based on phase cancellation of fat and water protons within the same voxel.

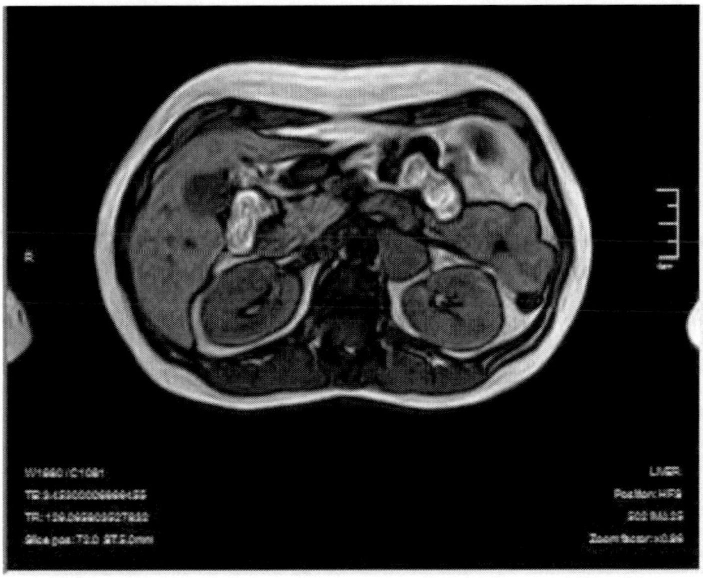

Figure 4. Adrenal adenoma. An axial T1-weighted in-phase MR image shows a large homogeneous mass in the left adrenal gland (arrow) with signal intensity similar to that of the paraspinal muscle or spleen.

II. Adrenal Myelolipoma

Adrenal myelolipoma is a rare non-malignant, non-secreting tumor usually appearing in the 5th-6th decade of life. In the majority of cases it is unilateral and represents 3-5% of all primary adrenal tumors [28].

Radiographic Approach

Ultrasound: Adipose tissue distribution in the lesion, determines its sonographic image. Most commonly they are depicted as a heterogeneous mass of both hyper- and hypoechoic components [28].

Computed Tomography (CT): Myelolipomas typically appear as relatively well-circumscribed adrenal masses. They contain fatty components, the amount of which may vary. In many cases, small punctate calcifications can be seen, as well as regions of higher attenuation (in cases of present hemorrhage - seen in larger lesions) [28-29].

Magnetic Resonance Imaging (MRI): T1: typically hyper-intense due to fat contents, T1 (FS): typically shows fat suppression, T1 + (Gd): shows striking enhancement, T2: intermediate to hyperintense (varies depending of hemorrhage products), in and out of phase: out of phase imaging may demonstrate signal loss in mixed components masses [28, 30].

III. Adrenal Cortical Carcinoma

Adrenal cortical adenoma is a very rare but aggressive tumor (incidents 1-2 cases pes million). Clinical manifestations are present in around 50-60% of all cases and are attributed most commonly to cortisol excess (Cushing syndrome). Fewer cases are presented with symptoms of hyper secretion of the remaining cortical hormones (aldosterone, sex hormones). Usually at the time of the diagnosis local spread or distant metastasis are already present [31-32].

Radiographic Approach

Focal extensions can occur into the renal vein, as wells as in the IVC and liver [31-32].

Ultrasound: A well-defined adrenal mass is usually observed, with small lesions being homogeneous and larger ones rather heterogeneous, because of necrosis or hemorrhage [31-32].

Computed Tomography (CT): Adrenal carcinomas are usually large masses (> 6 cm), variably enhanced in CT, because of their irregular shape and central hemorrhagic and necrotic areas. Smaller carcinomas look much similar to adenomas [31-32].

Magnetic Resonance Imaging (MRI): It is usually used to determine the presence of metastases where CT may be inconclusive. The administration of gadolinium reveals the heterogeneity of the mass due to the presence of hemorrhagic components [31-32].

Angiography: Selective arteriography can distinguish renal from adrenal tumors by identifying the source of the primary vascular supply, when the organ of origin cannot be identified [31-32].

IV. Pheochromocytoma

Pheochromocytoma is a neuroendocrine tumor of the adrenal medulla. Pathological origin can be traced to adrenal chromaffin cells which are derived from the neural crest. During embryological development, these cells migrate to the adrenal medulla (80-90%) and the rest can be found in the ganglia of the Autonomous Nervous System (ANS) [33]. Usually pheos follow the ''rule of 10'': 10% bilateral, 10% malignant, 10% are found in children 10% familial (associated with either MENII , Von Hippel-Lindau disease, Neurofibromatosis 1, familial types of pheochromocytomas), 10% located in the ANS ganglia (paragangliomas), 10% are not associated with hypertension [33].

Cardinal clinical manifestations are headaches and blood pressure disorders: 1) typically paroxysmal type, 2) constant severe hypertension is more common in malignant pheos,3) even hypotension can occur in tumor necrosis when large quantities of epinephrine are released in the circulation leading to massive vasodilation by β- receptor activation. Other clinical symptoms include tachycardia, palpitations, anxiety, dyspnea, diaphoresis, vomiting, weight loss and hyperglycemia [33].

Diagnostics tests include 24 hour urine collection and measurement of metanephrine-VMA-catecholamine levels [33].

Radiographic Approach

Adrenal tumors are usually larger than 3cm (~5 cm) and therefore easy to identify. However, small extra-adrenal tumors are quite challenging to find. Malignancy can be evaluated from the image only when local tissue invasion or metastases are present [34-35] *(Figure 5).*

Ultrasound: The appearance is variable (solid/cystic/mixed) [34-35].

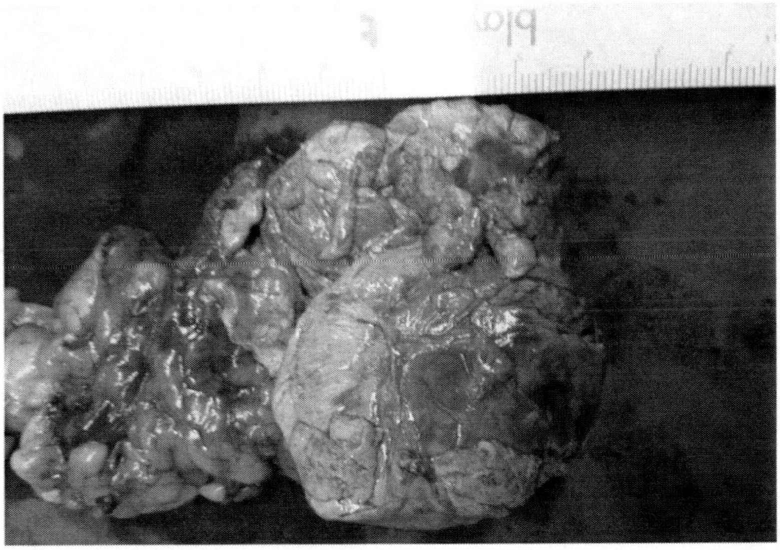

Figure 5. Pheochromocytoma. Surgical specimen.

Computed Tomography (CT): CT is highly sensitive and therefore the first imaging modality to be used. Pheochromocytomas are usually large and heterogeneous, with necrotic areas, cystic modifications and maybe calcifications. Rich enhancement is typically noted [34-35].

Magnetic Resonance Imaging (MRI): MRI demonstrates the highest sensitivity in identifying pheochromocytomas and most valuable in cases of extra-adrenal localization of tumors. T1 signal will be more heterogeneous in necrotic or hemorrhagic areas with the rest of the adrenal being slightly hypo-intense. T1 C+ (Gd): persistent heterogenous enhancement. T2 markedly hyper-intense: light bulb sign and areas of necrosis / haemorrhage /calcification would change the signal [34-35].

Nuclear medicine: Pheochromocytomas, even extra-adrenal ones, can be imaged using various agents. The specificity of this method is not very high though and its spatial resolution is limited [34].

Octreotide (somatostatin) scans: Somatostatin receptors are expressed in over 70% of pheochromocytomas. These method lacks specificity though as the same receptors can also be found in kidneys, areas of inflammation and other glands, making interpretation quite difficult. Imaging is executed 4 hours after intravenous infusion [34].

Positron Emission Tomography (PET): PET scan is considered to be highly sensitive [36].

V. Neuroblastoma

Neuroblastoma is the 4th most common malignancy in childhood [6]. Most children are diagnosed under the age of five. It's a malignancy that arises from nerves of the sympathetic system [6].

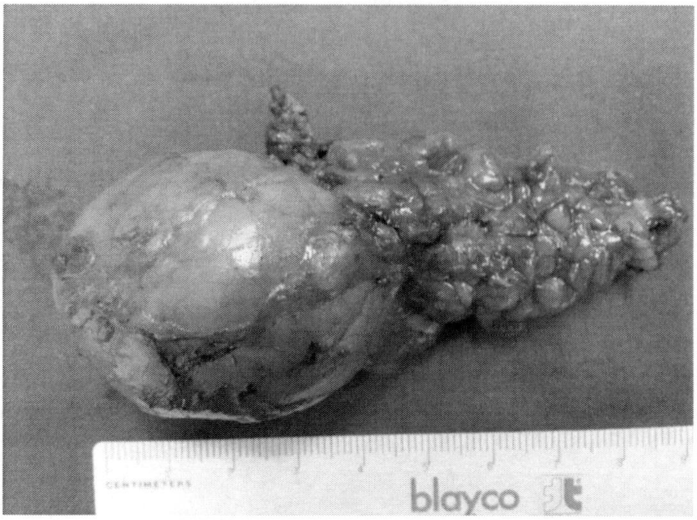

Figure 6. Ganglioneuroma. Surgical specimen.

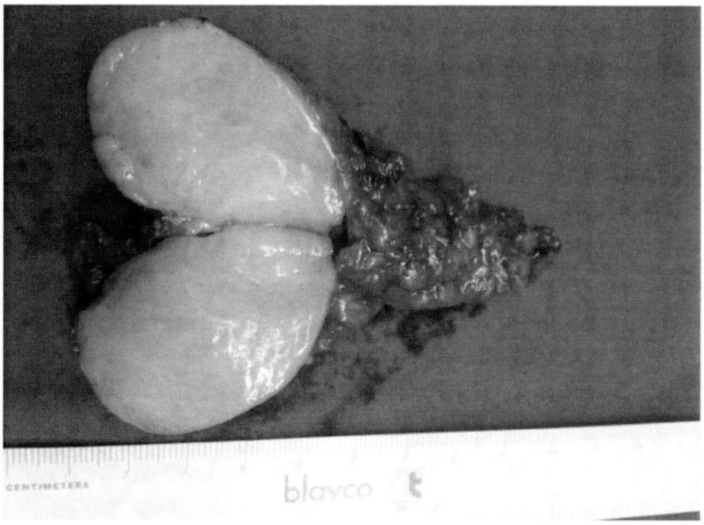

Figure 7. Ganglioneuroma. Surgical specimen (dissected).

They can be located anywhere along that path. Around 30% of these tumors are located in the adrenal glands. *(Figures 6, 7)* Other sites may include i) paraspinal ganglia, ii) thoracic cavity and pelvic cavity [6]. Symptoms and signs are usually restricted to a palpable abdominal mass which is only rarely accompanied with pain [6]. Less commonly, neuroblastomas are accompanied by: opsoclonus, Hutchinson syndrome due to bone metastases, Pepper syndrome which is in fact hepatomegaly due to extensive liver metastases, blueberry muffin syndrome presenting with multiple cutaneous lesions [37-38]. Diagnostic results include in 90% of cases elevated VMA, HVA in 24 hour urine collection sample [38].

Radiographic Approach

Ultrasound: Neuroblastoma is depicted as a heterogeneous mass with internal vascularity, necrotic areas and calcification [37-38].

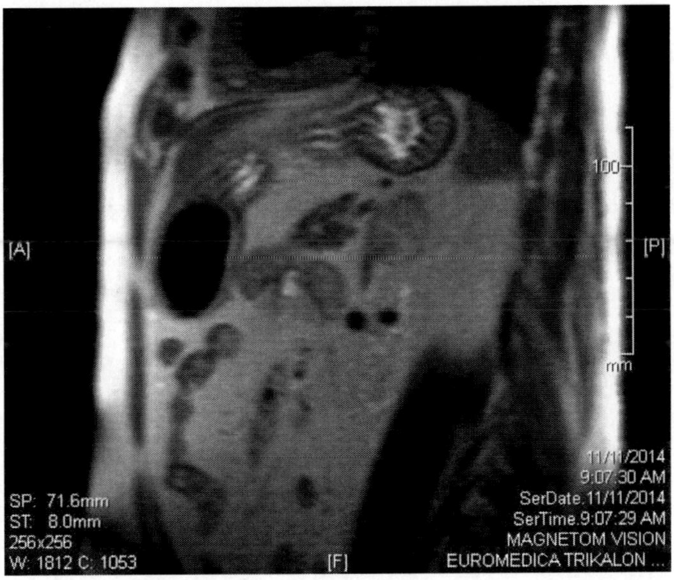

Figure 8. Ganglioneuroma. A coronal T1-weighted out-of-phase MR image shows no signal loss within the lesion, presence of intracellular lipid.

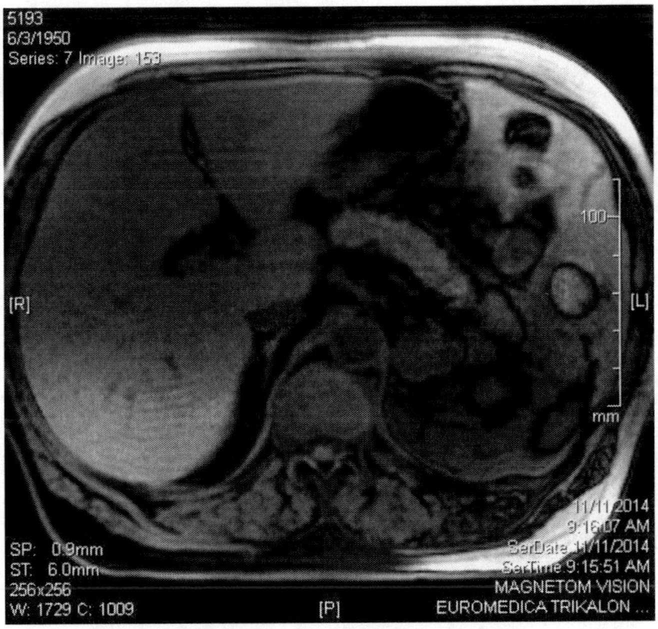

Figure 9. Ganglioneuroma. Axial T1weighted image heterogenously intermediate, distinguished mild capsule.

Nuclear medicine: Agents used for diagnosis and staging:

- pentetreotide labeled to Indium-In111 (somatostatin analog) – nonspecific
- MIBG (metaiodobenzylguanidine labeled to Iodine-123) – screening for metastatic recurrence.
- Tc-99m MDP-mostly used in evaluating metastases [37-38].

Computed Tomography (CT): A heterogeneous mass with calcifications is usually noticed. The tumor displaces, compresses or invades adjacent structures depending on its malignant potential [37-38].

Magnetic Resonance Imaging (MRI): MRI assesses CNS involvement, as well as determines the organ of origin.T1: heterogeneous and iso- to hypo- intense. T1+ (Gd): variable and heterogeneous enhancement. T2 heterogeneous and hyper-intense with cystic/necrotic areas of notably high intensity [37-38] (Figure 8, 9, 10).

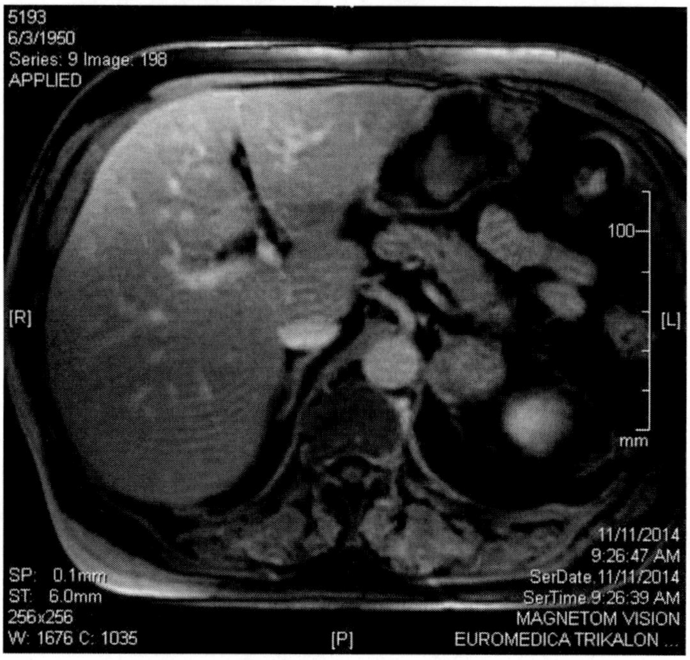

Figure 10. Ganglioneuroma. Axial T1 C+ (Gd) weighted image with heterogenous enhancement.

VI. Adrenal Metastases

Most common primary tumors which produce adrenal metastases are: lung cancer, colorectal cancer, breast cancer, pancreatic cancer and others like renal cell carcinoma, hepatocellular carcinoma, and malignant melanoma [39].

Radiographic Approach

Computed Tomography (CT): Metastases have variable appearance in a CT scan. The enhancement washout percentage is usually <50% and is similar to that of lipid-poor adrenal adenomas in cases of renal cell or hepatocellular carcinoma [32, 39]. *Magnetic Resonance Imaging (MRI):* Signal characteristics may vary; the most common ones include: T1: usually have a low signal intensity. T1 C+ (Gad): a progressive enhancement after administration of contrast material. T2: usually have a high signal intensity [32, 39].

VII. Other Rare Adrenal Lesions

Ganglioneuromas

These constitute benign tumors of the Sympathetic Nervous System (SNS). They are extremely rare and usually asymptomatic. Majority of cases are diagnosed incidentally [37].

Radiographic Approach

Computed Tomography (CT): Findings are compatible with well circumscribed, solid, encapsulated masses. Lesions tend to be iso- to hypo-attenuating compared to muscle signals. May demonstrate calcifications (~ 20%) [37].

Magnetic Resonance Imaging (MRI): T1 - tends to have homogeneously low or intermediate signal. T2 - tends to have heterogeneously intermediate or high signal. T1 C+ (Gd) - variable ranging from none to heterogeneous enhancement. ADC - ADC values tend to be higher to that of a neuroblastoma [37].

Adrenal Cysts and Pseudocysts

Adrenal cysts constitute rare (incidence of 0.06% to 0.18% in autopsy studies), benign, and usually nonfunctional lesions. They tend to be large at presentation (> 6 cm), and at times hard to distinguish from renal upper-pole cysts. They are often the outcome of prior adrenal trauma or hemorrhage. Adrenal pseudocysts do not contain an epithelial wall but rather a fibrous sheath. They compromise about 40% of adrenal cysts and more likely than simple cysts to be asymptomatic [26-28].

Radiographic Approach

Symptoms may develop if the lesion is very large or in the event of hemorrhage, infection, or rupture. Simple endothelial-lined cysts are more often well-defined cysts with thin or imperceptible walls that show fluid density on CT and are homogeneously hypointense on T1weighted images and hyperintense on T2-weighted images. No enhancement occurs after the administration of intravenous (IV) contrast. Pseudocysts may have a more heterogeneous appearance because of the presence of blood products, septations, and calcifications. On MRI, blood products present variable T1- and T2-weighted signal intensities, depending on the stage of degeneration. Calcifications are better appreciated on CT images [26-28].

Hemangiomas

Hemangiomas are benign lesions. Theoretically they can develop at any age in both sexes, but they do are more common in 40-70 year old female patients. As a rule these remain asymptomatic until and if they grow large.

Severe spontaneous bleeding is not a common phenomenon. Hemangiomas are predominantly solid tumors with cystic central areas and calcifications. Peripheral enhancement is noted after intravenous contrast administration [40].

CONCLUSION

In contemporary medicine, no one can function as a sole unit. Physicians need to cooperate, with each one offering their expertise for the benefit of the patient. In this spirit of holistic approach to healing, the surgeon acts a leading player of a team, which includes anaesthesiologists, internists, pathologists, surgical nurses and of course radiologists. It is with sophisticated imaging equipment and experienced diagnosticians that Surgeons acquire decisive information which help them understand the unique anatomical and physiological background of the patient's disease. Indeed, operating on adrenal lesions without detailed radiologic examinations could be catastrophic for a patient especially in cases of pheochromocytomas or malignancies. Indisputably, adrenal cysts and myelolipomas have characteristic imaging findings which lead to a safe diagnosis. Often, the specific diagnosis of adrenal adenoma can also be made based on CT attenuation measurements, CT washout criteria, or signal loss on opposed-phase MR imaging.

However, it is imperative to avoid blind adherence to imaging studies as they do have sensitivity and specificity limitations. surgeons should embrace this endogenous flaw and invest in their training. In order to be considered an endocrine surgeon one is obliged to master at least open and laparoscopic techniques, whilst maintaining a high-volume patient load per year. Taking everything into account, the quality of care offered to patients with adrenal disease will boost exponentially with the combination of in-depth surgical training and sincere cooperation with other medical specialties.

Conflict of interest: The authors report no conflict of interest.
Obtained funding: Not applicable.

REFERENCES

[1] Perrier, ND, Boger, MS. Surgical anatomy. In: Adrenal Glands: Diagnostic Aspects and Surgical Therapy, Linos, D, van Heerden, JA (Eds), Springer, New York 2005. p.7.

[2] Surgical embryology and anatomy of the adrenal glands. In: Textbook of Endocrine Surgery, 2nd edition, Clark, OH, Duh, QY, Kebebew, E (Eds), Elsevier Saunders, Philadelphia 2005. p.557.

[3] Hall JE, Guyton AC. Guyton and Hall Textbook of Medical Physiology, 12th edition. *Saunders*. ISBN 978-1416045748. 2010.

[4] Bland ML, Desclozeaux M, Ingraham HA. Tissue growth and remodeling of the embryonic and adult adrenal gland. *Ann. N. Y. Acad. Sci.* 2003; 995:59.

[5] Unsicker K, Huber K, Schober A, Kalcheim C. "Resolved and open issues in chromaffin cell development." *Mechanisms of Development* 130 (6–8): 324–329. 2013.

[6] Ramzi Cotran, Vinay Kumar, Tucker Collins (1999). Robbins Pathologic Basis of Disease, Sixth Edition. W.B. Saunders.

[7] Chaudhary V, Bano S. Anatomical and functional imaging in endocrine hypertension. *Indian J. Endocrinol. Metab.* 2012;16:713–21.

[8] Mayo-Smith WW, Boland GW, Noto RB, Lee MJ. State-of-the-art adrenal imaging. Radiographics. Jul-Aug 2001;21(4):995-1012.

[9] Liberati A, Altman DG, Tetzlaff J, Murlow C, Gøtzsche PC, et al. (2009) The PRISMA statement for reporting systematic reviews and meta-analyses of studies that evaluate health care interventions: explanation and elaboration. *Ital. J. Public Health* 4: 354–91.

[10] Gagner M, Lacroix A, Bolte E. Laparoscopic adrenalectomy in Cushing's syndrome and pheochromocytoma. *N. Engl. J. Med.* 1992;327:1033.

[11] M. Mellon, A.Sethi, C. Sundaram. Laparoscopic adrenalectomy: Surgical techniques. *Indian J. Urol.* 2008 Oct-Dec; 24(4): 583–589.

[12] Sung GT, Hsu THS, Gill IS. Retroperitoneoscopic adrenalectomy: Lateral approach. *J. Endourol.* 2001;15:505–11.

[13] Kiziloz H, Meraney A, Dorin R, Nip J, Kesler S, Shichman S. J .Prognostic indices of perioperative outcome following transperitoneal laparoscopic adrenalectomy. Laparoendosc *Adv. Surg. Tech. A.* 2014 Aug;24(8):528-33.

[14] Walz MK, Peitgen K, Walz MV, Hoermann R, Saller B, Giegler RM, et al. Posterior retroperitoneoscopic adrenalectomy: Lessons learned within five years. *World J. Surg.* 1998;20:769–74.

[15] Walz MK, Alesina PF, Wenger FA, Deligiannis A, Szuczik E, Petersenn S, Ommer A, Groeben H, Peitgen K, Janssen OE, Philipp T, Neumann HP, Schmid KW, Mann K. Posterior retroperitoneoscopic adrenalectomy--results of 560 procedures in 520 patients. *Surgery.* 2006 Dec;140(6):943-8.

[16] Berber E, Tellioglu G, Harvey A, Mitchell J, Milas M, Siperstein A. Comparison of laparoscopic transabdominal lateral versus posterior retroperitoneal adrenalectomy. *Surgery.* 2009 Oct;146(4):621-5.

[17] Chai YJ, Kwon H, Yu HW, Kim SJ, Choi JY, Lee KE, Youn YK. Systematic Review of Surgical Approaches for Adrenal Tumors: Lateral Transperitoneal versus Posterior Retroperitoneal and Laparoscopic versus Robotic Adrenalectomy. *Int. J. Endocrinol.* 2014;2014:918346.

[18] Gill IS, Meraney AM, Thomas JC, Sung GT, Novick AC, Lieberman I. Thoracoscopic transdiaphragmatic adrenalectomy: the initial experience. *The Journal of Urology.* 2001 Jun;165(6 Pt 1):1875-81.

[19] Lal G, Duh QY. Laparoscopic adrenalectomy--indications and technique. *Surg Oncol.* 2003 Aug;12(2):105-23.

[20] Piazza L ,Caragliano P,Scardilli M,Sgroi AV,Marino G,Giannone G. Laparoscopic robot-assisted right adrenalectomy and left ovariectomy (case reports). ChirItal1999;51:465–6.

[21] Hubens G,Ysebaert D,Vaneerdeweg W,Chapelle T,Eyskens E. Laparoscopic adrenalectomy with the aid of the AESOP2000 robot. *Acta Chir Belg.* 1999;99:125–7, discussion127–9.

[22] Hyams ES, Stifelman MD. The role of robotics for adrenal pathology. *Curr. Opin Urol.* 2009;19:89–96.

[23] Marescaux A., Leroy J., Gagner M., Rubino F., Mutter D., Vix M., Butner S., Smith M. Transatlantic robot-assisted telesurgery. *Nature* 413, 379-380 (27 September 2001).

[24] Brandao LF, Autorino R, Laydner H, Haber GP, Ouzaid I, De Sio M, Perdonà S, Stein RJ, Porpiglia F, Kaouk J. Robotic versus laparoscopic adrenalectomy: a systematic review and meta-analysis. *Eur. Urol.* 2014 Jun;65(6):1154-61.

[25] Boland GW, Blake MA, Hahn PF et-al. Incidental adrenal lesions: principles, techniques, and algorithms for imaging characterization. *Radiology*. 2008;249 (3): 756-75.

[26] Blake MA, Holalkere NS, Boland GW. Imaging techniques for adrenal lesion characterization. *Radiol. Clin. North Am*. 2008;46 (1): 65-78, vi.

[27] Elsayes KM, Mukundan G, Narra VR et-al. Adrenal masses: mr imaging features with pathologic correlation. *Radiographics*. 2004;24 Suppl 1 (suppl 1): S73-86.

[28] Brant WE, Helms CA. Fundamentals of Diagnostic Radiology. *Lippincott Williams & Wilkins*. (2007) ISBN:0781761352.

[29] Kenney PJ, Wagner BJ, Rao P et-al. Myelolipoma: CT and pathologic features. *Radiology*. 1998;208 (1): 87-95.

[30] Cyran KM, Kenney PJ, Memel DS et-al. Adrenal myelolipoma. *AJR Am. J. Roentgenol*. 1996;166 (2): 395-400.

[31] Fishman EK, Deutch BM, Hartman DS et-al. Primary adrenocortical carcinoma: CT evaluation with clinical correlation. *AJR Am. J. Roentgenol*. 1987;148 (3): 531-5.

[32] Mayo-smith WW, Boland GW, Noto RB et-al. State-of-the-art adrenal imaging. *Radiographics*. 21 (4): 995-1012.

[33] Tsirlin A, Oo Y, Sharma R et-al. Pheochromocytoma: a review. *Maturitas*. 2014;77 (3): 229-38.

[34] Leung K, Stamm M, Raja A et-al. Pheochromocytoma: the range of appearances on ultrasound, CT, MRI, and functional imaging. *AJR Am. J. Roentgenol*. 2013;200 (2): 370-8.

[35] Blake MA, Kalra MK, Maher MM et-al. Pheochromocytoma: an imaging chameleon. *Radiographics*. 2004;24 Suppl 1 (suppl_1): S87-99.

[36] Hoegerle S, Nitzsche E, Altehoefer C et-al. Pheochromocytomas: detection with 18F DOPA whole body PET--initial results. *Radiology*. 2002;222 (2): 507-12.

[37] Lonergan GJ, Schwab CM, Suarez ES et-al. Neuroblastoma, ganglioneuroblastoma, and ganglioneuroma: radiologic-pathologic correlation. *Radiographics*. 22 (4): 911-34.

[38] David R, Lamki N, Fan S et-al. The many faces of neuroblastoma. *Radiographics*. 1989;9 (5): 859-82.

[39] Choi YA, Kim CK, Park BK et-al. Evaluation of adrenal metastases from renal cell carcinoma and hepatocellular carcinoma: use of delayed contrast-enhanced CT. *Radiology*. 2013;266 (2): 514-20.

[40] Johnson PT, Horton KM, Fishman EK. Adrenal imaging with MDCT: Nonneoplastic disease. *AJR Am. J. Roentgenol*. 2009;193 (4): 1128-35.

In: The Role of Imaging Technology …
Editor: Georgios Tsoulfas

ISBN: 978-1-63483-490-2

Chapter 7

THE ROLE OF IMAGING IN HEPATOBILIARY SURGERY

Polyxeni Agorastou*[1]*, MD, PhD, Andreas Tooulias*[2]*, MD and Georgios Tsoulfas*[2,*]*, MD, PhD, FACS

[1]Department of Gastroenterology, Aristoteleion University of Thessaloniki, Greece
[2]Department of Surgery, Aristoteleion University of Thessaloniki, Greece

ABSTRACT

The increasing complexity of hepatobiliary diseases, benign or malignant, that a surgeon is called to treat, has led to a deeper understanding of the importance of a multidisciplinary approach. Imaging, with its various modalities, plays a central role in the diagnosis and management of hepatobiliary malignancies. An integral part of this remains the communication between the surgeon and the radiologist regarding the exact findings, as well as the different types of management, ranging from surgery to interventional radiology. The goal remains to find the best treatment for the patient. This chapter will present the existing preferences regarding the diagnosis and management of one of the main primary hepatobiliary malignancies, which is hepatocellular carcinoma (HCC). Additionally, we will examine certain special cases (such as the imaging of the early lesion or standardization of imaging reporting), as well as report on the possibilities offered by newer imaging developments. Finally, we will also address the identification and management of a focal hepatic lesion. Overall, the goal is for this chapter to be part of the interplay and the dialogue between the surgeon and the radiologist, in terms of information that needs to be communicated and the best way to do that.

* Corresponding author: Georgios Tsoulfas, 66 Tsimiski Street, Thessaloniki 54622, Greece. Tel: 306971895190. Fax: 302310342094. E-mail: tsoulfasg@gmail.com.

THE ROLE OF IMAGING IN THE MANAGEMENT OF HEPATOCELLULAR CARCINOMA (HCC)

Introduction

Hepatocellular carcinoma (HCC) continues to increase in incidence, becoming the fifth most common cancer worldwide and responsible for slightly less than 10% of all cancers [1]. The major risk factor for HCC remains cirrhosis, irrespective of its etiology.

Specifically, a variety of causes, such as alcoholic liver disease, viral hepatitis, cholestatic liver diseases, autoimmune and metabolic disorders and the nonalcoholic steatohepatitis, all represent chronic liver insults, which in due time will change the liver architecture and physiology and lead to cirrhosis, if left untreated. Once cirrhosis occurs, irrespective of the causative factor, it is a risk factor for HCC. This process of carcinogenesis in the liver is a progressive one, and as such there would be great value in being able to recognize it at an early stage, something which is made harder by the presence of the cirrhotic nodules.

Additionally, these patients now have to face the dual threat of a hepatic malignancy, with the background of a declining liver function. The importance of HCC worldwide and the need for early diagnosis and successful treatment, have placed a heavy burden on the different imaging modalities. The role of hepatobiliary imaging is critical in the management of HCC, as it can make the difference when deciding whether a hepatic resection or an orthotopic liver transplantation (OLT) will be needed for treatment.

An example of the importance of accurate radiological diagnosis for HCC, is its role in deciding the need and the urgency for OLT for a patient. Specifically, currently in the United States and in many other countries, the place in the waiting list for a liver transplant is determined by the Model for End-Stage Liver Disease (MELD) score, which is basically an approximation of the patient's hepatic synthetic function by including the INR, serum bilirubin and serum creatinine into an equation. This will lead to a score of 6-40, with 6 representing normal liver function and anything over 30 representing an over 90% possibility of mortality in the next 3 months. Although this type of calculation is a relatively objective one, it does represent a problem for patients with cirrhosis and HCC. The reason is that in these patients, their hepatic function is usually well-preserved (and thus their MELD score is relatively low), whereas the more imminent danger for them is the HCC. If the disease progresses beyond certain criteria (usually the Milan criteria are the ones quoted most frequently with one lesion 5cm or less or 3 lesions none bigger than 3cm and no metastatic disease), then the patient cannot be transplanted and expect good results.

Based on this, the decision has been made in many countries using the MELD system to give extra points to patients with cirrhosis and HCC (if it is within criteria), in order to get them to an OLT sooner rather than later. However, in order to do that it is important to accurately diagnose the presence of HCC and liver biopsy is not an easy task for a small lesion in a cirrhotic patient. As a result, in over 95% of patients receiving these HCC exception points, the diagnosis of HCC was made using a good quality MDCT or MRI, thus underscoring the importance of radiological imaging for these patients. Additionally, advances in interventional radiology have added significant weapons (such as percutaneous radiofrequency or microwave ablation or chemoembolization) to the armamentarium of the hepatobiliary multidisciplinary management team.

As part of the overall progress, there are currently international guidelines, whereby dynamic cross-sectional hepatic imaging is considered diagnostic to the extent that a liver biopsy may not be needed [2]. Having said all that, we should stress that more questions have arisen, with the critical one being, what is the role of all this different radiologic modalities within the spectrum of therapeutic modalities for HCC. However, before answering this question, we need to review the existing radiological modalities, including their advantages and disadvantages and the future prospects.

THE ROLE OF DIFFERENT IMAGING MODALITIES IN THE DIAGNOSIS AND MANAGEMENT OF HCC

Ultrasound

The key to achieving long-term success in the management of HCC is early diagnosis. The majority of international societies have agreed that a major step towards this goal is the development of ultrasound surveillance programs, especially in patients who are at higher risk, such as cirrhotics [3, 4]. The major challenge is identifying a dysplastic lesion in the background of a cirrhotic liver, and then following it closely with serial exams, as approximately a third of them will develop into a malignancy [5]. Ultrasound offers the advantage of a practical, easily repeatable, cost-conscious method of being able to follow these patients, without the complications that can (rarely) arise in the other more complex methods. The disadvantage is the subjective nature of ultrasound, as it is very much dependent on the experience of the person performing it. One of the improvements has been the use of contrast-enhanced ultrasound, which used a variety of microbubble-based contrast agents to correctly diagnose HCC. These agents offer the advantage of being able to visualize and evaluate tumor hemodynamics, including the hypervascularity which is frequently associated with HCC in the arterial phase [6]. The increasing experience and aptitude with contrast-enhanced ultrasound may very soon challenge the primacy of dynamic CT for the diagnosis of HCC.

Mutlidetector Computed Tomography (MDCT)

One of the most frequent challenges in making the diagnosis of a liver lesion, is deciding between a primary HCC or a metastatic lesion. The way to make this differentiation is through the use of a triple-contrast CT, with an arterial, a portal venous and an equilibrium phase. The rationale is that HCC is characterized by hypervascularity during the arterial phase and contrast washout during the portal venous and equilibrium phases. On the other hand, hepatic metastatic disease will be more prominent during the portal venous phase, thus allowing the differentiation between HCC and liver metastatic disease. The significance of the hypervascularity of HCC is that for the majority of associations, such as the American Association for the Study of Liver Diseases (AASLD) and the European Association for the Study of the Liver (EASL), this pattern of contrast uptake (the arterial phase "wash in" and the portal venous phase "wash out") is considered diagnostic for HCC, when the lesions are

2cm in diameter or bigger. The problem and the debate is for smaller lesions. Specifically, whereas for the AASLD the MDCT is sufficient for all lesions > 1cm, the EASL guidelines and for lesions 1-2cm require a second study for the confirmation, based on data from prospective studies [3, 4]. This is where Magnetic resonance imaging (MRI) comes into play, as it can offer a slightly improved accuracy or at least confirmation for lesions < 2cm. Adding to this problem is the fact that smaller lesions, such as early HCC or borderline ones, may not exhibit the typical HCC contrast uptake pattern and show isoattenuation or even low attenuation to the liver parenchyma in the arterial phase, thus making the MDCT less helpful.

Magnetic Resonance Imaging

Although there is a "typical" pattern for HCC in MRI, with lesions being hypointense on T1-weighted and hyperintense on T2-weighted images, this also depends on the degree of lesion differentiation, as early HCC may often exhibit hyperintensity on T-1 weighted images and iso- to hypointensity on T2-weighted images. Although it may seem counterintuitive, international guidelines do not support MRI over MDCT, as in most studies the diagnostic accuracy of both is similar [7]. The one area where there may be an advantage for the use of MRI, is for the smaller nodules (< 2cm) as it was mentioned before, as well as the fact that there are newer MRI techniques, such as the diffusion-weighted imaging (DWI) and newer hepatobiliary (HB) contrast agents, such as gadopentetate dimeglumine (Gd-EOB-DTPA), which allow for greater diagnostic capability [8-10].

These hepatobiliary agents use a delayed hepatobiliary phase, as they are transported into the hepatocytes. The use of Gd-EOB-DTPA, which is a T1-shortening, extracellular and hepatocyte contrast agent, with its increased accuracy have made it extremely useful in the case of lesions smaller than 2cm and for borderline lesions, such as those represented by hypovascular HCC [11, 12]. This increased sensitivity using the hepatobiliary contrast agents (such as Gd-EOB-DTPA) can be critical in patients with early HCC, as it was shown in a recent paper where treatment was modified in up to 12% of the included patients, based on information obtained by HB-enhanced MRI [13]. The value of MRI increases even more if we consider DWI MR sequences, which evaluate the random motion of water in biological tissues. This way, and because of the restriction of water molecules in the tumor, those areas appear brighter, and have made DWI a valuable resource for borderline and hypovascular lesions [14, 15]. Overall, the MRI is an excellent and safe study for HCC, and liver lesions in general. However, it remains an expensive imaging modality, and as such it is important to ensure that it is used wisely and that both the referring physician and the radiologist know what to ask for and what to look for, respectively.

Positron Emission Tomography

Positron Emission Tomography (PET) differs from CT and MRI, in the sense that it is more dependent on the molecular changes that occur in the tumor and normal tissue cells, versus anatomical changes.

The basis for the emphasis on these molecular changes has to do with the fact that tumors are metabolically different from normal tissue and, as such, the uptake and metabolism of certain molecules (glucose for example) can be used to identify cancerous changes.

Although PET is not an anatomic study, it is used in combination with CT (PET-CT), in order to locate "geographically" in the liver the area with the higher uptake. Despite its many promises, a recent review study of available literature, has shown that PET may not be ideal for identifying primary hepatic malignancies [16].

Challenges in the Role of Imaging for HCC

The different imaging techniques that were described above represent the main ones involved in the diagnosis, staging and treatment of HCC. However, the deeper we delve into the variety of these imaging techniques, it becomes obvious that the more questions arise, which essentially point out the finer nuisances of these techniques, as well as the opportunities that they may offer. Next, we will discuss some of these challenges and opportunities that are presented by these current imaging methods.

Hepatocarcinogenesis

The presentation of a HCC is the result of the progression from a dysplastic nodule in a cirrhotic liver, to one with overt malignancy. This evolution is characterized by the development of new arteries, which are not accompanied by bile ducts, which allows the differentiation between a regenerative and a dysplastic nodule [17, 18]. It is interesting that there appears to be a correlation between the number of new arteries and the degree of HCC differentiation, especially in the case of smaller lesions. This, combined with the decrease in the number of Kupffer cells, has enabled current imaging techniques to observe and define the different phases and steps of hepatocarcinogenesis, thus playing a critical role in earlier detection [2].

Limitations of the Different Management Systems and the Need for Standardization

There are approximately a total of 19 diagnostic systems and guidelines published or presented between 2001 and 2013 for the diagnosis and management of HCC [19, 20]. The majority of these guidelines contain imaging-based diagnostic systems, which have become increasingly more detailed and sophisticated, given the corresponding progress and accuracy in imaging technology. In the earlier systems the hypervascular appearance of a lesion was sufficient, whereas in the more recent ones issues such as capsule appearance or contrast washout appearance play a more important role.

Some of the issues between the different systems have to do with terminology, whereas others have to do with more basic disagreements regarding the importance of different factors in the diagnosis and management.

These systems may reflect differences in clinical practice, contrast agents used, tumor biology, cultural preferences and geographical patterns. Additionally, these systems may not be detailed enough to help radiologists make the proper diagnosis, as they may place more emphasis on the classical appearance of HCC and not include the various subtypes, whose appearance may be more perplexing. Also, the European and the US systems, ask for a biopsy in cases of hypo- or iso-enhancing arterial phase lesions, given the fact that a 100% positive predictive value for these features does not exist. On the other hand, in 2008 the American College of Radiology came up with the Liver Imaging Reporting and Data System (LI-RADS), which would classify such lesions (hypo- or iso-enhancing) as LR 4, which is possible HCC [21]. Finally, most systems, with the exception of the Japan Society of Hepatology, do not include hepatobiliary phase MRI, thus making it harder, possibly, to diagnose smaller lesions. The reason is that HB phase MRI provides functional data on a lesion, such as water molecule motion and hepatobiliary cellular function, thus making the identification of hypovascular lesions possible.

No matter what these differences, the fact remains that we are lacking a common language to discuss the diagnosis, staging and management of HCC. This problem becomes an even bigger challenge, if we consider the continuous evolution of imaging techniques and the need to find the proper place for the newer methods by recognizing their advantages, as well as their limitations.

Assessing Response to Locoregional and Systemic Therapy for HCC

Locoregional treatments for HCC represent an important part of the armamentarium of the multidisciplinary team of physicians caring for the patient. The two main locoregional treatments include transarterial chemoembolization (TACE) and ablation methods, which include radiofrequency ablation or microwave ablation among others. TACE can be used in patients with hepatocellular carcinoma at various stages of the disease. Specifically, it can be used as first line treatment for unresectable intermediate stage HCC, or as a bridge to liver transplantation (avoid an increase in the tumor, while the patient is on the waiting list), or as a downstaging method. In the case of the latter, the goal is to reduce the tumor burden through the use of TACE, thus making the patient eligible for resection of liver transplantation [22-24]. Additionally, in patients with advanced disease, TACE can be used as a temporizing measure, in the sense that it can control the growth of the tumor or the symptoms caused by it and do that in a manner that does not affect hepatic function significantly (and thus quality of life for the patient) and can be repeated.

Radiofrequency ablation (RFA) is one of the main tumor ablation methods and can be done either percutaneously or surgically (open or laparoscopic surgery), depending on the size and location of the lesion. It is usually performed on patients with small HCCs, stage A1 to A3 by Barcelona Clinic Liver Cancer (BCLC), in order to avoid surgical resection [25]. It can also be used for resection of lesions, as well as in combination with other invasive techniques such as microwave ablation [26]. According to the American Association for the Study of Liver Diseases (AASLD) guidelines, RFA is a safe and effective method to treat patients with advanced liver tumors. For up to 4-5 hepatic lesions, less than 3cm in diameter, initial complete response rates of more than 90% and local tumor progression rates between 10-20% have been reported [27, 28].

Both of these types of locoregional treatment have proven to be a valuable tool for the management of patients at different stages of HCC and for different purposes. One of their most critical advantages, is the fact that they can be repeated with acceptable safety margins.

However, in order for this to be meaningful, it is essential to be able to evaluate the result of these treatments radiologically. The methods used most frequently are cross-sectional imaging with MRI and CT. The information needed in order to accurately assess the response to the therapy includes evaluation of the tumor size (including the margins involved and the areas of necrosis), the presence of any embolization agents used or not, and the detection either of remaining tumor (with the challenge being to identify whether it is active or not) or of tumor recurrence [29].

Portal Vein Embolization

Portal vein embolization (PVE) represents an extension of the role of embolization in the management of HCC. Specifically, there are patients where a hepatectomy to remove the HCC, may leave behind a liver remnant that is less than 40% (in a healthy liver) or 20-25% (in a cirrhotic liver), thus placing the patient's survival in jeopardy, as there is a significant risk of hepatic decompensation.

In order to improve on this predicament, one option is PVE, whereby interventional radiologists embolize the portal vein branch on the side of the tumor. In approximately 4-6 weeks, this leads to a hypertrophy of the healthy liver lobe, which will become the liver remnant after the resection, of about 10-30%, thus potentially allowing the liver resection to proceed [30]. Obviously, the overall process is significantly more complicated as it has to be performed with accuracy and there are several factors that play a role including the experience of the radiologist performing it, the type of embolization agent used, managing the complications that can occur and identifying the optimal timing to proceed with the resection.

Image-Guided Surgery

One of the challenges, which is more evident with the use of neoadjuvant treatment for hepatic metastatic disease, is the fact that although the lesions may disappear on the CT, cancer cells may still be present in approximately one third of the patients [31]. These patients may end up with recurrent disease, and as a result many favor a liver resection for the potentially involved segment. Another situation which may require delicate maneuvers, is that of a non-anatomic hepatectomy, where the involved part of the liver is resected, but not along the division of Quinaud, and essentially leaving behind as much parenchyma as possible. To be able to do this successfully, it is important to have accurate imaging of the liver "topography," which is not very easy with the routine cross-sectional methods, such as CT and MRI, given the complex 3-D anatomy of the liver with all its variations.

The answer to these problems could be the use of image-guided surgery, whereby preoperative medical images are registered with intraoperative landmarks, in order to provide a 3-D image of the liver that will allow the surgeon to proceed with the resection in an interactive manner, that is be aware at every point of the resection of the relation to the vascular and biliary structures that may be encountered [32].

The steps required include the preoperative processing of the CT or MRI images, obtaining information on the specific liver anatomy and matching the pre- and intra-operative data [33]. This last part, the matching or registration process, which essentially involves the linking of the preoperative imaging information with the real-time location of the resection plane during the surgery, is the hardest one to accomplish. There is significant interest in this endeavor, including several commercial programs, and so the hope is that there will continue to be improvements of the system. It is important to point out that the majority of the planning regarding the resection plane and strategy is done preoperatively using the 3-D imaging.

Conclusion

We have examined in this chapter the current techniques used for imaging of the liver, with special emphasis on the diagnosis, staging and treatment of hepatocellular carcinoma. Additionally, we have examined some of the developments in this field that represent significant achievements, as well as future challenges.

Obviously, the role of imaging techniques in hepatic surgery is critical and it continues to evolve as technology progresses. However, it is essential to identify for all the new techniques their proper place in the armamentarium of the multidisciplinary team dealing with this complex disease. The reason is that by knowing their advantages, as well as their limitations, only then can we offer our patients the best, all-around care and do that in a sensible manner.

References

[1] Ferlay, J., Shin, H. R., Bray, F., Forman, D., Mathers, C., Parkin, D. M. Estimates of worldwide burden of cancer in 2008: GLOBOCAN 2008. *Int. J. Cancer* 2010; 127: 2893-2917.

[2] International Consensus Group for Hepatocellular Neoplasia. Pathologic diagnosis of early hepatocellular carcinoma: a report of the International Consensus Group for Hepatocellular Neoplasia. *Hepatology* 2009; 49: 658-664.

[3] European Association for the Study of the Liver, European Organisation for Research and Treatment of Cancer. EASL-EORTC clinical practice guidelines: management of hepatocellular carcinoma. *J. Hepatol.* 2012; 56:908-943.

[4] Bruix, J., Sherman, M. American Association for the Study of Liver Diseases. Management of hepatocellular carcinoma: an update. *Hepatology* 2011; 53: 1020-1022.

[5] Terasaki, S., Kaneko, S., Kobayashi, K., Nonomura, A., Nakanuma, Y. Histological features predicting malignant transformation of nonmalignant hepatocellular nodules: a prospective study. *Gastroenterology* 1998; 115: 1216-1222.

[6] Burns, P. N., Wilson, S. R. Microbubble contrast for radiological imaging: Principles. *Ultrasound Q.* 2006; 22: 5-13.

[7] Sangiovanni, A., Manini, M. A., Iavarone, M., et al., The diagnostic and economic impact of contrast imaging techniques in the diagnosis of small hepatocellular carcinoma in cirrhosis. *Gut* 2010; 59: 638-644.

[8] Noguchi, Y., Murakami, T., Kim, T., et al., Detection of hepatocellular carcinoma: comparison of dynamic MR imaging with dynamic double arterial phase helical CT. *AJR Am. J. Roentgenol.* 2003; 180: 455-460.

[9] Imai, Y., Murakami, T., Yoshida, S., et al., Superparamagnetic iron oxide-enhanced MR images of hepatocellular carcinoma: correlation with histological grading. *Hepatology* 2000; 32: 205-212.

[10] Saito, K., Kotake, F., Ito, N., et al., Gd-EOB-DTPA enhanced MRI for hepatocellular carcinoma: quantitative evaluation of tumor enhancement in hepatobiliary phase. *Magn. Reson. Med. Sci.* 2005; 4: 1-9.

[11] Di Martino, M., De Filippis, G., De Santis, A., et al., Hepatocellular carcinoma in cirrhotic patients: prospective comparison of US, CT, and MR imaging. *Eur. Radiol.* 2010; 23: 887-896.

[12] Inoue, T., Kudo, M., Komuta, M., et al., Assessment of Gd-EOB-DTPA-enhanced MRI for HCC and dysplastic nodules and comparison of detection sensitivity versus MDCT. *J. Gastroenterol.* 2012; 47: 1036-1047.

[13] Yoo, S. H., Choi, J. Y., Jang, J. W., et al., Gd-EOB-DTPA-enahnced MRI is better than MDCT in decision making of curative treatment for hepatocellular carcinoma. *Ann. Surg. Oncol.* 2013; 20: 2893-2900.

[14] Xu, P. J., Yan, F. H., Wang, J. H., Shan, Y., Ji, Y., Chen, C. Z. Contribution of diffusion-weighted magnetic resonance imaging in the characterization of hepatocellular carcinomas and dysplastic nodules in cirrhotic liver. *J. Comput. Assist. Tomogr.* 2010; 34: 506-512.

[15] Wu, L. M., Xu, J. R., Lu, Q., Hua, J., Chen, J., Hu, J. A pooled analysis of diffusion-weighted imaging in the diagnosis of hepatocellular carcinoma in chronic liver diseases. *J. Gastroenterol. Hepatol.* 2013; 28: 227-234.

[16] Lan, B. Y., Kwee, S. A., Wong, L. L. Positron emission tomography in hepatobiliary and pancreatic malignancies: a review. *Am. J. Surg.* 2012; 204: 232-241.

[17] Hiimeno, H., Enzan, H., Saibara, T., Onishi, S., Yamamoto, Y. Hitherto unrecognized arterioles within hepatocellular carcinoma. *J. Pathol.* 1994; 174: 217-222.

[18] Matsui, O. Analysis of intranodular hemodynamics of dysplastic nodules in cirrhotic livers. *Radiology* 2001; 218: 603-605.

[19] Song, P., Tobe, R. G., Inagaki, Y., et al., The management of hepatocellular carcinoma around the world: a comparison of guidelines from 2001 to 2011. *Liver Int.* 2012; 32: 1053-1063.

[20] Cruite, I., Tang, A., Sirlin, C. B. Imaging-based diagnostic systems for hepatocellular carcinoma. *Am. J. Roentgenol.* 2013; 201: 41-55.

[21] American College of Radiology. Liver imaging reporting and fata system, version 1.0. *Amercian College of Radiology website.* www.acr.org/Quality-Safety/Resources/LIRADS/Archive/. Published 2011. Accessed May 28, 2015.

[22] Yao, F. Y., Breitenstein, S., Broelsch, C. E., Dufour, J. F., Sherman, M. Does a patient qualify for liver transplantation after the down-staging of hepatocellular carcinoma? *Liver Transpl.* 2011;17: S109-S116.

[23] Majno, P., Lencioni, R., Mornex, F., Girard, N., Poon, R. T., Cherqui, D. Is the treatment of hepatocellular carcinoma on the waiting list necessary? *Liver Transpl.* 2011;17: S98-S108.

[24] Pomfret, E. A., Washburn, K., Wald, C., Nalesnik, M. A., Douglas, D., Russo, M., et al., Report of a national conference on liver allocation in patients with hepatocellular carcinoma in the United States. *Liver Transpl.* 2010;16: 262-78.

[25] Fontana, R. J., Hamidullah, H., Nghiem, H., et al., Percutaneous radiofrequency thermal ablation of hepatocellular carcinoma: a safe and effective bridge to liver transplantation. *Liver Transplant.* 2002;8:1165-74.

[26] Yin, X. Y., Xie, X. Y., Lu, M. D., Xu, H. X., Xu, Z. F., Kuang, M., Liu, G. J., Liang, J. Y., Lau, W. Y. Percutaneous thermal ablation of medium and large hepatocellular carcinoma: long-term outcome and prognostic factors. *Cancer* 2009; 115:1914-23.

[27] Cho, Y. K., Kim, Y., Rhim, H. Pitfalls in the radiological and pathological correlation of tumour response rates of hepatocellular carcinoma following radiofrequency ablation. *J. Clin. Pathol.* 2009; 62: 1071-3.

[28] Elias, D., Baton, O., Sideris, L., Matsuhisa, T., Pocard, M., Lasser, P. Local recurrence after intraoperative radiofrequency ablation of liver metastases: a comparative study with anatomic and wedge resections. *Ann. Surg. Oncol.* 2004;11: 500-5.

[29] Yaghmai, V., Besa, C., Kim, E., Gatlin, J. L., Siddiqui, N. A., Taouli, B. Imaging Assessment of hepatocellular carcinoma response to locoregional and systemic therapy. *Am. J. Roentgenol.* 2013; 201: 80-96.

[30] Madoff, D. C., Hicks, M. E., Vauthey, J. N., et al., Transhepatic portal vein embolization: anatomy, indications, and technical considerations. *Radiographics* 2002; 22: 1063-1076.

[31] Auer, R. C., White, R. R., Kemeny, N. E., Schwartz, L. H., et al., Predictors of a true complete response among disappearing liver metastases from colorectal cancer after chemotherapy. *Cancer* 2010; 116: 1502-1509.

[32] Kingham, T. P., Jayaraman, S., Clements, L. W., Scherer, M. A., Stefansic, J. D., Jarnagin, W. R. Evolution of image-guided liver surgery: transition from open to laparoscopic procedures. *J. Gastrointest. Surg.* 2013; 17: 1274-1282.

[33] Oldhafer, K. J., Stavrou, G. A., Prause, G., Peitgen, H. O., Lueth, T. C., Weber, S. How to operate a liver tumor you cannot see. *Langenbecks Arch. Surg.* 2009; 394: 489-494.

In: The Role of Imaging Technology …
Editor: Georgios Tsoulfas

ISBN: 978-1-63483-490-2

Chapter 8

THE ROLE OF IMAGING IN PANCREATIC SURGERY

A. Mastoraki[1], MD, N. Economopoulos[2], MD, I. Papanikolaou[3], MD and N. Arkadopoulos[1,*], MD

[1]4th Department of Surgery, National and Kapodistrian University of Athens, "Attikon" University Hospital, Athens, Greece

[2]2nd Department of Radiology, National and Kapodistrian University of Athens, "Attikon" University Hospital, Athens, Greece

[3]2nd Department of Internal Medicine, National and Kapodistrian University of Athens, "Attikon" University Hospital, Athens, Greece

ABSTRACT

The pancreas is an organ that has presented surgeons with significant challenges as both benign and malignant lesions, given the location and physiology of the organ, require significant expertise for both diagnosis and treatment. This chapter will present the most current imaging technology available for pancreatic disease and provide examples of how the surgeon and the medical team can choose the best one for each possible situation.

INTRODUCTION

The pancreas is a retroperitoneal organ that lies in an oblique position, sloping upward from the C-loop of the duodenum to the splenic hilum. In an adult, the pancreas weighs 75 to 100 g and is about 15 to 20cm long. The fact that the pancreas is situated so deeply in the abdomen and is sealed in the retroperitoneum explains the poorly localized and sometimes ill-defined nature with which pancreatic pathology presents.

* Corresponding author: N. Arkadopoulos. 4th Department of Surgery, National and Kapodistrian University of Athens, "Attikon" University Hospital, 1 Rimini str. 12462 Chaidari-Athens, Greece. E-mail: narkado@hotmail.com.

In this chapter, we start with a brief overview of basic pancreatic anatomy and then we present thirteen common pancreatic conditions that may require surgical intervention and analyze the role of the various imaging modalities in the diagnosis and planning for surgery. All images used in this chapter originate from the authors' personal archives.

Pancreatic Anatomy

An understanding of embryology is required to appreciate the common variations in pancreatic duct anatomy. The pancreas is formed by the fusion of a ventral and dorsal bud. The duct from the smaller ventral bud connects directly to the common bile duct (CBD) while the duct from the larger dorsal bud drains directly into the duodenum. The duct of the ventral anlage becomes the duct of Wirsung, and the duct from the dorsal anlage becomes the duct of Santorini. With gut rotation, the ventral anlage rotates to the right and around the posterior side of the duodenum to fuse with the dorsal bud. The ventral anlage becomes the inferior portion of the pancreatic head and the uncinate process, while the dorsal anlage becomes the body and tail of the pancreas. The ducts from each anlage usually fuse together in the pancreatic head such that most of the pancreas drains through the duct of Wirsung, or main pancreatic duct (MPD), into the common channel formed from the bile duct and pancreatic duct. In 10% of patients, the ducts of Wirsung and Santorini fail to fuse. This results in the majority of the pancreas draining through the duct of Santorini and the lesser papilla, while the inferior portion of the pancreatic head and uncinate process drains through the duct of Wirsung and major papilla. This normal anatomic variant, which occurs in one out of 10 patients, is referred to as pancreas divisum. The MPD is usually only 2-3mm in diameter and runs midway between the superior and inferior borders of the pancreas. The MPD joins with the CBD and empties at the ampulla of Vater or major papilla, which is located on the medial aspect of the second portion of the duodenum. When the accessory pancreatic duct or lesser duct drains into the duodenum, a lesser papilla can be identified approximately 2cm proximal to the ampulla of Vater.

The blood supply to the pancreas comes from multiple branches from the celiac and superior mesenteric arteries (SMA). The common hepatic artery (CHA) gives rise to the gastroduodenal artery (GDA) before continuing toward the porta hepatis as the proper hepatic artery. The GDA becomes the superior pancreaticoduodenal artery as it passes behind the first portion of the duodenum and branches into the anterior and posterior superior pancreaticoduodenal arteries. As the SMA passes behind the neck of the pancreas, it gives off the inferior pancreaticoduodenal artery at the inferior margin of the neck of the pancreas. This vessel quickly divides into the anterior and posterior inferior pancreaticoduodenal arteries. The superior and inferior pancreaticoduodenal arteries join together within the parenchyma of the anterior and posterior sides of the head of the pancreas along the medial aspect of the C-loop of the duodenum to form arcades that give off numerous branches to the duodenum and head of the pancreas. Therefore, it is impossible to resect the head of the pancreas without devascularizing the duodenum, unless a rim of pancreas containing the pancreaticoduodenal arcade is preserved. Variations in the arterial anatomy occur in one out of five patients. The right hepatic artery, CHA, or gastroduodenal arteries can arise from the SMA. In 15 to 20% of patients, the right hepatic artery will arise from the SMA and travel upwards toward the liver along the posterior aspect of the head of the pancreas.

It is important to look for this variation on preoperative computed tomographic (CT) scans and in the operating room so the replaced hepatic artery is recognized and injury is avoided. The body and tail of the pancreas are supplied by multiple branches of the splenic artery. The splenic artery arises from the celiac trunk and travels along the posterior-superior border of the body and tail of the pancreas toward the spleen. The inferior pancreatic artery usually arises from the SMA and runs to the left along the inferior border of the body and tail of the pancreas, parallel to the splenic artery.

Three vessels run perpendicular to the long axis of the pancreatic body and tail and connect the splenic artery and inferior pancreatic artery. They are, from medial to lateral, the dorsal, great, and caudal pancreatic arteries. These arteries form arcades within the body and tail of the pancreas, and account for the rich blood supply of the organ.

The venous drainage of the pancreas follows a pattern similar to that of the arterial supply. The veins are usually superficial to the arteries within the parenchyma of the gland. There is an anterior and posterior venous arcade within the head of the pancreas.

The superior veins drain directly into the portal vein (PV) just above the neck of the pancreas. The posterior inferior arcade drains directly into the inferior mesenteric vein (IMV) at the inferior border of the neck of the pancreas. The anterior inferior pancreaticoduodenal vein joins the right gastroepiploic vein and the middle colic vein to form a common venous trunk, which enters into the superior mesenteric vein (SMV).

I. Annular Pancreas

Definition

Annular pancreas refers to a ring of pancreatic tissue that encircles mainly the second part of the duodenum. This congenital anomaly of the pancreas usually manifests in neonates or remains asymptomatic until adulthood [1].

Associated congenital abnormalities consist of intestinal malrotation, imperforate anus, esophageal atresia, duodenal stenosis, Down syndrome and cardiovascular disorders.

Surgical Interventions

- ✓ Retrocolic duodenojejunostomy/gastrojejunostomy in pediatric population
- ✓ Surgical and interventional endoscopic procedures in adult population

Imaging Modalities

The role of imaging modalities in case of annular pancreas is to establish the diagnosis and differentiate other causes which can produce "narrow duodenal lumen."

Radiographic Findings

Plain x-ray of the abdomen reveals narrowing of descending duodenum. The classic "double-bubble" sign refers to a large proximal bubble describing the dilated stomach and a small distal one indicative of concomitant dilation of the duodenal bulb.

Fluoroscopic guided Barium Study depicts an extrinsic, eccentric defect on medial margin of the second part of the duodenum with concentric narrowing and dilation of the proximal duodenum [2]. Periampullary duodenal ulcer due to reverse peristalsis may be encountered in adults implying the presence of Zollinger-Ellison syndrome (ZES).

Ultrasonography

Real time U/S is only indicative of a nonspecific enlargement of pancreatic head.

Computed Tomography

CT findings are often non-specific suggesting pancreatic head enlargement along with central area of increased attenuation representing contrast within narrowed duodenal segments. Parallel gastric and duodenal dilatation with circumferential thickening of the wall as well as obstructing band of pancreatic tissue and dilated MPD, CBD and intrahepatic ductal system may be detected [3].

Magnetic Resonance Imaging

Fat-suppressed T1WI images describe normal pancreatic tissue encircling the duodenum. Subsequent MRCP depicts course and drainage pattern of pancreatic duct [4].

Angiography

Celiac angiography often reveals an anomalous branch from posterior pancreaticoduodenal artery that courses in a right and inferior direction supplying annular moiety.

Endoscopic Retrograde Cholangiopancreatography

ERCP describes a normal MPD in the body and tail of the pancreas communicating with small duct of pancreatic head encircling the duodenum.

On occasion, a small duct of the head originating on right anterior surface of duodenum, passing posteriorly around the organ and entering the MPD may be recognized.

Differential Diagnosis

- ✓ Duodenal carcinoma
- ✓ Postbulbar peptic ulcer
- ✓ Pancreatic carcinoma
- ✓ Duodenal hematoma

II. Acute Pancreatitis

Definition

Acute pancreatitis is described as an acute inflammatory process of the pancreas with variable involvement of relevant regional tissues or remote organ systems. It can be initiated by several factors including biliary tract disease, alcohol, severe trauma, infectious disorders, ischemia, pancreatic duct obstruction and post-operative inflammation. Cases of hereditary pancreatitis have also been reported. Associated complications implicate fluid collection, extended edema, tissue destruction, fat necrosis and hemorrhage. Potential formation of pseudocyst, abscess or vascular pseudoaneurysm along with porto-splenic thrombosis or Disseminated Intravascular Coagulation (DIC) and sepsis has been suggested as major determinants of the outcome [5].

Surgical Interventions

- ✓ Drainage of infected pseudocyst
- ✓ Surgical debridement of infected necrosis

Imaging Modalities

The role of imaging modalities in case of acute pancreatitis is to establish the diagnosis and assess disease severity. Additional surgical intervention in case of necrotizing pancreatitis is also imaging dependent. If there is an indication of infection, then a CT- or US-guided fine-needle aspiration (FNA) should be performed for Gram's stain and culture of the fluid or tissue, and the indicated antibiotic therapy initiated.

Ultrasound

Abdominal U/S examination is the best imaging technique in confirming the presence of gallstones in suspected biliary pancreatitis. It may also determine extrapancreatic ductal dilations, pancreatic edema, swelling or fluid selection. Nevertheless, in the majority of affected patients U/S does not provide satisfactory results due to the presence of bowel gas which tends to obscure sonographic imaging of the pancreas.

Thus real time U/S could only reveal an enlarged hypoechoic gland or elucidate the formation of a pseudocyst or abscess. Therefore, additional CT is always implemented in order to distinguish milder categories of the disease from severe cases of necrotizing or infected pancreatitis and provide optimal care to the patient [6].

Computed Tomography

CT scanning with bolus intravenous contrast has become the gold standard for assessing the severity of acute pancreatitis. While clinically mild inflammation of the pancreas is correlated with interstitial edema with the microcirculation remaining intact and the gland presenting with uniform enhancement. In necrotizing pancreatitis, the microcirculation is disrupted. Therefore, the enhancement of the gland on contrast-enhanced CT (CECT) scan is considerably decreased (Figure 1). The presence of air bubbles is an indication of infected necrosis or abscess (Figure 2).

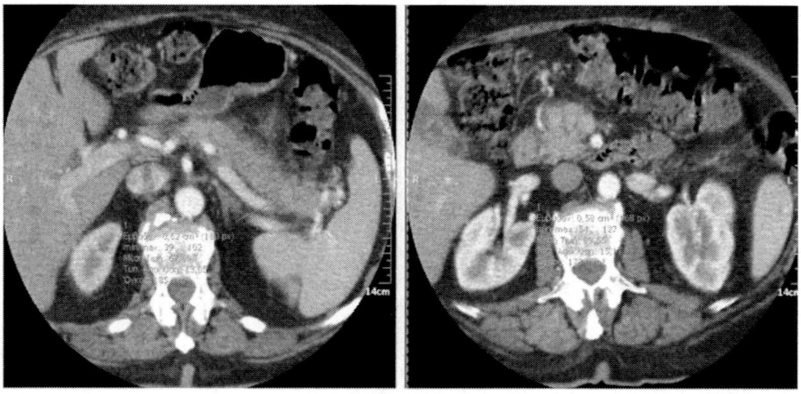

Figure 1. Abdominal CT in acute pancreatitis:-Pancreatic phase of enhancement: Decreased enhancement of the pancreas (less than 100HU) (green ROI).

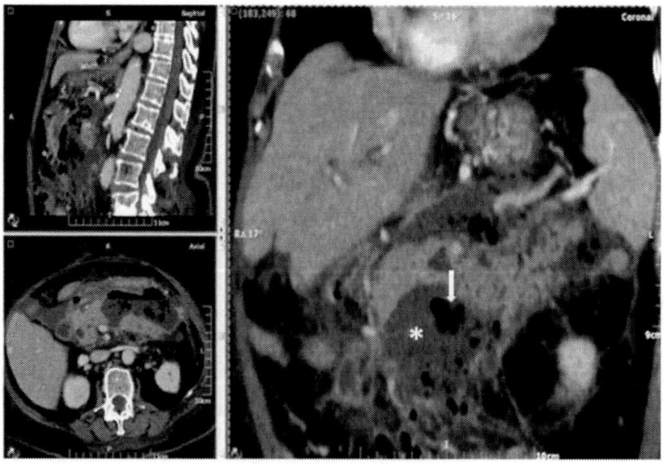

Figure 2. Abdominal CT in acute pancreatitis - Pancreatic phase of enhancement: Air containing (arrow) peripancreatic fluid collection (asterisk) in a septic patient.

In conclusion, focal or diffuse enlargement of the pancreas along with heterogenous enhancement and infiltration of peripancreatic fat are major CT findings indicative of acute pancreatitis [7, 8]. The formation of pseudoaneurysm may also be apparent (Figure 3). Chest CT may reveal concomitant pleural effusions and basal atelectasis. Currently, intravenous, contrast-enhanced CT scanning is routinely performed on patients who are suspected of harboring severe pancreatitis, regardless of Ranson's criteria or APACHE scores. Imaging of acute pancreatitis necessitates not only an understanding of the disease subtypes and the myriad of associated complications but also familiarity with the appropriate radiologic nomenclature as defined by the Atlanta symposium and recently revised by the Acute Pancreatitis Classification Working Group. The use of standardized terminology will hopefully improve the communication between radiologists, gastroenterologists and surgeons to facilitate treatment schedule and lead to favorable outcomes for patients with acute pancreatitis as well as create uniformity for enrollment into research surveys [9, 10].

CT revised Atlanta classification: Five grades based on severity

- Grade A: Normal pancreas
- Grade B
  - Focal or diffuse enlargement of the gland
  - Contour irregularities and heterogeneous attenuation (Figure 4)
  - Absence of peripancreatic inflammation
- Grade C: Intrinsic pancreatic abnormalities and associated inflammatory changes in peripancreatic fat (Figure 5)
- Grade D
  - Small and usually single, ill-defined fluid collection
- Grade E
  - Two or more large fluid collections
  - Presence of gas in pancreas or retroperitoneum
  - Most important criterion: Presence and extent of necrotizing pancreatitis (non-enhancing parenchyma) (Figure 6)

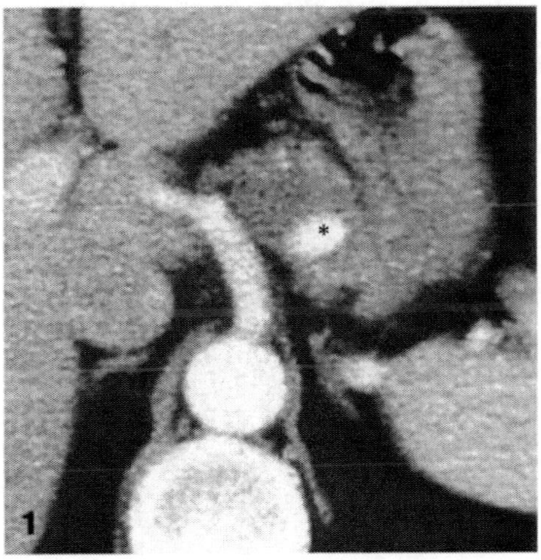

Figure 3. Abdominal CT in acute pancretitis: Pseudoaneurysm of the splenic artery (asterisk).

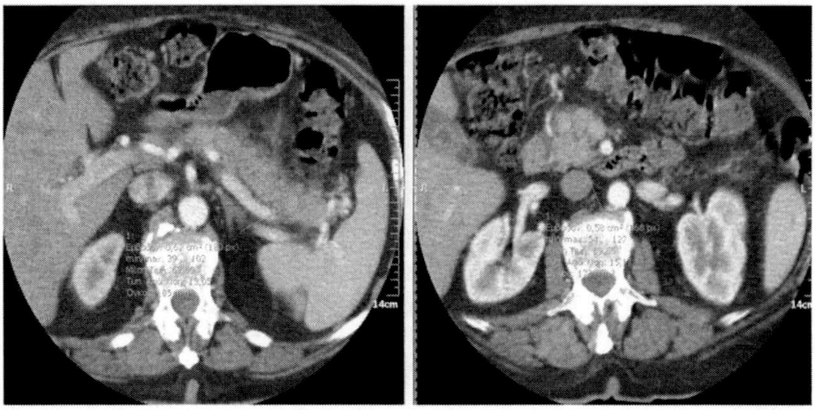

Figure 4. Abdominal CT in acute pancreatitis: Contour irregularity, heterogeneous attenuation of the pancreas.

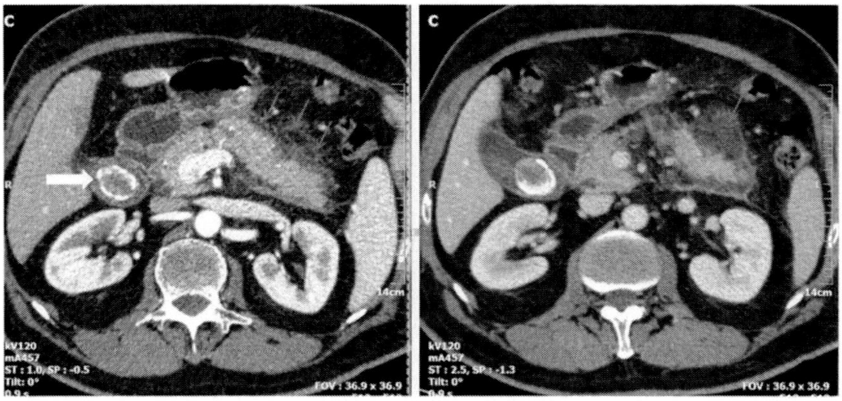

Figure 5. Abdominal CT in acute pancreatitis: Intrinsic pancreatic abnormalities and associated inflammatory changes in peripancreatic fat (blue arrows). Cholelithiasis (thick white arrow).

Magnetic Resonance Imaging – Magnetic Resonance Cholangiopancreatography

MR findings refer to variable decreased signal intensity and gland enlargement on T1WI images. A heterogenous enhancement pattern along with the detection of a pancreatic pseudocyst contiguous with the MPD and potential vascular occlusion may be easily demonstrated. On fat suppressed T2WI images fluid collections as well as pseudocysts and necrotic areas are depicted hyperintense contrary to hypointense lesions including gallstones or intraductal calculi [11].

Furthermore, MRCP provides evidence of a dilated MPD or an associated pseudocyst. Finally, it is important to differentiate between an acute pseudocyst and walled-off pancreatic necrosis (WOPN) by accurate definition and characterization of the solid necrotic debris. Patients presenting with WOPN require more aggressive endoscopic intervention, in contrast to simple transmural drainage, which may prove adequate for therapeutic approach of pseudocysts [12].

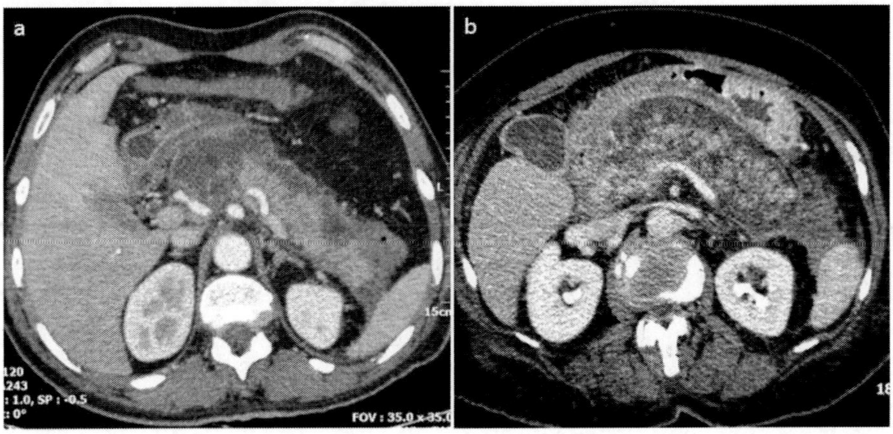

Figure 6. a) Abdominal CT in acute pancreatitis: Necrotizing pancreatitis (non enhancing parenchyma > 30%) (asterisks), b) More than 50%.

In addition, morphological features of WOPN determine treatment strategy since collections with greater amounts of solid necessitate direct endoscopic necrosectomy as well as aggressive surgical procedures for successful clinical outcome. WOPNs contain both liquid and solid necrotic debris and it is usually difficult to distinguish them from pure liquid collections on contrast-enhanced CT. MRI and endoscopic U/S (EUS) have been shown comparable sensitivity in the detection of the solid necrotic debris. Nevertheless, EUS is an invasive diagnostic modality that causes patient discomfort.

Angiography

Conventional angiography is performed when a pseudoaneurysm is suspected or for the detection of a vascular cause of pancreatitis with regard to polyartiritis nodosum, lupus or vasculitis.

Endoscopic Retrograde Cholangiopancreatography

ERCP is an invasive endoscopic technique which may be useful in the identification of a dilated or normal MPD. Additional communication with a pseudocyst could be acutely elucidated. Moreover, ERCP is warranted for the depiction of a narrowed or tapered distal CBD with prestenotic biliary dilatation.

Differential Diagnosis

- ✓ Infiltrating pancreatic carcinoma
- ✓ Perforated gastric ulcer
- ✓ Trauma
- ✓ Lymphoma and metastases

III. Pancreatic Pseudocyst

Definition

The formation of a pseudocyst refers to a chronic collection of pancreatic fluid surrounded by a nonepithelialized wall of granulation tissue and fibrosis. Pseudocysts occur in up to 10% of patients presenting with acute pancreatitis and 20-38% of chronic pancreatitis affected patients. They may occur intrapancreatically or extend beyond the region of the pancreas into other cavities or compartments.

The lesions may become secondarily infected, in which case they behave as abscesses. They can compress or obstruct adjacent organs or structures, leading to superior mesenteric – portal vein or splenic vein thrombosis. In addition, they can erode into visceral arteries and provoke intracystic hemorrhage or pseudoaneurysm formation [13].

Surgical Interventions

- ✓ Percutaneous drainage of a symptomatic or increase in size pseudocyst
- ✓ Surgical internal (usually into the stomach) or external drainage of a pseudocyst

Imaging Modalities

The role of imaging modalities in case of pancreatic pseudocyst detection is to establish the diagnosis and assess potential necessitation of surgical intervention. Drainage of infected or obstructing pseudocysts is also based on imaging techniques.

If infection is suspected, the pseudocyst should be aspirated by CT- or US-guided FNA, and the contents examined for organisms by Gram's stain and culture. If infection is present, and the contents resemble pus, external drainage is employed, using either surgical or percutaneous techniques.

Finally, although pseudocysts comprise roughly two thirds of all pancreatic cystic lesions, they resemble cystadenomas and cystadenocarcinomas radiographically and therefore differential diagnosis is based on advanced imaging modalities and related diagnostic procedures.

Ultrasound

Real-time U/S usually depicts a solitary unilocular cystic mass at the body or the tail of the pancreas. Multilocular lesions are apparent in 6% of affected patients. Parallel description of fluid-debris level and internal echoes due to autolysis along with blood clots or cellular debris is common U/S finding.

Rarely, septations as well as signs of infection or hemorrhage are defined. Additional dilation of CBD and CPD and calcification of the gland in cases with chronic pancreatitis may be reported.

Computed Tomography

CT characteristic findings of a mature pseudocyst refer to a round or oval, homogeneous, hypodense lesion with a near water density. On the contrary, a hemorrhagic, infected pseudocyst appears as a lobulated, heterogeneous, mixed density lesion. Intense pancreatic calcification as well as MPD and CBD involvement are adequately detected. Enhancement of thin rim of fibrous capsule associated with absence of similar finding of pseudocyst contents is common in contrast-enhanced CT (Figure 7).

The presence of gas within pseudocyst suggests superimposed infection or decompression of pseudocyst into pancreatic duct, stomach or bowel.

Finally, pseudoaneurysms caused by or simulating a pseudocyst could be depicted [14]. Pitfalls in the management of pseudocysts result from the presumptive diagnosis of a cystic neoplasm masquerading as a pseudocyst, a failure to appreciate the solid or debris-filled contents of the lesion which appears fluid filled on CT scan and incompetence to document potential adherence with an adjacent portion of the stomach before attempting transgastric internal drainage. If infection is suspected, the pseudocyst should be aspirated (not drained) by CT- or U/S-guided Fine Needle Aspiration (FNA) and the content examined for organisms by Gram's stain and culture. If infection is identified and the content resembles pus, external drainage is employed using either surgical or percutaneous modalities [15, 16].

Magnetic Resonance Imaging – Magnetic Resonance Cholangiopancreatography

MR findings are indicative of a hypointense lesion with parallel enhancement of fibrous capsule on T1WI images. On the contrary on T2WI images the pseudocyst presents hyperintense or with mixed intensity containing both fluid and debris.

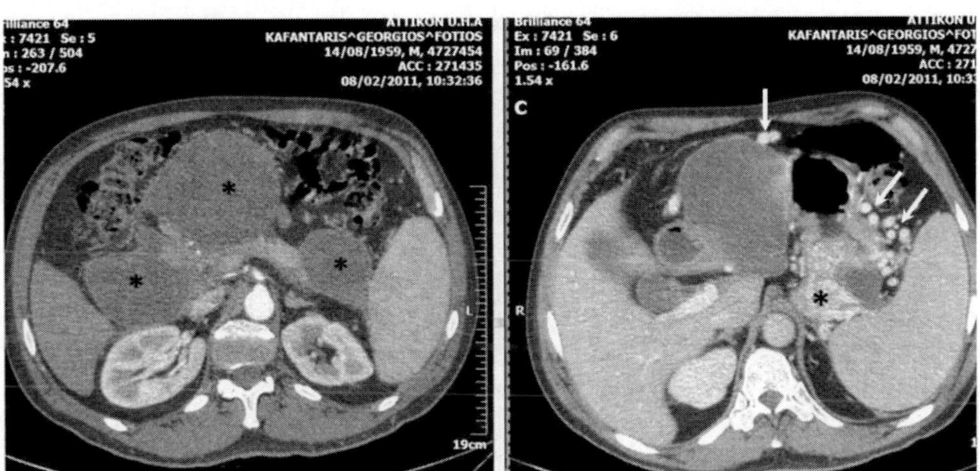

Figure 7. Abdominal CT: Smooth wall cystic lesions in the lesser sac and the transverse mesocolon (black asterisks). Splenic vein obstruction, gastrosplenic (thick white arrows) and gastric fundus varices.

Subsequent MRCP reveals a hyperintense cyst contiguous with dilated CPD. Similar findings are confirmed on ERCP with the communication of pseudocyst with CPD depicted in 70% of the cases.

Angiography

Conventional angiography is only performed in order to elucidate the diagnosis of pseudoaneurysm. Splenic artery is most frequently involved, followed by inferior and superior pancreatico-duodenal arteries.

Differential Diagnosis

- ✓ Serous microcystic cystadenoma
- ✓ Mucinous cystic tumor of pancreas
- ✓ Intraductal papillary mucinous tumor of the pancreas
- ✓ Cystic islet cell tumor
- ✓ Congenital cysts

IV. Chronic Pancreatitis

Definition

Chronic pancreatitis is an incurable, chronic inflammatory condition that is multifactorial in its etiology, highly variable in its presentation, and a challenge to treat successfully. Alcohol consumption and abuse is associated with chronic pancreatitis in up to 70% of cases.

Other major causes worldwide include tropical and idiopathic disease as well as metabolic disorders, hereditary cases and trauma. Radiologic imaging of chronic pancreatitis contributes in four areas including diagnosis, evaluation of severity of the disease, detection of complications and assistance in determining treatment options.

With the advent of cross-sectional imaging techniques such as CT and MRI, the contour, content, ductal pattern, calcifications, calculi and cystic disease of the pancreas are all readily discernible [17, 18].

Surgical Interventions

- ✓ Surgical internal or external drainage of a symptomatic or increase in size pseudocyst
- ✓ Pancreatic duct decompression for chronic obstructive pancreatitis
- ✓ Partial distal pancreatectomy for patients with focal inflammatory changes localized to the body and tail of the gland

- ✓ Radical distal pancreatectomy described by Fry and Child intended for patients with sclerotic small duct disease and preserving the rim of pancreas in the pancreaticoduodenal groove
- ✓ Pancreatoduodenectomy procedure with or without pylorus preservation for symptomatic chronic pancreatitis and pain relief
- ✓ Duodenum-preserving pancreatic head resection described by Beger for the treatment of chronic pancreatitis
- ✓ Extended lateral pancreaticojejunostomy with excavation of the pancreatic head for the complete decompression of the entire pancreatic ductal system described by Frey.

Imaging Modalities

The role of imaging modalities in case of chronic pancreatitis is to establish the diagnosis and differentiate from other conditions which may cause MPD dilatation and glandular atrophy. Additional assessment of potential necessitation of endoscopic or surgical intervention is also imaging dependent. Drainage of infected or obstructing pseudocysts is always based on imaging techniques.

Ultrasound

Transabdominal U/S is frequently employed as an initial imaging method in patients with abdominal symptoms and modifications consistent with pancreatic duct dilatation, intraductal filling defects, cystic changes and heterogeneous texture are encountered in chronic pancreatitis. The sensitivity of transabdominal U/S ranges from 48 to 96% and is operator dependent. Nevertheless, the contour, texture and ductal pattern are usually quite detectable and it is a reliable modality for periodic re-examination to determine the efficacy of therapeutic intervention.

Therefore, major U/S indications of chronic inflammation of the pancreas are the depiction of an atrophic gland along with a tubular anechoic structure consistent with a dilated MPD in up to 90% of the cases and the identification of calcifications appearing as echogenic foci with posterior acoustic shadowing and pseudocyst formation [19].

Computed Tomography

CT scanning has affected diagnostic approach of pancreatic disease more broadly than any other method. Prior to its widespread introduction, pancreatic imaging was largely a matter of detecting the displacement of adjacent, contrast-filled viscera by mass lesions of the pancreas. Since the application of cross-sectional techniques and with the advent of contrast-enhanced CT scanning and CT angiography, visualization of the nature, extent, location and relative relationships of pancreatic structures and lesions is accomplished with great clarity. CT scanning presents a false-negative rate of less than 10% for chronic pancreatitis, but early or mild chronic abnormalities may be undetected [20]. Another drawback of CT scanning is its lower sensitivity for identifying small neoplasms, which may be invisible to all modalities apart from EUS. Nevertheless, major CT findings indicative of chronic pancreatitis are the presence of an atrophic gland along with an occasionally focal or diffuse enlargement of the pancreas, dilated MPD with ductal calculi, intra and peri-pancreatic cysts formation and extensive thickening of peri-pancreatic fascia (Figure 8).

Additional splenic vein thrombosis implied by splenomegaly and varices confirmation could be depicted. Moreover, a hypodense focal mass with fibrosis and fat necrosis usually in the pancreatic head may simulate neoplastic transformation.

Magnetic Resonance Imaging – Magnetic Resonance Cholangiopancreatography

MRI, in both the cross-sectional mode and the coronally-oriented heavily weighted T2 or high spin ratio imaging (MRCP) have added heavily to the imaging options of chronic pancreatitis. The resolution of MRI scanning is now approaching that of CT, although its availability and the complexity of the images produced have limited its large-scale use for routine imaging of the pancreas.

A heterogeneous enhancement pattern along with nonenhancing decreased signal areas implying necrosis, and pseudocyst formation usually contiguous with dilated MPD are well depicted. Vascular occlusions may also be demonstrated [21]. Moreover, MRCP has been shown to be an effective screening technique for disclosing ductal abnormalities possessing the advantage of noninvasive methodology and the ability to image obstructed ducts that are not opacified by ERCP injection. Parallel dilatation of MPD with radicles and CBD with smooth distal tapering is the pathognomonic MRCP finding of chronic pancreatitis (Figure 9). Therefore, MRCP remains a useful screening modality to determine duct abnormalities and confirm the need for interventional procedures. Oral, intravenous and intraductal contrast administration are not implemented. Thus, its lack of ionizing radiation makes this imaging technique the safest method to image the ductal system in high-risk patients [22, 23].

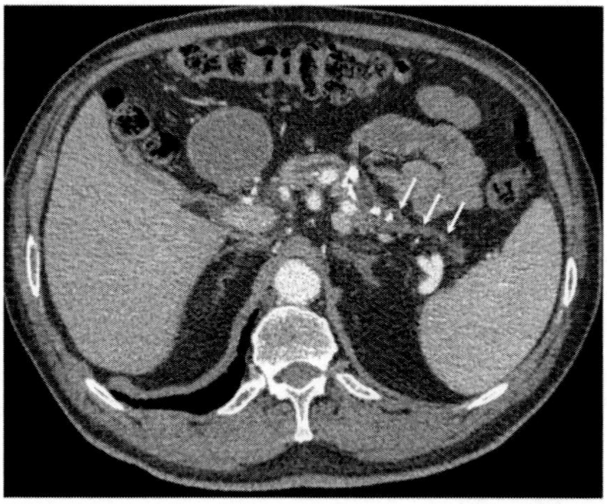

Figure 8. Abdominal CT in chronic pancreatitis: Calcification of the pancreatic parenchyma following the course of the main pancreatic duct and its branches (red arrowheads). Mild dilatation of main pancreatic duct and parenchymal atrophy (thick white arrows).

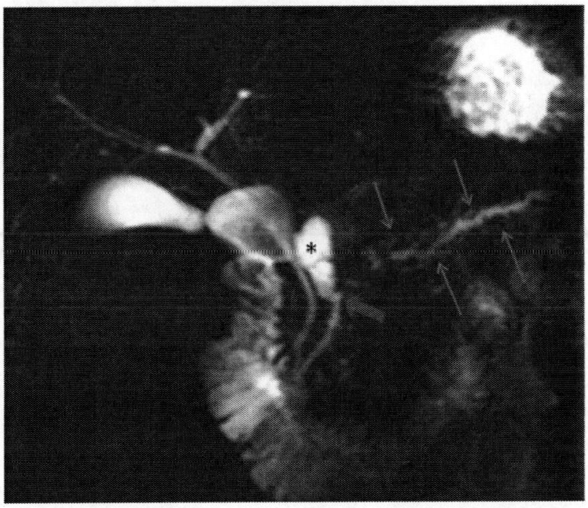

Figure 9. MRCP in chronic pancreatitis: Irregularly dilated main pancreatic duct and its branches (thin blue arrows), communicating (thick red arrow) with a pseudocyst (asterisk).

Endoscopic Ultrasonography

EUS has heavily impacted the evaluation and management of patients with chronic pancreatitis. Although it is more operator dependent and less widely available than transabdominal U/S, EUS provides not only imaging capability, but adds the capacity to obtain cytological and chemical samples of tissue and fluid aspirated with linear array monitor [24, 25]. EUS images obtained through a high-frequency transducer are to evaluate subtle changes in 2- to 3-mm structures within the pancreas, and detect indolent neoplasms in the setting of chronic inflammation. Small intraductal lesions and mucus as well as subtle ductular abnormalities and cystic disorders are also recognizable with EUS [26]. This allows ERCP to be reserved for these patients who require therapeutic maneuvers or for the identification of more problematic nosologic entities (Figure 10). EUS is comparable to ERCP in the detection of advanced changes in chronic pancreatitis and may be more sensitive in the confirmation of mild disease.

Endoscopic Retrograde Cholangiopanceatography (ERCP)

ERCP is considered to be the gold standard for the diagnosis and staging of chronic pancreatitis. It also serves as a vehicle that enables other diagnostic and therapeutic maneuvers such as brushing for cytology or the employment of stents to relieve obstruction or drain a pseudocyst. Dilated and beaded MPD with radicles along with MPD filling defects indicating the presence of intraductal calculi are common ERCP findings of chronic pancreatitis [27]. In addition, CBD may appear dilated with distal narrowing. Unfortunately, ERCP carries a risk of procedure-induced pancreatitis that occurs in approximately 5% of patients. Post-ERCP pancreatitis occurs after uncomplicated procedures as well as after those that require prolonged manipulation. Patients at increased risk include those with documented sphincter of Oddi dysfunction.

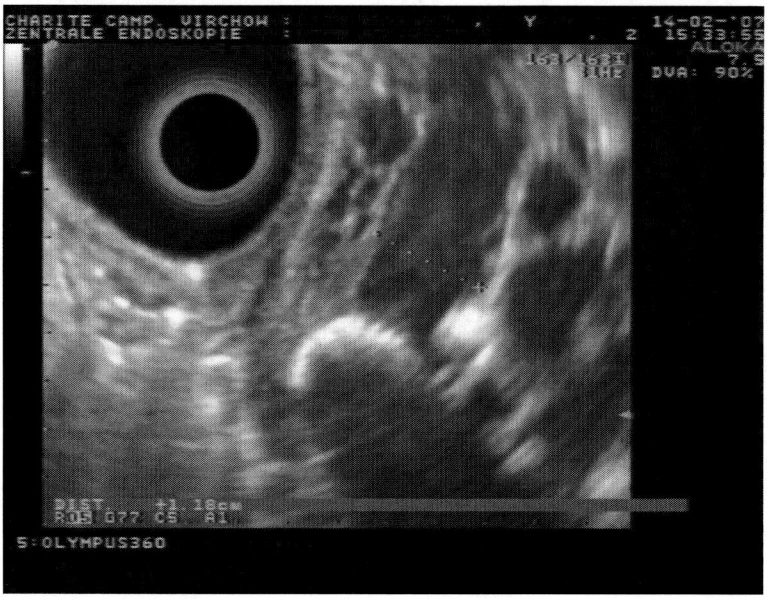

Figure 10. EUS in chronic pancreatitis identifying a dilated main pancreatic duct with filling defects indicative of the presence of intraductal calculi.

Therefore, this method should be reserved for patients with unclear diagnosis or in whom a diagnostic and therapeutic intervention is crucial [28].

Differential Diagnosis

- ✓ Pancreatic carcinoma
- ✓ Intraductal papillary mucinous tumor of the pancreas

V. Traumatic Pancreatitis

Definition

Blunt pancreatic transection at the neck of the pancreas can occur with a direct blow to the abdomen. As an isolated injury it is difficult to detect. Since the MPD is transected the patient will develop a pseudocyst or pancreatic ascites, but there is little inflammation since the pancreatic enzymes remain inactivated. Diagnostic approach can occasionally be accomplished with CT using fine cuts through the pancreas. Nevertheless, CT will not identify a significant number of transections if performed within 6 hours of injury. Optimal management of pancreatic trauma is determined by the location of the injury and whether or not the MPD is involved. In case of an intact MPD treatment may be accomplished only by drainage. In contrast, traumatic pancreatitis associated with a ductal injury always requires therapeutic intervention in order to prevent pancreatic ascites or a major external fistula. Direct exploration of perforations or lacerations will confirm the diagnosis in most instances [29, 30].

Surgical Interventions

- ✓ Surgical drainage in case of pancreatic trauma with an intact MPD
- ✓ Distal pancreatectomy with or without splenectomy for severe injury of the neck, body and tail of the pancreas with parallel MPD transection
- ✓ Limited resection from the site of the injury to the head of the pancreas with preservation of pancreaticoduodenal vessels and CBD in case of severe traumatic lesion of the head and MPD involvement

Imaging Modalities

The role of imaging modalities in case of traumatic pancreatitis is to establish the diagnosis and assess the pancreatic duct integrity. Conservative treatment can also be selected with imaging evaluation at regular intervals.

Ultrasound

Transabdominal U/S findings in traumatic pancreatitis may be similar to those of non-traumatic inflammation of the gland. In addition U/S depiction is not as sensitive and accurate as CT in diagnosing acute injury of the pancreas.

Computed Tomography

Focal or diffuse pancreatic enlargement with irregularity of pancreatic contour is always indicative of traumatic pancreatitis. The presence of edema as well as fluid collection in peri-pancreatic fat with concomitant heterogeneous parenchymal attenuation is often apparent. Thickening of anterior renal fascia may be an additional indirect CT finding. Nevertheless, peri-pancreatic soft tissue changes of traumatic pancreatitis are often subtle and become more evident within 24-48 hours. In case of laceration an area of low attenuation is usually revealed while its actual size is difficult to visualize.

Moreover, potential pancreatic fracture or transection is detected as an ill-defined low density area which results in clear separation of two ends of the gland and nearly always extends through pancreatic neck (Figure 11).

However, lacerations and fractures may produce non-specific changes in parenchymal density and become undetectable on CT scanning. Extra-pancreatic fluid collections around major vascular structures, transverse mesocolon, pararenal space, lesser sac, and the root of mesentery are usually well depicted along with concomitant injury to left lobe of the liver [31]. In conclusion, CT remains the most accurate method of detecting extra-pancreatic fluid collections, pancreatic lacerations or fractures taking into thorough consideration the protocol advice about performing 24-48 hours delayed scans that may uncover findings not present earlier.

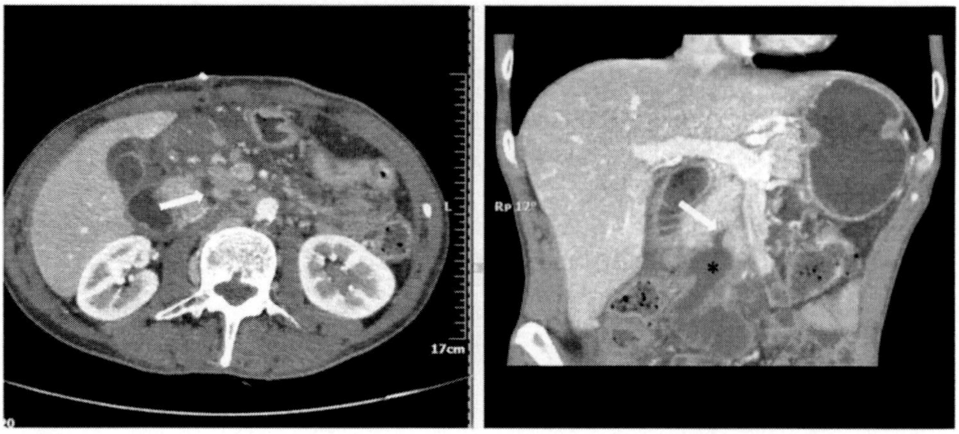

Figure 11. Abdominal CT in pancreatic trauma (axial and coronal reformation): Interruption of the pancreatic head (thick white arrow) associated with peripancreatic fluid collection (asterisk).

Magnetic Resonance Imaging – Magnetic Resonance Cholangiopancreatography

Variable decreased signal intensity with heterogeneous enhancement pattern and non-enhancing hypointense areas indicative of fluid collection, pseudocyst formation and necrosis are often defined in T1W1 images. On the other hand, on fat suppressed T2WI images liquid selections or pseudocysts are demonstated as hyperintense lesions. Subsequent MRCP reveals possible rupture of MPD (23%) or potential communication with post-traumatic pseudocyst.

Endoscopic Retrograde Cholangiopanceatography (ERCP)

It is obvious based on the above options that no ideal method exists for identifying pancreatic ductal injuries that cannot be ruled out by direct exploration. Alternative method is the use of ERCP. Nevertheless, this modality is very helpful in the delayed diagnosis of a ductal pancreatic injury. Potential transection of MPD reveals an abrupt duct termination or contrast extravasation.

Additional communication of pseudocyst with pancreatic duct may be apparent. However, procedure-induced pancreatitis may also be invoked.

Differential Diagnosis

- ✓ "Shock" pancreas
- ✓ Intramural duodenal hematoma
- ✓ Duodenal rupture

VI. SEROUS CYSTADENOMA OF THE PANCREAS

Definition

The term usually refers to a benign glycogen-rich pancreatic tumor that arises from acinar cells with mainly microcystic appearance. It is encountered most frequently incidentally in middle-aged women. Best diagnostic clue is the depiction of a honeycomb or sponge-like mass in pancreatic head with calcification and innumerable small cysts varying from 1-20mm within large cystic lesion.

Tumors show increased frequency in patients with von Hippel-Lindau disease. Based on WHO classification two types of serous cystadenoma are recognized including the microcystic adenoma and the less common oligocystic (macrocystic) variant [32].

Surgical Interventions

- ✓ Complete surgical excision of a symptomatic and large tumor

Imaging Modalities

The role of imaging modalities in cases of serous cystadenoma of the pancreas is to establish the diagnosis and assess whether surgical resection should be implemented.

Differential diagnosis of other cystic tumours categories and pseudocysts is only accomplished on the basis of specific imaging features as well as examination of fluid aspirated under imaging guidance.

Ultrasound

Real-time U/S usually depicts a hyperechoic mass with tiny cystic lesions. Less commonly, a tumor with large cysts defined as discrete anechoic areas with thin walls is described. Additional calcifications are detected as highly reflective echoes with acoustic shadowing.

Computed Tomography

Honeycomb pattern remains the pathognomonic CT finding indicative of a microcystic adenoma. Additional enhancement of septa delineating small cysts or calcification within central scar may be encountered (Figure 12). CBD and/or MPD dilatation as well as atrophy of pancreas distal to the tumor is common among cystic epithelial neoplastic lesions.

Furthermore, macrocystic (usually unilocular) serous cystadenoma is located in the pancreatic head and is depicted with one or few cystic components (locules) covered by thin non enhancing imperceptible wall. Therefore, differential diagnosis from mucinous cystic lesions remains problematic [33, 34].

Magnetic Resonance Imaging – Magnetic Resonance Cholangiopancreatography

T1W1 MRI images usually elucidate the presence of a hypointense tumor with central scar enhancement on delayed scan and calcification while blood within cysts is often depicted with varied intensity (Figure 13). Capsular enhancement is also commonly observed. Relevant findings are detected on T2WI images. Subsequent MRCP confirms potential MPD and CBD dilatation. Displacement, narrowing and dilatation of adjacent MPD and/or CBD are also mentioned in ERCP.

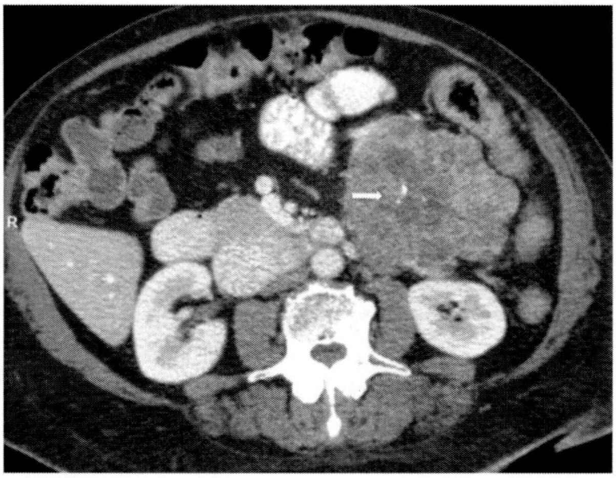

Figure 12. Abdominal CT showing a multicystic lesion that contains tiny cysts and central calcification at the pancreatic tail (thick white arrow).

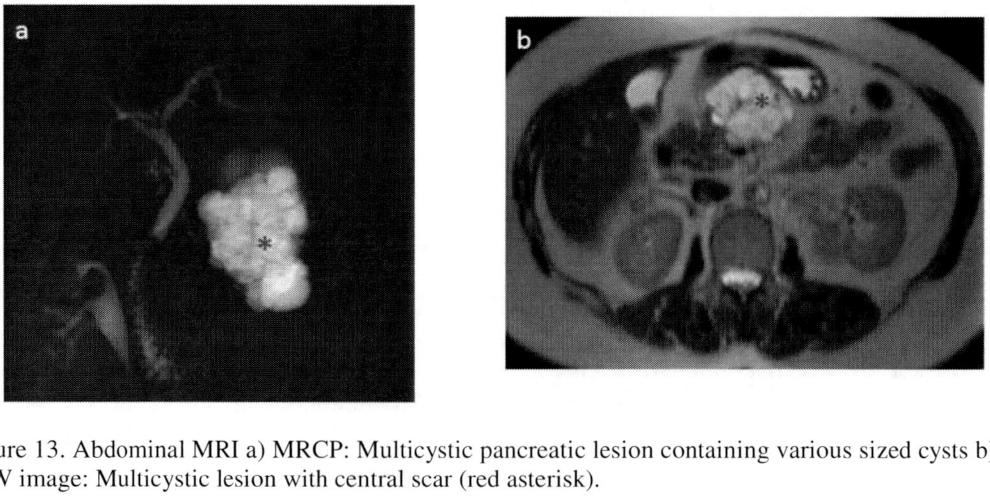

Figure 13. Abdominal MRI a) MRCP: Multicystic pancreatic lesion containing various sized cysts b) T2W image: Multicystic lesion with central scar (red asterisk).

Angiography

Conventional angiography reveals a highly vascular tumor due to extensive capillary network within septa with neovascularity and dense blush. Large cysts produce lucent regions with dilated feeding arteries and prominent draining veins.

Nevertheless, exclusive angiographic characteristics are absent.

Endoscopic Ultrasonography

The unequivocal diagnosis of a pancreatic cystic lesion without a clear association to acute or chronic pancreatitis should always raise a tumor suspicion, reinforced by other factors such as female gender, higher age and location in the gland. Among the tumors, the mucinous types have to be taken more seriously with surgery being considered in all of them, whereas the rate of malignancy in serous cystadenomas seems to be very low [35, 36]. Early papers suggested specific EUS image features to be more frequent among different types of cystic tumors, but this may not be helpful in the individual case (Figure 14).

Furthermore, agreement among endosonographers was only fair in this differential diagnosis. It is assumed that the risk of malignancy is very low for serous cystadenoma, which was confirmed recently in a series of 158 such cases undergoing surgery, with only two malignancies, one diagnosed initially, the other one on follow-up due to metastases after an initial benign diagnosis from the resection specimen.

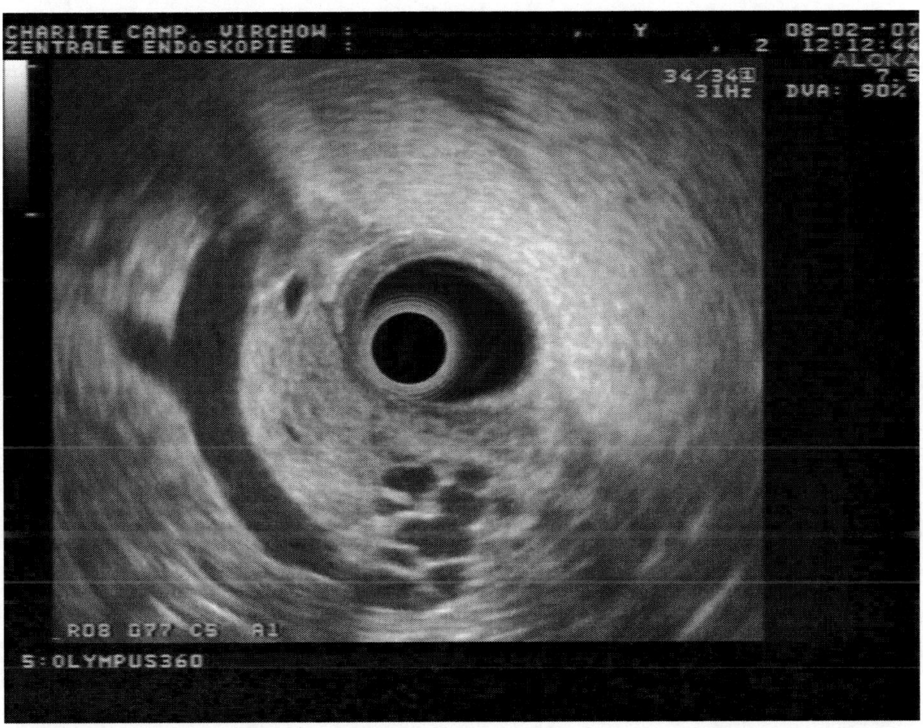

Figure 14. EUS depiction of serous cystadenoma of the pancreas with multiple small compartments within a cystic mass (honeycomb appearance).

Studies evaluating EUS-FNA with different parameters to be assessed from the aspirated fluid (amylase, mucin, CEA, cytology) also reached contradictory conclusions [37]. EUS potentially with FNA in general contributes limited information to the management of patients with indeterminate cystic lesions.

Clinical parameters including absence of pancreatitis, gender and age add at least as much important information as morphology (EUS and/or CT) and FNA results do. Surgery should be considered in all operable patients with incidental cysts located at the head of the gland. Specific parameters with regard to morphology suggesting serous cystadenoma may lead to FNA in individual cases, if the results have an impact on the patient's management.

Differential Dagnosis

- ✓ Mucinous cystadenoma of pancreas
- ✓ Intraductal papillary mucinous tumor (IPMT)
- ✓ Pseudocyst
- ✓ Pancreatic carcinoma
- ✓ Congenital pancreatic cysts
- ✓ Cystic islet cell tumor

VII. Mucinous Cystic Pancreatic Tumor (MCPT)

Definition

The terminology refers to an uncommon primary enhancing multiseptated mass in the body or tail of the pancreas. It is recognized as a large smooth encapsulated lesion with thick fibrous capsule and lobulated surface.

The presence of multi-/unilocular large cysts is obvious. Cystic cavity may be filled with thick mucoid material or clear, green blood-tinged fluid. Otherwise, solid papillary projections protrude into interior of the tumor indicating the malignant potential of the neoplasm which shares both clinical and pathologic characteristics of biliary and ovarian tumors.

Rarely MCPT may manifest with local invasion or distant metastases or symptoms of mass effect on adjacent structures. Laboratory data including increased levels of serum CEA and elevated cyst fluid levels of CA 19-9 and CA 72-4 present 80% sensitivity and 95% specificity for tumor identification [38].

Surgical Interventions

- ✓ Complete surgical excision

Imaging Modalities

The role of imaging modalities in case of mucinous cystic pancreatic tumor is to establish the diagnosis and confirm the need for subsequent complete surgical resection. Differential diagnosis of other cystic tumours categories and pseudocysts is only accomplished on the basis of specific imaging features as well as estimation of fluid aspirated with image-guided diagnostic procedures.

Ultrasound

Real Time U/S usually detects a multilocular cystic mass with echogenic internal septa. Alternatively, a unilocular anechoic lesion is frequently depicted with limited contribution to the differential diagnosis among cystic pancreatic neoplastic disorders.

Computed Tomography

NECT reveals a hypodense unilocular or multilocular cyst with focal calcifications.

Subsequent CECT describes a multilocular cystic lesion with enhancement of thin internal septa and cyst wall [39].

Magnetic Resonance Imaging – Magnetic Resonance Cholangiopancreatography

On T1W1 images variable signal intensity based on cyst content is documented. Fluid-like material as well as focal calcifications are characterized as hypointense while proteinaceous or hemorrhagic elements are hyperintense.

On the other hand, cystic lesions are depicted as hyperintense areas with hypointense internal septations and focal calcifications on T2WI images (Figure 15).

MRCP as well as ERCP is indicative of extensive displacement, narrowing and prestenotic dilatation of MPD adjacent to tumor [40].

Angiography

Conventional angiography often reveals a predominantly avascular cystic mass with solid components and small areas of vascular blush and neovascularity. Additional displacement of surrounding major vascular structures is identified.

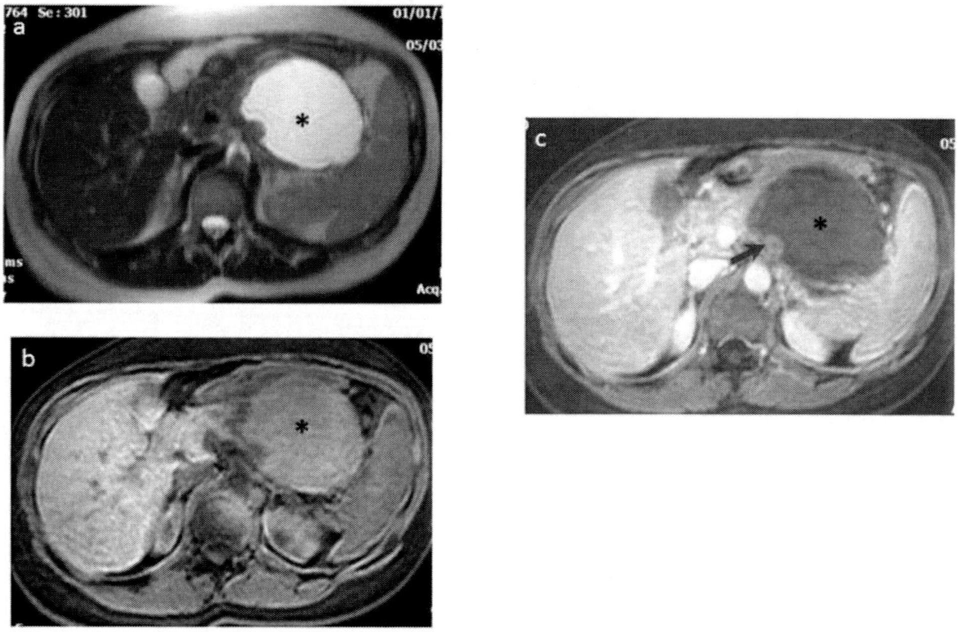

Figure 15. Abdominal MRI of a mucinous pancreatic tumor: a) T2W image: Unilocular cystic lesion with hypointense mural nodule (black asterisk) b) 3D T1 fat suppressed image: Hyperintensity of the cystic content indicating the presence of mucin (black asterisk) c) 3D T1 fat suppressed image after contrast medium administration: Enhancement of the mural nodule (red thick arrow).

Endoscopic Ultrasonography

Several EUS findings have been evaluated to diagnose pancreatic cystic lesions. Small cyst size does not exclude malignancy; one series reported 20% of lesions 2cm or smaller to be malignant and 45% possessed malignant potential.

However, only 3.5% among asymptomatic lesions with tumor size less than 2cm were malignant [41]. Certain features do appear to be more predictive in diagnosing particular types of cystic pancreatic lesions (Figure 16, 17). The finding of multiple small compartments within a cystic mass is suggestive of a serous cystadenoma, with an accuracy of 92% to 96%, and is not encountered in mucinous cystadenomas [42].

In addition, a cystic tumor without septations or solid components and detected within a pancreas having parenchymal abnormalities suggests a pseudocyst formation with a sensitivity of 94% and a specificity of 85%.

EUS findings may also help identify those patients with mucinous lesions with malignant potential who might benefit from surgical resection. One study reported that the presence of any one of the following had a sensitivity of 91% but a specificity of 60% for detecting a lesion with malignant potential: (1) cyst-wall thickness greater than 3mm, (2) intracystic compartments larger than 10mm ("macroseptations"), (3) intramural masses, or (4) cystic dilatation of the MPD [43]. Another study found the accuracy for detecting those lesions with malignant potential varied from 40% to 93%.

This suggests that, whereas EUS findings may add some diagnostic information, results may not be reliable enough for making management decisions [44].

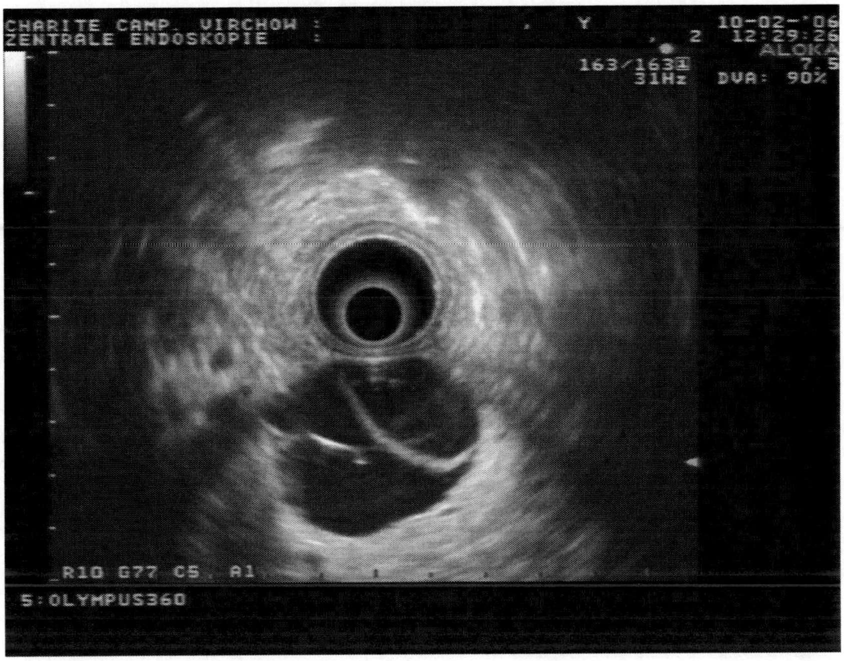

Figure 16. EUS showing a mucinous cystic tumor of the tail of the pancreas with characteristic cyst-wall thickness.

Differential Diagnosis

- ✓ Serous cystadenoma of the pancreas
- ✓ Intraductal papillary mucinous tumor (IPMT)
- ✓ Pseudocyst
- ✓ Variant of ductal adenocarcinoma
- ✓ Congenital pancreatic cysts
- ✓ Cystic islet cell tumor
- ✓ Lymphangioma

VIII. Intraductal Papillary Mucinous Tumor

Definition

IPMT is a subdivision of mucin producing tumors along with mucinous macrocystic neoplasm and is classified into three types:

- Branch pancreatic duct (BPD) type with focal lobulated "multicystic" dilatation of branch ducts
- Main pancreatic duct (MPD) type with diffuse dilatation of MPD
- Combined type with parallel dilatation of both BPD and MPD which is the most common variety.

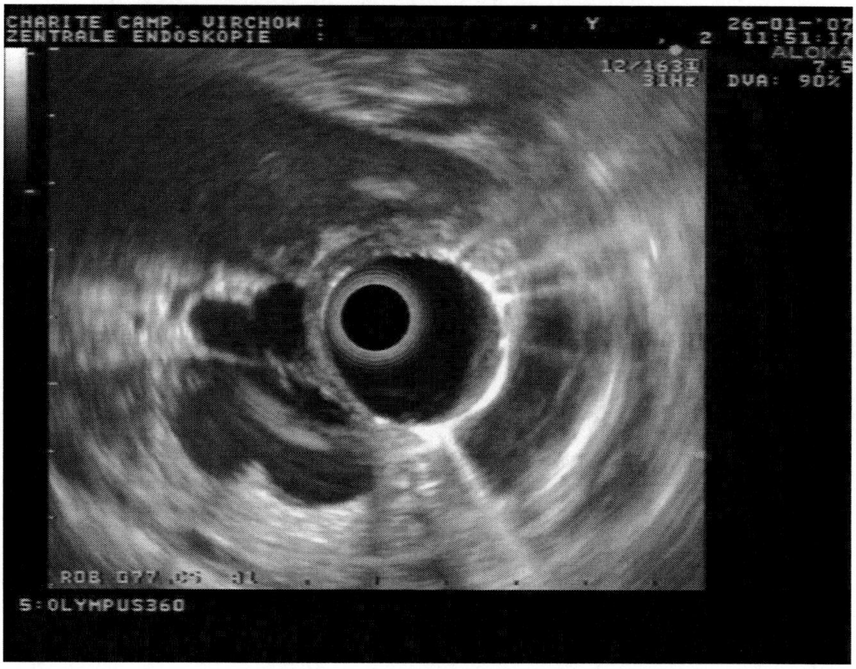

Figure 17. EUS showing a mucinous cystic tumor of the pancreas with intracystic compartments, intramural masses and associated cystic dilatation of the main pancreatic duct.

Tumors are typically papillary lesions ranging in size from a few millimeters to panductal with varying proportions of dysplasia and in situ cancer. Papillary projections protrude into and expand BPD and MPD as well. Excessive mucin production combined with obstruction and dilatation of BPD and MPD is also noted. Most specific predictive signs of malignant transformation refer to diabetes mellitus, detection of a solid mass on imaging or a dilated MPD more than 10mm, diffuse or multifocal involvement and presence of attenuating or calcified intraluminal content. Associated laboratory data refer to increased serum and urinary amylase and altered pancreatic function tests [45].

Surgical Interventions

- ✓ Laparoscopic distal pancreatectomy with or without splenic preservation may be employed for cystic lesions located in the tail of the pancreas
- ✓ Duodenum-preserving pancreatic head resection for isolated lesions in the head of the pancreas
- ✓ Total pancreatectomy in case of multi-focal disease

Imaging Modalities

The role of imaging modalities in case of intraductal papillary mucinous cystic tumor of the pancreas is to establish the diagnosis and confirm the necessity of concomitant complete surgical excision.

Differential diagnosis of other cystic tumours categories and pseudocysts is only accomplished on the basis of specific imaging features as well as estimation of fluid aspirated with advanced imaging guided diagnostic procedures.

Therefore, imaging methods potentially with FNA contributes significant information to the management of patients with indeterminate cystic lesions of the pancreas.

Ultrasound

Real-time U/S usually defines the presence of a septated cystic lesion along with a dilated MPD and occasionally punctate calcifications. Nevertheless, intra-operative or endoscopic sonography affords superior visualization of ductal system of the pancreas.

Computed Tomography

Differential diagnosis among pancreatic cystic lesions as well as specific types of IPMTs is always attempted with CECT scanning. BPD type is described as a thin, lobulated, irregular, peripheral ring-enhancing "multicystic" lesion.

A bulging ampulla at duodenal sweep with thin rim enhancement is often apparent [46]. On the contrary, MPD type is related to a markedly dilated tortuous MPD. Additional punctate calcifications along with polypoid lesions lining MPD may be visualized.

Magnetic Resonance Imaging – Magnetic Resonance Cholangiopancreatography

On axial TlWI images hypointense branch duct cysts associated with a dilated MPD are always revealed. In addition, clustered cystic lesions with thin septa are depicted on coronal T1W1 images. On T2WI depictions relevant disorders are hyperintense with parallel detection of papillary excrescence in cystic lesion of pancreatic head or along MPD.

Subsequent MRCP is mainly indicative of lobulated clustered cysts, dilated MPD and possible communication between cystic tumors and ductal system (Figure 18). Intraductal mucin and papillary lesions may be also described as nodular filling defects [47].

Endoscopic Retrograde Cholangiopanceatography

ERCP confirms the diagnosis of IPMT of pancreas contributing to the detection of a dilated MPD with thick intraductal mucinous secretions. Mucin and papillary tumors are clearly defined as elongated, nodular or band-like filling defects in MPD. Concomitant real-time visualization of patulous ampulla and increased mucus production is warranted.

Endoscopic Ultrasonography

EUS cannot accurately determine the extent of involvement of IPMT and is not reliable in distinguishing malignant from benign forms of this neoplasm (Figure 19).

Intraductal U/S may suggest malignant IPMT by the presence of protruding lesions ≥ 4 mm (Figure 20). Areas of uncertainty likely reflect the only fair to moderate agreement among experienced endosonographers about the presence or absence of particular EUS findings or specific diagnoses [48, 49]. EUS-guided FNA (EUS-FNA) of pancreatic cystic lesions yields fluid for cytological and chemical analyses.

Moreover, any solid components associated with a lesion or regional lymph nodes can be aspirated for cytology or histological evaluation. Dilated pancreatic ducts can be safely targeted for FNA when IPMT is suspected. Knowledge of patient's clinical history may help improve the accuracy of EUS for diagnosing IPMTs [50].

Differential Diagnosis

- ✓ Serous cystadenoma of the pancreas
- ✓ Mucinous cystic neoplasm
- ✓ Pancreatic pseudocyst
- ✓ Pancreatic carcinoma
- ✓ Chronic pancreatitis

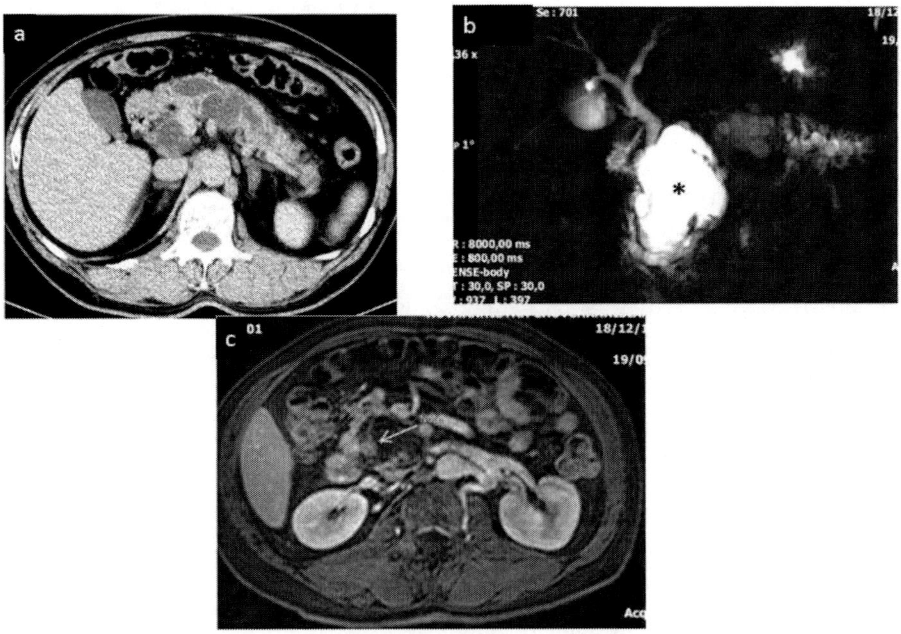

Figure 18. Intraductal papillary mucinous tumor of the pancreas a) Abdominal CT: Irregular dilatation of the main pancreatic duct with associated cystic branches dilatation b) MRCP: Large cystic lesion at the pancreatic head (black asterisk), cystic dilatation of main pancreatic duct and its branches c) 3D T1 Fat Suppressed image after contrast medium administration: Enhancement of the solid component of the cystic lesion, indicating malignant transformation (green arrow).

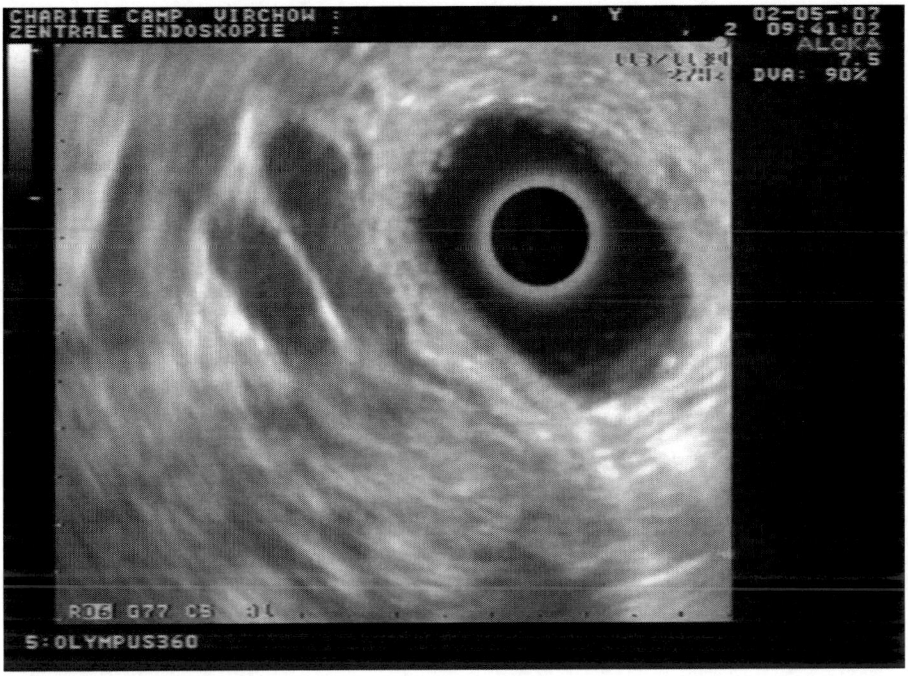

Figure 19. EUS detection of double duct sign associated with main branch intraductal papillary mucinous tumor of the pancreas.

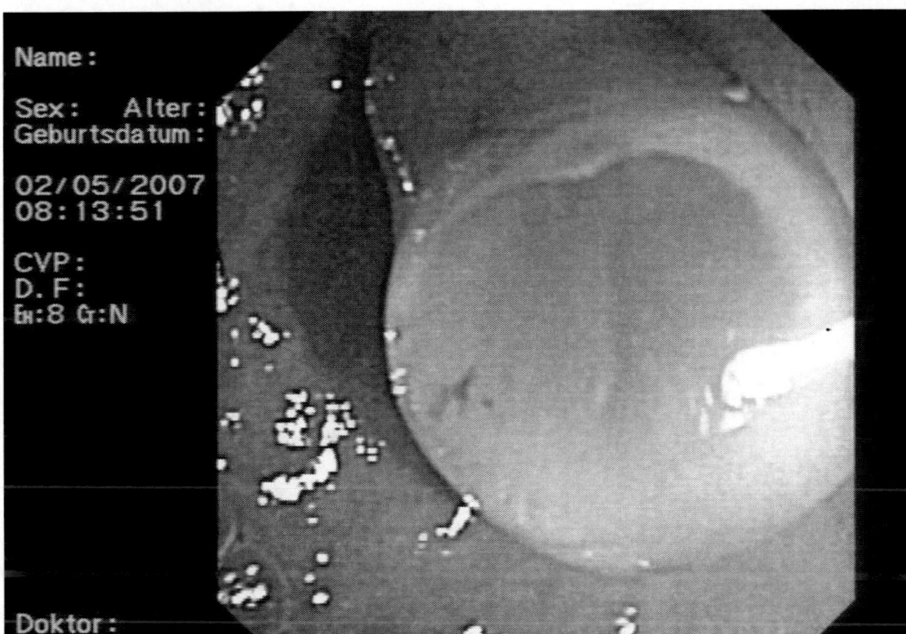

Figure 20. EUS detection of a dilated main pancreatic duct with thick intraductal mucinous secretions indicative of the presence of intraductal papillary mucinous tumor of the pancreas.

IX. Pancreatic Ductal Carcinoma

Definition

Pancreatic adenocarcinoma is the most common type of pancreatic cancer accounting for more than 80% of all pancreatic malignancies. About two thirds of pancreatic adenocarcinomas arise within the head or uncinate process of the pancreas; 15% are located in the body, and 10% in the tail, with the remaining tumors demonstrating diffuse involvement of the gland [51]. Tumors in the pancreatic body and tail are generally larger at the time of diagnosis, and therefore, less commonly resectable.

Tumors in the head of the pancreas are typically diagnosed earlier because they cause obstructive jaundice. Ampullary carcinomas, carcinomas of the distal bile duct, and periampullary duodenal adenocarcinomas present in a similar fashion to pancreatic head cancer but possess a slightly better prognosis, probably because early obstruction of the bile duct and jaundice leads to the prompt diagnosis. Exact pathologic staging of pancreatic cancer is important because it allows accurate quantitative assessment of results and comparisons between institutions. Surgery with margin negative resection also known as R0 resection is the only potentially curative approach in pancreatic carcinoma.

However, only 15-20% of affected patients present with potentially resectable disease. Due to the high morbidity of the surgical procedure, accurate selection of patients in the preoperative setting who will proceed to operation is critical [52].

Surgical Interventions

- ✓ Distal pancreatectomy with splenectomy may be employed for pancreatic adenocarcinomas located in the body and the tail of the gland
- ✓ Pancreaticoduodenectomy, also called "Whipple operation," for complete resection of isolated malignant lesions in the head of the pancreas
- ✓ Palliative endoscopic stenting for obstructive jaundice relief
- ✓ Palliative gastric by-pass in case of duodenal obstruction of unresectable tumor
- ✓ Palliative celiac nerve block for abdominal pain

Imaging Modalities

The role of imaging modalities in cases of pancreatic ductal carcinoma is to establish the diagnosis and assess tumor resectability. The accuracy of imaging techniques for predicting unresectable disease is about 90 to 95%.

Specific imaging findings that indicate a tumor is unresectable include invasion of the CHA or SMA, enlarged lymph nodes outside the boundaries of resection, ascites, and distant metastases mainly to the liver. Invasion of the SMV or PV remain relative contraindications to resection as long as the veins are patent.

Ultrasound

One of the common presentations of patients with pancreatic adenocarcinomas of the head of the pancreas is painless jaundice. The initial imaging modality is typically an ultrasound to evaluate the intrahepatic biliary system, the common duct and the gallbladder.

Presence of CBD dilatation along with intrahepatic and MPD involvement is a strong indication for further meticulous investigation with cross sectional imaging. Real-time U/S often reveals a hypoechoic mass combined with contour deformity of the gland. Due to overlying bowel gas and differences in operator scanning technique and experience, U/S in not typically used as the modality of choice in staging pancreatic adenocarcinoma.

Computed Tomography

CT is usually the cross sectional imaging modality of choice for staging in pancreatic cancer patients. Parallel administration of oral and iodinated contrast intravenously injected prior to the CT scan is implemented. Dual phase imaging is performed. The first phase refers to the pancreatic parenchymal process of enhancement while the second one describes the portal venous phase. The pancreatic tumor is best detected during the first phase of enhancement due to optimal depiction of the pancreas with greatest attenuation difference between the tumor and the normal gland (Figure 21).

Liver metastatic disease is best elucidated in the second portal phase of enhancement. The images are reconstructed at either 0.625 or 1.25mm slice thickness. These thin section images can help in multiplanar reconstructions and in improved detection of small tumors. Associated secondary signs of malignancy as well as potential vascular involvement are always assessed. Pancreatic adenocarcinomas are typically low attenuation, infiltrative masses on the pancreatic parenchymal phase of enhancement.

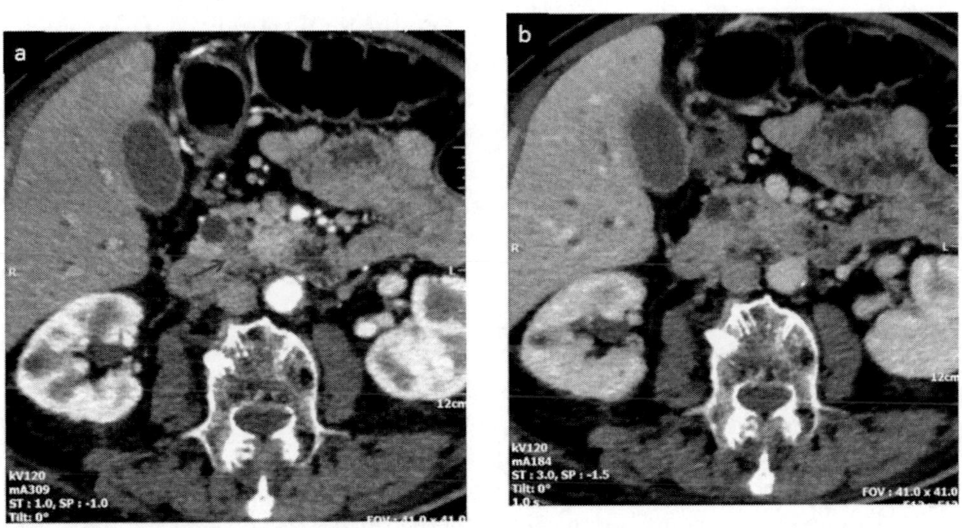

Figure 21. Abdominal CT in pancreatic ductal carcinoma: a) Pancreatic phase of enhancement: Small pancreatic cancer causing obstruction of the common bile duct and the main pancreatic duct (red arrow) b) Portal phase of enhancement: The pancreatic lesion is not visible.

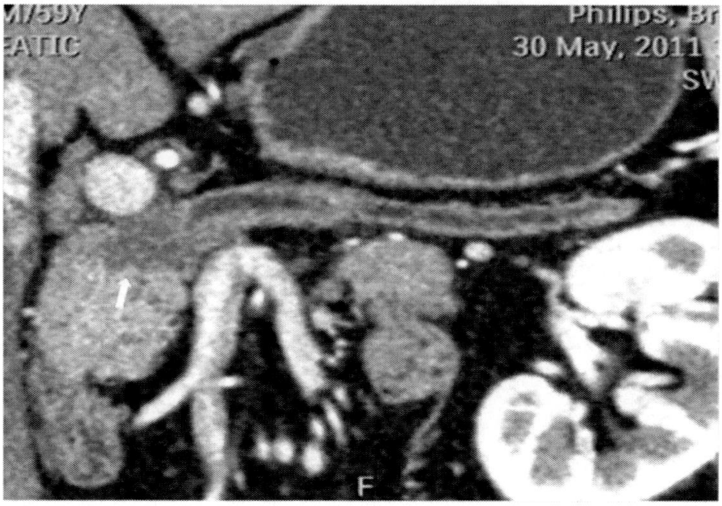

Figure 22. Abdominal CT in pancreatic ductal carcinoma: Pancreatic phase of enhancement, curved reconstruction along the course of MPD: Hypoattenuating lesion (pancreatic cancer) obstructing the main pancreatic duct (white arrow), causing upstream dilatation and distal atrophic changes.

Secondary signs of malignancy include loss of normal lobulation of the pancreatic parenchyma along with CBD and MPD narrowing or obstruction with upstream dilatation and distal pancreatic atrophic changes (Figure 22) [53, 54].

Vascular involvement may be related to venous or arterial infiltration. The most commonly affected veins are the SMV, portal and splenic vein respectively depending on the primary tumor location (Figure 23). The most commonly involved arteries can include the GDA, SMA, inferior pancreaticoduodenal artery (IPDA), splenic artery, CHA and celiac trunk as well. The T3 stage refers to extension of the tumor outside the pancreas with respect to the celiac trunk or the SMA.

On the contrary, T4 stage suggests involvement of relevant vascular structures (Figure 24). The location of the pancreatic tumor determines its local spread and potential infiltration of major vessels. Gradual development of pancreatic tail lesions often involves the splenic vessels and the splenorenal ligament (Figure 25).

Moreover, a tumor that is located in the body of the pancreas may spread to involve the celiac trunk and its branches. A body tumor if large enough can extend caudally to involve the SMA. A tumor located in the anterior head and neck of the pancreas may spread to involve the GDA, CHA and the gastrocolic trunk respectively. A tumor of the posterior neck and head of the pancreas typically can involve the PV as well as the portal venous confluence, the SMV and the SMA.

Finally, an uncinate tumor tends to typically track along the IPDA and may secondarily involve the jejunal and the mesenteric vessels [55].

A relatively new category is emerging from pancreatic cancer staging called "borderline resectable" tumors. The amount of extension or involvement of the celiac artery or SMA can vary on CT evaluation [56]. The term "abutment or involvement" has been designated to correspond to extension of tumors that involve less than 180° of the circumference of the vessel while the term "encasement" has been proposed to refer to development of the tumor more than 180° of the circumference of the vessel.

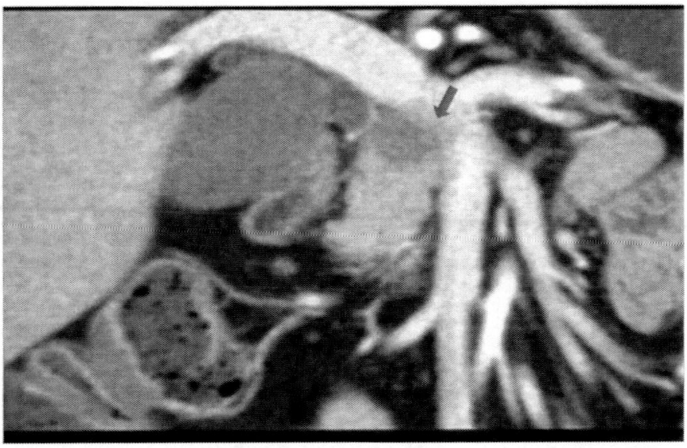

Figure 23. Abdominal CT in pancreatic ductal carcinoma: Portal phase of enhancement coronal reconstruction: Pancreatic neck cancer invading the splenomesenteric confluence and the proximal portal vein (thick blue arrow).

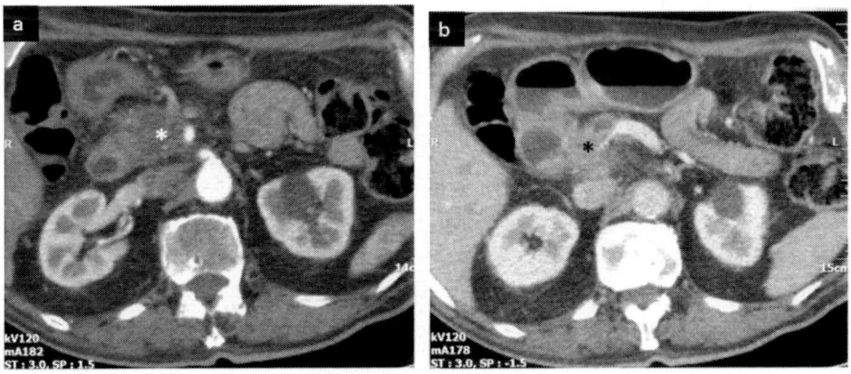

Figure 24. Abdominal CT in pancreatic ductal carcinoma: Pancreatic phase of enhancement: a) Pancreatic tumor encasing the superior mesenteric artery (white asterisk) b) Encasing of the superior mesenteric vein and the splenomesenteric confluence (black asterisk).

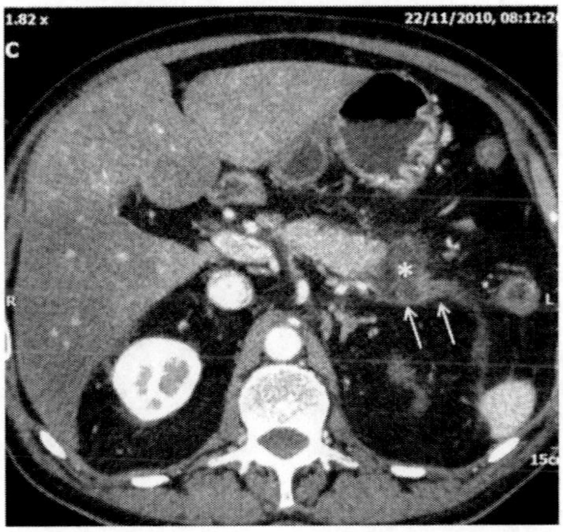

Figure 25. Abdominal CT in pancreatic ductal carcinoma: Pancreatic phase of enhancement: Inhomogeneous necrotic lesion at the pancreatic tail (blue circle), invading the perirenal fascia (white arrows).

Borderline resectable tumors are defined as lesions that abut or encase a short segment of the common hepatic artery without involvement of the celiac artery, abut the SMA or may cause short segment occlusion of the SMV, PV or the portal venous confluence with suitable veins above and below the level of the occlusion for venous reconstruction (Figure 26).

The importance of the borderline resectable category is that affected patients appear with CT findings that preclude immediate surgery due to high risk for a margin positive resection [57]. These patients are typically treated with neoadjuvant chemotherapy or combined chemoradiation therapy. Advantages of neoadjuvant chemoradiation include optimal patient selection for surgical intervention by excluding those patients with progressive disease on therapy and by initiating immediate treatment to prevent systemic spread.

Recently defined CT criteria for vascular involvement in pancreatic adenocarcinoma in comparison with surgical results confirm that identification of fat plane (type A) or normal pancreatic parenchyma (type B) separating the tumor from adjacent vessels predict tumor resectability in 95% of selected patients. When the tumor is inseparable from the vessels but the points of contact form a convexity against the vascular structure (type C), CT is not reliable in predicting vascular involvement.

When the tumor is partially encircling (type D) the vessel, the tumor is fixed against the vessels in the majority of the cases. Forty seven percent of these patients are resectable but relevant procedure usually involves venous resection as well.

When the tumor is completely encircling (type E) or occluding (type F) the vessel, 100% of the lesions could not be resected with a negative margin. This yielded a sensitivity of 84% and a specificity of 98% [55].

Detailed anatomy of the peripancreatic lymph nodes was originally described by the Japanese Pancreatic Society. The T, N, and M categories all independently influence survival of pancreatic carcinoma [58]. Nevertheless, nodal involvement has been reported the strongest predictor of poor survival after pancreatic resection for invasive pancreatic adenocarcinoma. The presence of GDA node positivity shares a poor prognosis similar to that of metastatic disease spread to the peritoneum or liver. The incidence of nodal involvement is 72-83% on autopsy series [59].

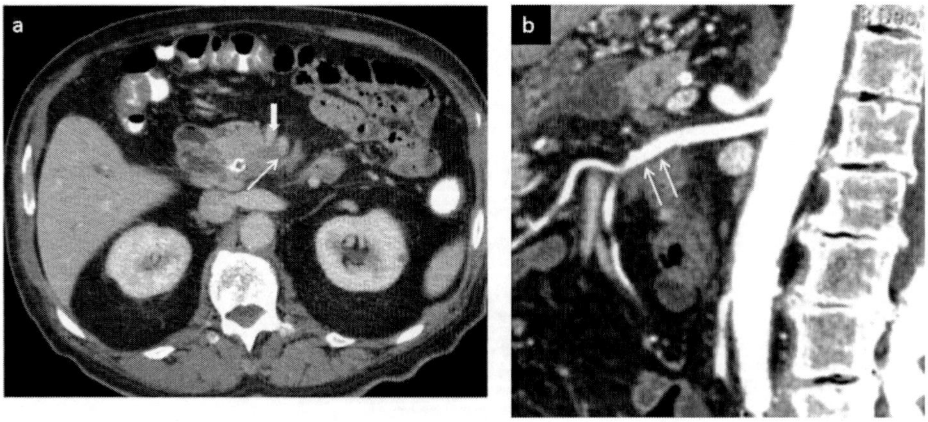

Figure 26. Abdominal CT in pancreatic ductal carcinoma: Abdominal CT: a) Portal phase of enhancement: Pancreatic tumor abutting the superior mesenteric artery, tear drop sign of the superior mesenteric vein (thick white arrow) b) Pancreatic phase of enhancement sagittal reformation: Pancreatic tumor abutting the superior mesenteric artery (thin white arrows).

CT accuracy for nodal staging is 44-47% after meticulous correlation of imaging findings with pathology results. In addition, detection of ovoid nodal shape, clustering of nodes and the absence of a fatty hilum are not useful predictors of malignancy on CT [60]. Moreover, the incidence of con-peritoneal involvement is between 40-55%. While the most common CT finding is that of peritoneal thickening, small nodules and ascites, larger peritoneal implants and omental caking may be encountered. Additional liver metastases are typically low attenuation lesions and may present perilesional enhancement on the pancreatic parenchymal phase, which fades on the portal phase of enhancement.

Nevertheless, detection of small volume liver metastases and peritoneal implants remains challenging despite the use of CT in the preoperative staging of pancreatic adenocarcinoma [61, 62]. Finally, the most common appearance of pulmonary metastases is lung nodules with irregular or speculated borders. However, lung metastases with a diffuse air space pattern or with lymphangitic carcinomatosis may be recognized [63].

Magnetic Resonance Imaging – Magnetic Resonance Cholangiopancreatography

Pancreatic ductal adenocarcinoma typically manifests as an infiltrating poorly defined mass, desmoplastic in nature, with sparse vascularity. This histology contrasts with that of normal pancreatic parenchyma. For this reason, small tumors are well seen as relatively low signal intensity poorly defined lesions on fat suppressed T1 weighted images against the normal high signal intensity of uninvolved pancreatic parenchyma (Figure 27) [64].

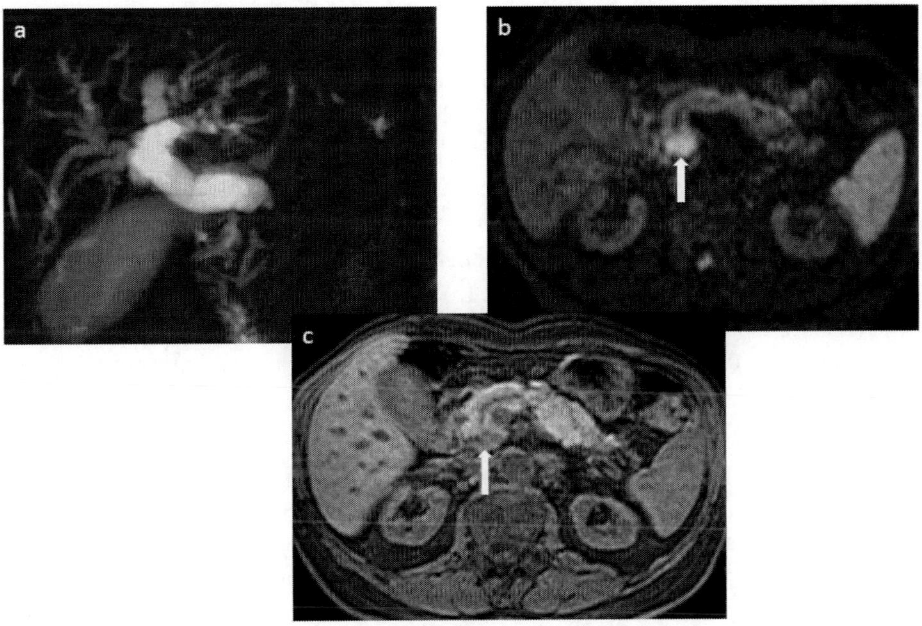

Figure 27. Abdominal MRI demonstrating a small pancreatic ductal carcinoma: a) MRCP: Obstruction of the common bile duct with proximal dilatation of the billiary ducts b) Diffusion Weighted Image: Hyperintense lesion (restricted diffusion pattern) at the pancreatic head (thick white arrow) c) 3D T1 Fat Suppressed image: Hypointense lesion at the pancreatic head (thick white arrow).

Pancreatic cancer is most conspicuous on the arterial phase of dynamic gadolinium imaging against the prominently enhancing capillary rich uninvolved surrounding pancreatic parenchyma. Close attention to technique, particularly timing, is vital [65].

On delayed, interstitial phase images, the appearance of pancreatic cancer can be very variable. Small pancreatic tumors can present a variable enhancement pattern, ranging from hypointense to slightly hyperintense on delayed images and may actually show rim enhancement. In contrast, large pancreatic ductal adenocarcinomas tend to remain low in signal intensity on delayed images [66].

Often pancreatic tissue proximal to pancreatic cancer may be lower in signal intensity than the normal gland. This typically occurs as a consequence of tumor associated pancreatitis secondary to the obstruction of the MPD. The greater the resultant progression to fibrosis and glandular atrophy from long standing pancreatic ductal obstruction, the less conspicuous the pancreatic carcinoma. For this reason, all sequences must be carefully evaluated to define the true extent of the tumor. The combined MRI features of a focal pancreatic mass, pancreatic duct dilatation and parenchymal atrophy are highly suggestive of ductal adenocarcinoma. However, it should be noted that it may be impossible to accurately differentiate pancreatic adenocarcinoma from focal chronic pancreatitis [67]. Comparing MR imaging with CT, several studies suggest that MRI is comparable to the detection and staging of pancreatic cancer. Recent meta-analysis of 68 studies revealed the sensitivity of MRI to be 84% versus 91% for helical CT in the evaluation of pancreatic adenocarcinoma. The sensitivity to resectability was equal for both MR and helical CT (82 and 81%). It has been suggested that due to MRI's inherently higher soft tissue contrast, the recognition of subtle pancreatic lesions could be potentially improved over CT [68].

Because of the heavily T2 weighted nature of MRCP imaging, what is visualized on this diagnostic modality is the effect of tumor on a fluid filled duct. The lesion itself is not commonly seen. For this reason, a comprehensive workup of a pancreatic mass typically includes additional sequences including dynamically enhanced imaging. The double duct sign indicating the obstruction of both the CBD and the MPD was described initially on ERCP, but this sign can also be identified with other modalities such as MRCP. More commonly depicted are ductal stenoses or associated obstruction. Nevertheless, although the double duct sign, when confirmed at MRCP, is highly suggestive of pancreatic head malignancy, it is not pathognomonic [69]. On MRCP, the "duct penetrating sign" has been suggested as a means to distinguish an inflammatory pancreatic mass from pancreatic carcinoma.

This sign is encountered in 85% of chronic pancreatitis and only 4% of patients with cancer and refers to the visualization of the MPD penetrating an inflammatory pancreatic mass rather than the complete obstruction seen commonly with pancreatic carcinoma (Figure 28) [64]. Some studies have reported the specificity of this sign being as high as 100% for benign stricture. Therefore, it has been suggested that MRCP may provide a benefit in differentiating benign lesions from malignancy [70]. Another important factor to consider is that seeing a normal sized pancreatic duct on MRCP in the setting of extrahepatic biliary obstruction should not be interpreted as excluding the possibility of pancreatic carcinoma. Indeed, it has been reported that the caliber of the MPD can be normal in up to 20% of patients with pancreatic malignancy causing bile duct obstruction. Finally, when MRCP is used in combination with a dynamic MR examination of the pancreas, comprehensive preoperative imaging can be accomplished to facilitate the detection and preoperative staging of a pancreatic cancer.

Meticulous evaluation of the combined use of MRI and MRCP in the diagnostic procedures of pancreatic neoplastic disease showed a sensitivity of 87%, a specificity of 97%, and an accuracy of 95% [71]. It is also important to note that the isolated obstruction of the pancreatic duct, even in the absence of a pancreatic mass, should be viewed with great suspicion for the possibility of an underlying tumor. Accurate staging is of particular importance for pancreatic cancer because of the aggressive nature of the disease.

Overstaging can prevent patients from potentially curative surgical intervention. On the contrary, understaging can subject patients to unnecessary morbidity from futile surgery. Complete surgical resection is only possible in the absence of metastatic disease and in those patients in whom the tumor can be removed in its entirety with negative surgical margins (R0 resection) [72]. Patients with locally advanced ductal adenocarcinoma of the pancreas subjected to surgery with macroscopic positive margins (R2 resection) have no survival benefit over those who receive palliative care.

Therefore, accurate pretreatment staging is crucial to correctly identify surgical candidates and differentiate them from patients with unresectable disease [73]. Recent advances in surgical technique with venous interposition grafts has impacted on patients previously considered with unresectable disease and moved them into the potentially resectable category. Advances in chemotherapy, surgery, and radiation, including protocols of combined preoperative therapeutic approach, can potentially result in downstaging of patients with previously unresectable tumors. The demand for accurate preoperative evaluation of treatment planning has placed added responsibility on radiology to precisely assess the local extent of disease. Furthermore, in those patients who are considered resectable, imaging is also expected to provide an accurate roadmap in order to facilitate surgical planning.

Accurate preoperative staging of pancreatic cancer requires a careful evaluation of tumor infiltration into the major peripancreatic arteries. The same principles and grading system have been applied in the literature to contrast enhanced CT and MRI [74].

Most studies have shown MRI to be comparable to CT regarding the accuracy of staging. Early investigations comparing MRI with helical CT showed MRI to be equal to, or even possibly slightly better than, helical CT.

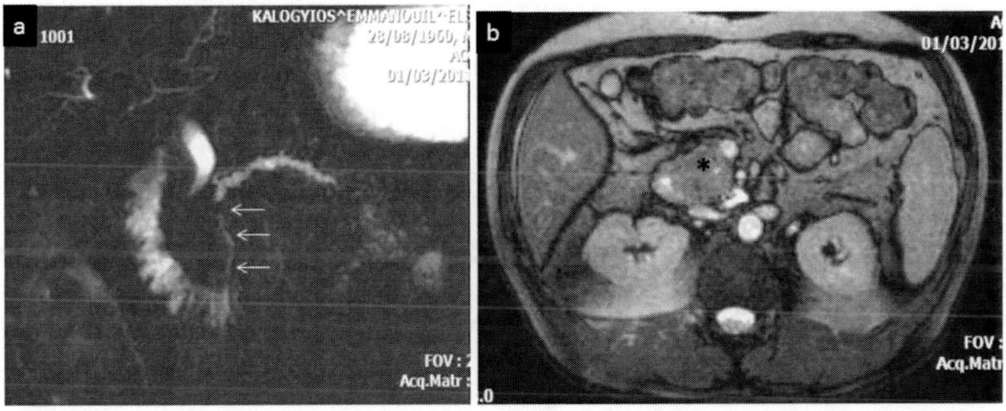

Figure 28. Abdominal MRI: a) MRCP, b) T2W image: Irregular dilatation with segmental stenoses of the main pancreatic duct, penetrating a solid lesion (black asterisk) at the pancreatic head with concomitant dilatation of the common bile duct (thin white arrows). This is a penetrating duct sign in a case of focal pancreatitis.

Recently, with the major advance of multidetector CT (MDCT) technology, which continues to evolve, the difference between MRI and CT has narrowed. In the past, the involvement of the PV or SMV was considered a contraindication to surgery. However, with the development of venous bypass grafts, venous involvement is no longer considered necessarily unresectable disease, but this is not necessarily the case at all institutions [75]. Careful description by radiologists of the extent of venous involvement is therefore necessary for surgical planning. The signs of venous vascular invasion are similar on both CT and MR imaging and refer to occlusion, deformity of the vascular contour including "beaking" and tumor vessel contiguity greater than half the circumference of the vessel.

With recent advances in surgical technique, particularly in venous resection and reconstruction with interposition venous grafts, tumor involvement limited to the PV or SMV can be considered for potentially curative resection. It is now possible in certain institutions to resect and reconstruct the SMV and PV as long as the vessel remains patent with normal flow and adequate distal (PV) and proximal (SMV) margins free of tumor can be obtained [76]. Vascular encasement is best demonstrated on MR imaging with contrast enhanced 3D spoiled gradient echo images with thin sections, which may be reviewed in the axial plane or reconstructed in the coronal or sagittal planes. Coronal and sagittal reconstructions may be of value to illustrate the length of tumor involvement of the vessel in question as this information has important implications for surgical planning [77].

In certain institutions, long segment (more than 2cm) encasement or occlusion of the SMV or PV is a relative contraindication to vascular reconstructive surgery, although the boundaries of resectable disease appear to be continually changing. In addition, attention to variant venous anatomy is now important, and certain anatomic variations may render venous reconstructions difficult or even impossible. As an illustration, multiple jejunal branches inserting high on the SMV near the PV may preclude an adequate proximal surgical margin for an interpositioned venous graft.

It is important to note that the location of the pancreatic tumor determines the primary route of spread and the regional nodal groups involved. The secondary drainage usually describes the nodal stations in the porta hepatis, celiac axis, and nodes along the root of the small bowel mesentery. The para-aortic nodal stations represent third order lymphatic drainage and are considered distant nodal metastases. Cross sectional imaging modalities such as CT and MRI traditionally rely on size to discriminate between normal and metastatic lymph nodes, and therefore both techniques suffer from poor sensitivity and specificity for the detection of nodal metastases. The high prevalence of nodal micrometastases in pancreatic cancer makes nodal enlargement a poor predictor of nodal involvement. Using a criterion of greater than 1cm in short axis diameter for metastatic nodes on helical CT yields a sensitivity of only 14%, specificity of 85%, positive predictive value (PPV) of 17%, and negative predictive value (NPV) of 82% [78]. Another confounding factor is that of superimposed inflammatory changes. Pancreatitis can complicate the diagnosis of pancreatic cancer, particularly, following invasive diagnostic procedures such as ERCP. The inflammatory changes may result in reactive peripancreatic lymphadenopathy, contributing to an overall low staging accuracy for CT and MRI.

On MRI, lymph nodes are well demonstrated on T2 weighted sequences with fat suppression and interstial phase gadolinium enhanced fat suppressed images. Lymph nodes appear as well defined moderately hyperintense oval masses against a background of low signal intensity with both techniques.

On T1 weighted images without fat saturation lymph nodes appear as low signal intensity oval masses in a background of high signal intensity fat. Imaging in the coronal plane may be helpful for the identification of mesenteric and peripancreatic nodes.

Pancreatic cancer frequently metastasizes to the liver and the detection and the characterization of hepatic lesions in the setting of pancreatic malignancy are of paramount importance and are achieved through differences in signal intensity between the metastatic implants and the adjacent liver parenchyma. High sensitivity for lesion assessment and specificity for lesion characterization are achieved by selecting the appropriate imaging protocol consisting of T2 weighted sequences, T1 weighted gradient echo images pre-contrast, and dynamic gadolinium enhanced gradient echo images with fat suppression. Most hepatic metastases are of lower signal than the surrounding hepatic parenchyma on T1 weighted sequences, which is in contradistinction to lesions of hepatocellular origin, such as focal nodular hyperplasia (FNH) or well differentiated hepatocellular carcinoma (HCC), which appear isointense to normal liver.

Furthermore, T1 weighted gradient echo in and out of phase sequences are very helpful to demonstrate focal fatty infiltration and sparing as well. These entities are known to decrease lesion conspicuity on CT, contributing to the lower sensitivity of this imaging modality for lesion detection in the setting of hepatic steatosis. T2 weighted sequences possess higher sensitivity to hepatic metastases than unenhanced T1 weighted images. Metastases usually appear as focal areas of moderately high signal on T2 weighted images in comparison with the remainder of the hepatic parenchyma.

Moreover, a broad range of MR imaging sequences and MR specific contrast agents is available to detect and characterize liver lesions. Finally, the appearance of peritoneal metastases on MR imaging ranges from small well demarcated nodules to diffuse thickening of the peritoneal lining, both of which usually show enhancement on T1 weighted fat suppressed sequences. The detection of small peritoneal nodules on cross sectional imaging involves a meticulous evaluation of the peritoneal cavity and its many recesses. Several studies have shown that dynamic contrast enhanced MR imaging is equal to or superior to contrast enhanced CT for the detection of peritoneal metastases [79].

Positron Emission Tomography

Currently CT is the modality of choice for diagnosing and staging pancreatic adenocarcinoma, because of its better spatial resolution and the ability to generate 3D images and multiplanar reformations. However, sometimes it is difficult to differentiate mass forming chronic pancreatitis, post treatment fibrosis from pancreatic adenocarcinoma and tumors less than 2cm in diameter [80].

Therefore, the utility of PET imaging is being explored to overcome some of these limitations. PET is an imaging technique that provides exclusive information about the molecular and metabolic changes associated with disease. The last years, remarkable improvements in technology, the routine availability of medical cyclotrons (to produce the necessary short lived positron emitters), and favorable reimbursement decisions have led to an increase in the use of this technology. The currently available agent for clinical use in published reports to evaluate pancreatic cancer with PET is the FDG. PET is a noninvasive method of tissue characterization based on specific tissue metabolism.

There are a few other investigational radiotracers available to image pancreatic cancer such as (18)F fluorothymidine (FLT) PET/CT, 11C harmine (a MAO A inhibitor) and (1 11C) acetate as well [81, 82].

In 1956, Warburg described that, malignant cells demonstrated increased glucose consumption. This high gylcolytic rate in malignant cells forms the basis of PET imaging. Several early comparative studies have shown FDG PET to be more accurate than conventional imaging techniques in diagnosing pancreatic carcinoma [83]. However, more recent surveys have shown that the role of FDGPET is still very controversial and suggest that there may be a complementary role of FDG PET to conventional CT imaging. A well-documented meta-analysis demonstrated that in the 387 patients studied, the weighted average sensitivity and specificity of FDG PET were 94 and 90% respectively compared with 82 and 75% for CT [84]. Nevertheless, a more recent investigation elucidates that FDG PET presents a lower sensitivity than CT and does not add additional information to the contrast enhanced CT. Therefore, FDG PET is helpful in the diagnostic approach of patients in whom CT does not identify a mass and in detection of metastatic disease [85].

Due to the high quality of cross sectional imaging, increasing number of patients are being diagnosed with cystic lesions the pancreas. However the conventional imaging techniques are limited in their ability to confidently distinguish benign from malignant cystic neoplasms. The presence of mural nodularity, internal septations, wall thickening and calcification is considered a predictor of malignancy on CT depiction. The presence of focal FDG activity within these lesions, irrespective of lesion morphology therefore provides a significant advantage to detect malignancy [86]. The importance of this finding lies in the fact that when FDG PET is used in the proper clinical setting of asymptomatic and high risk patients, lack of activity within a known cystic mass can reliably exclude malignancy and may help prevent unnecessary surgery.

Due to its low spatial resolution, FDG PET has a limited role in the T staging of pancreatic cancer. The extent of the tumor into the peripancreatic tissues and the adjacent vessels cannot be outlined. Therefore, conventional cross sectional imaging modalities, particularly multiphasic contrast enhanced multi detector helical CT and MRI can better demonstrate the relationship between the tumor, the adjacent organs, and the vascular structures. Currently no data supports the routine use of dual modality PET CTor FDG PET in the local T staging of pancreatic adenocarcinoma. In N staging of disease, both FDG PET and CT perform poorly. Reported sensitivities and specificities for FDG PET are 46% and 63% respectively [87]. The low sensitivity of FDG PET to detect locoregional adenopathy is attributed to the close proximity of the peripancreatic lymph nodes to the primary tumor, which can lead to a partial volume averaging effect and thereby obscure tumor in the nodal structures [88]. In addition, FDG uptake in the peripancreatic lymph nodes is nonspecific; particularly, reactive adenopathy can be avid or "hot" on FDG PET and may be encountered after biopsy of the primary pancreatic neoplasm.

FDG PET has the ability to identify distant metastases. In a large series of patients with pancreatic malignancies, reported sensitivity and specificity of FDG PET for detecting hepatic metastases > 1cm was respectively 68% and 95%. Smaller lesions could be detected with the same specificity but lower sensitivity of 43% [89].

The most important cause of false positives in these studies was intrahepatic cholestasis. FDG PET may detect occult peritoneal metastases, but only with difficulty. In approximately 25% of cases, however, poorly localized and microscopic disease may not be confirmed.

The utility of PET still remains controversial as some authors suggest that does not provide any additional information whereas other investigators support that it is complementary to conventional imaging in detecting distant metastases [90]. In conclusion, FDG PET has not yet been shown to be a valid population wide screening tool or to have a clear role in routine imaging related to the management of pancreatic cancer, including diagnosis, staging or prognostication.

As FDG PET has poor anatomical definition and spatial resolution capabilities, CT and EUS may be best suited to local staging of pancreatic disease to determine if the patient is a surgical candidate. To achieve this modality's full potential, combined PET CT should be performed, with the CT component optimized with intravenous contrast to provide full diagnostic information. However, the best use of PET CT must be further investigated to clearly define the criteria where the addition of FDG PET to CT would be additive. The existing evidence suggests that FDG PET has limited utility in initial staging. The strength of functional imaging lies in its ability to detect pathology, irrespective of lesion morphology.

This innate property gives FDG PET its strength in detecting small as well as cystic lesions and in differentiating benign from malignant disease. Thus, FDG PET may sometimes change the management strategy by providing a more precise diagnosis.

Endoscopic Ultrasonography

Pancreatic cancers are usually visualized on EUS as more or less well demarcated echo poor lesions, which depending on their exact morphology and size are homogeneous or inhomogeneous, with echo rich spots or even cystic spaces (Figure 29, 30) [91]. Nevertheless, small pancreatic carcinomas can also be recognized as echo poor and well demarcated lesions, thus resembling pancreatic tumors of the endocrine type, or display a pattern of focal inhomogeneity. With more advanced tumor stages, pancreatic cancers become more inhomogeneous and start to infiltrate into neighboring organs and major vascular structures [92]. Various criteria have been initiated to demonstrate vascular involvement in pancreatic cancer including lack of the hyperechoic interface between the vessel wall and the tumor, tumor infiltration in the vascular lumen, lack of visualization of a major vessel in the presence of collateral ones, or other indirect signs such as proximity of the tumor mass to vessels, or even mass size [93]. The accuracy and usefulness of these criteria remains under debate. In most cases of pancreatic cancer, some suspicion has already been raised by other imaging modalities before EUS is performed to visualize and stage the disease.

As previously mentioned, patients presenting with clinical evidence of a pancreatic neoplasm are initially imaged with transabdominal U/S. If the suspicion is further confirmed, a CT and/or EUS are usually suggested. Which examination should be performed first remains a topic of dispute. Despite attempts to gather objective data to answer the question, constant advancements in imaging technology render this a difficult task. Thus, despite existing reports (which are evolving and ambiguous anyway), the decision of the imaging procedure of choice for the management of pancreatic tumors is mostly dependent on test availability, local expertise, and referral patterns in everyday practice. Therefore, due to the wide access to helical CT scanners, CT is usually proposed prior to EUS in most centers. Combining clinical and laboratory data, together with initial imaging procedures in many cases is enough to confirm the diagnosis; further diagnostic evaluation is then unnecessary.

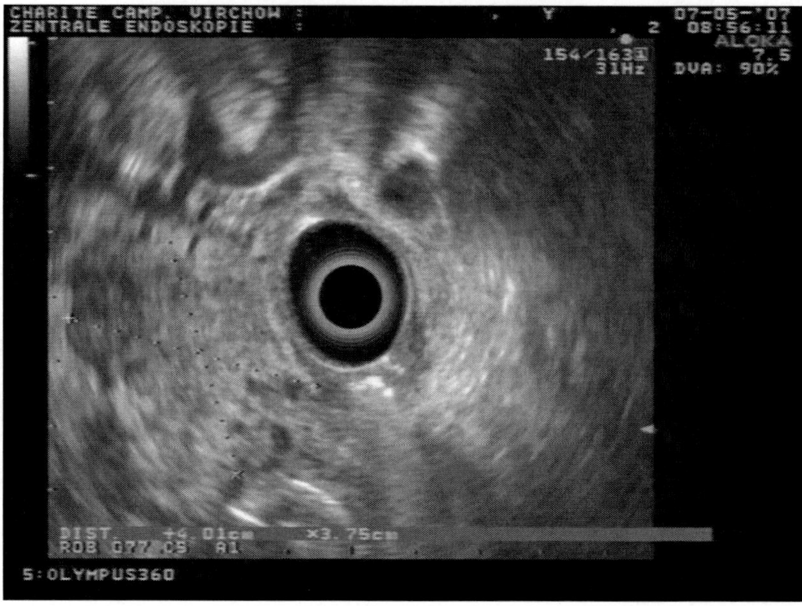

Figure 29. Radial EUS depiction of a relatively well demarcated echo poor lesion with inhomogeneous, echo rich spots indicative of a ductal adenocarcinoma of the pancreas.

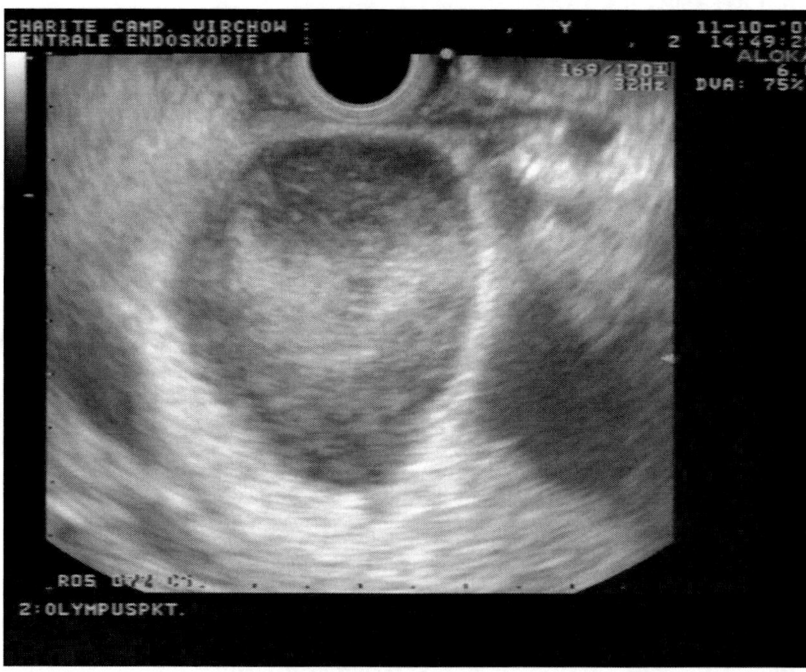

Figure 30. Linear EUS detection of a less demarcated echo poor pancreatic adenocarcinoma with cystic spaces within.

There are cases, however, in which diagnosis of a pancreatic neoplasm may be less clear cut, especially when the original nature of a pancreatic mass remains vague. The frequent situation of questionable pancreatic head enlargement on routine CT remains an important indication for EUS [94].

Multiple imaging tests including EUS, CT, MRI, and perhaps PET compete as to which examination or combination of diagnostic modalities is the most preferable in these settings. Several studies have supported superiority of EUS in comparison with other imaging techniques, especially when small tumors are concerned, beginning from the method's initial steps [95]. The ability of performing FNA during the diagnostic procedure has to be regarded as an additional advantage of EUS (Figure 31). Tumor detection with EUS has remained consistently high throughout the years, as long as we are dealing with focal masses outside of full blown chronic pancreatitis [96]. On the other hand, the pancreas is screened stepwise from several stations in duodenum and stomach and there is no systematic study that has actually evaluated the real ability of EUS to fully cover the pancreas. Image quality probably also plays a pivotal role in the detection of subtle pancreatic malignancy. Additionally, electronic EUS scanning also provides the expanded diagnostic possibilities of modern U/S technologies. Pancreatic EUS images acquired by tissue harmonic imaging were assessed as significantly clearer compared with those obtained by standard imaging. In the difficult issue of differential diagnosis between benign and malignant pancreatic mass lesions, good sensitivity and specificity values were reported for the clinical use of power Doppler and contrast enhanced EUS. However, it is apparent that these results need to withstand the test of time and be further assessed by well-documented surveys [97].

The major advantage of EUS for pancreatic cancer detection even in the era of recent imaging advances seems to be its high negative predictive value. Recent data support that absence of a circumscript mass on EUS performed by an expert endosonographer can reliably exclude pancreatic cancer, especially when the pretest probability is low or indeterminate [98]. Comparisons of EUS with other imaging modalities show that, although it is not a 100% foolproof method, EUS still remains one of the best choices to detect a pancreatic neoplasm.

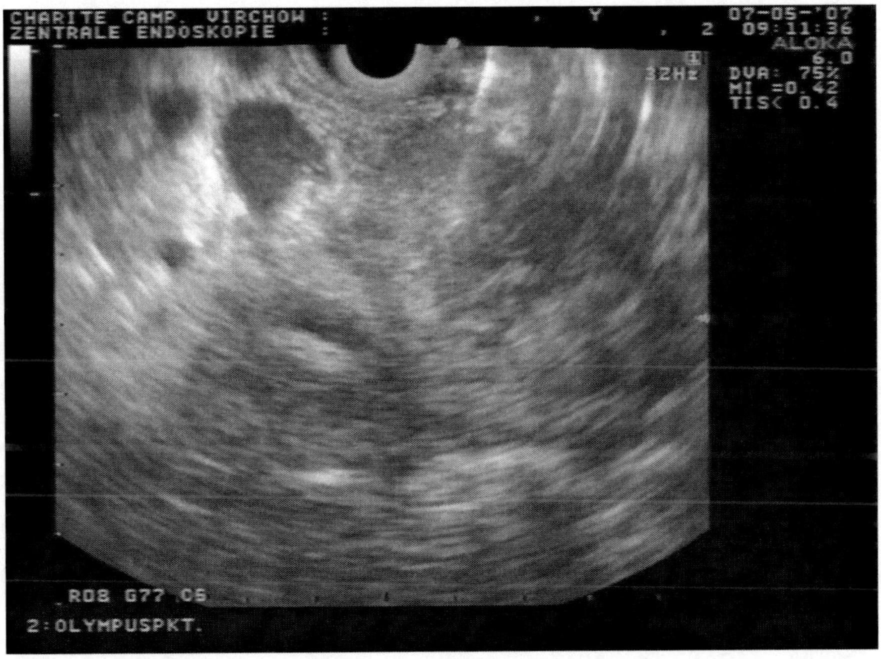

Figure 31. EUS FNA diagnostic procedure for pancreatic adenocarcinoma.

However, it should be emphasized that many of the studies comparing EUS and other cross sectional imaging techniques are characterized by the absence of blinding amongst examiners, and therefore, an objective evaluation of superiority of one test over another is inaccurate [99]. In everyday clinical practice, the role of CT, EUS, and the other imaging tests that might be available is rather complementary concerning the diagnosis and staging of pancreatic cancer.

EUS FNA is currently an established minimally invasive means of tissue acquisition, the implementation of which decisively broadened the spectrum of EUS by allowing direct transmural diagnosis (Figure 32). EUS FNA can therefore be extremely useful for various indications such as suspected pancreatic cancer, diagnosis of pancreatic carcinoma, or differential diagnosis of a pancreatic mass or smaller lesion [100]. Although criteria of EUS FNA remain rather controversial, the palliative setting where tissue confirmation is required prior to commencing chemotherapy or combined radiochemotherapy is a definitely undisputed indication of EUS FNA.

In contrast, in most cases of resectable tumors histological proof of pancreatic carcinoma it is not useful, since complete resection of the tumor is the only potentially curative approach [101]. The sensitivity, specificity, diagnostic accuracy, positive predictive value, and negative predictive value of EUS FNA, vary in published studies, but are generally high (e.g., 83%, 90%, 85%, 100% and 80% respectively in one multicenter study) [102]. Major complications after EUS FNA are rare. The rate of false positive diagnoses from EUS FNA is low in most papers.

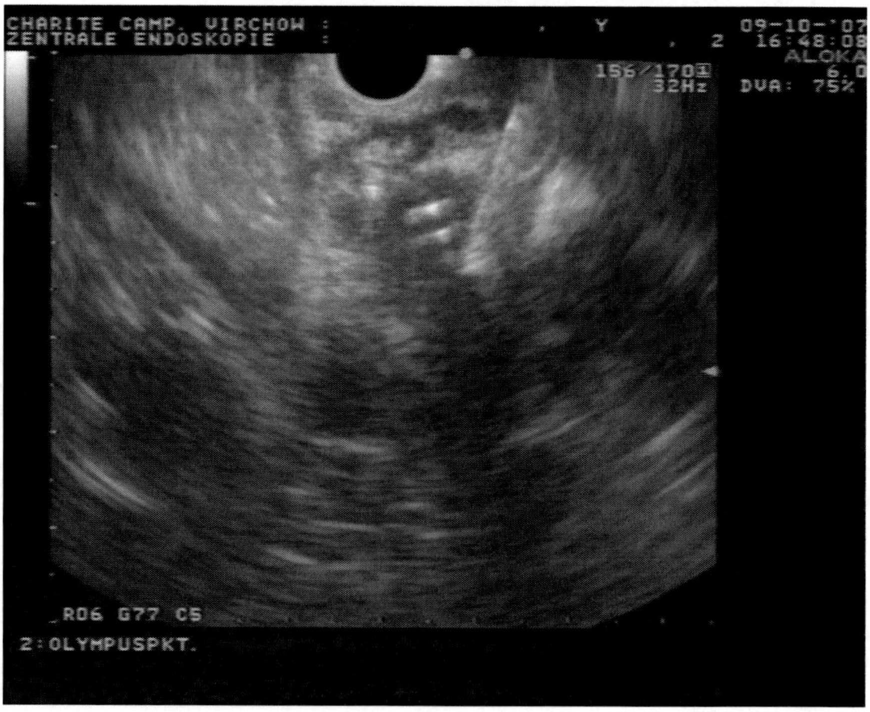

Figure 32. EUS FNA procedure for histological confirmation of an advanced ductal adenocarcinoma with previous stenting of the common bile duct.

It has been reported that false positive diagnoses are attributed to interpretation errors. It is also evident that in most cases, only a positive diagnosis of malignancy counts.

It is obvious as with other puncture techniques that EUS guided FNP is mainly established to differentiate between benign and malignant conditions, or to allow parallel cytological and histological characterization of a lesion that is strongly suspected to be malignant, but in which different tissue diagnoses result in variable treatment approaches. In principle, clinical consequences must be clear and weighted against potential procedure associated risks before a EUS FNP is performed.

If a pancreatic mass is resectable and will also be operated on even if EUS guided FNP is negative, the procedure is not clinically implemented. EUS guided FNP is, however, also beneficial when other puncture methods have failed or when they are more invasive or risky. Pancreatic malignancy can be proved with a lower sensitivity, between 70% and 85%, and the influence on outcome is less clear.

In unresectable tumors, EUS FNA is obligatory when radiochemotherapy regimens are applied, and can be performed in one step with staging and perhaps celiac plexus blockade in case of severe pain [103]. In this occasion EUS is in competition with percutaneous puncture, but it seems that EUS FNA is preferable, not only because of its high diagnostic accuracy but also due to a possibly lower tumor seeding risk due to the shorter puncture canal.

Another interesting issue is to compare the value of EUS FNA with the other most available types of tissue sampling including CT guided and ERCP based. In order to address this question, recent prospective survey performed EUS FNA in 185 patients with known or suspected pancreatic masses.

Besides displaying the superiority of EUS in tumor detection (99% sensitivity to detect a mass for EUS vs. 57% for CT, $p < 0.0001$), EUS FNA proved superior compared with both CT and ERCP based tissue sampling, even in cases when the alternative acquisition methods were negative. Equally important, these results were achieved at a very low toll of complications [104]. Performance of EUS guided FNA of local lymph nodes in pancreatic cancer also makes sense only if a positive diagnosis would alter the management.

The role of EUS in locoregional staging of pancreatic cancer has been seen throughout the years both enthusiastically reaching levels of 93% for correct T staging and 88% for N staging, as well as more skeptically, even by groups which had previously published very optimistic results.

In a retrospective review of a cohort of 89 patients who were evaluated preoperatively with EUS for pancreatic adenocarcinoma, it was concluded that EUS was finally not as accurate as previously reported and not predictive for respectability [105]. This deterioration of results over time seems somewhat peculiar in view of the advances in EUS imaging.

However, it can partially be interpreted by carefully observing the populations examined in more recent studies. Patients with evidence of unresectable disease on high quality cross sectional imaging tests are increasingly not referred for EUS. This can be displayed when noticing the relative paucity of known T4, M1 lesions. Moreover, many patients with clearly resectable disease do not always undergo EUS.

In other words, the typical patients referred for EUS staging are cases with possibly marginal indications of curative surgery without clear cut evidence of irresectability [106].

Endoscopic Retrograde Cholangiopanceatography

ERCP indicates the presence of an irregular, nodular, rat-tailed eccentric ductal obstruction. Additional localized encasement with prestenotic dilatation may be depicted. Nevertheless, parallel obstruction of MPD and CBD at the same level referring to the "Double duct" sign remains the most common indication of the presence of a pancreatic tumor.

Angiography

Conventional angiography may be effective in detecting carcinomas of the body and tail of the pancreas indicating the presence of a hypovascular tumor with concomitant narrowing of major vascular structures as a result of displacement or occlusion by the malignant lesion.

Differential Diagnosis

- ✓ Islet cell carcinoma
- ✓ Chronic pancreatitis
- ✓ Metastases
- ✓ Lymphoma

X. Pancreatic Islet Cells Tumors

Definition

Neoplasms of the endocrine pancreas (neuroendocrine tumors-NETs) are relatively uncommon. Tumors arise from pancreatic endocrine cells including islet and Langerhans cells. Some NETs are functional, secreting peptide products that produce interesting clinical presentations.

NETs that are not associated with excess hormone levels and a recognizable clinical syndrome are considered nonfunctional. Multiple endocrine neoplasia (MEN) syndromes occur when related cells cause tumors in multiple sites.

Special immunohistochemical stains allow pathologists to confirm the peptide products being produced within the cells of a NET. However, the histologic characteristics of these neoplasms do not predict their clinical behavior, and malignancy is usually determined by the presence of local invasion and lymph node or hepatic metastases.

Unfortunately, most NETs are malignant, but the course of the disease is far more favorable than that encountered with pancreatic exocrine cancer.

The key to diagnosing these rare tumors is recognition of the classic clinical syndrome; confirmation is achieved by measuring serum levels of the elevated hormone. Localization of the tumor can be a challenging step, but once accomplished, the surgery is relatively straightforward [107, 108].

Surgical Interventions

- ✓ Complete surgical excision, often accomplished with insulinomas and in a minority of gastrinomas
- ✓ Complete surgical resection or embolization for nonfunctional NETs
- ✓ Debulking procedures to controlling symptoms
- ✓ Unresectable disease in the liver is often addressed with transarterial chemoembolization

Imaging Modalities

The role of imaging modalities in cases of pancreatic NETs is to establish the diagnosis and assess tumor resectability. Advanced imaging techniques are also recommended in localizing already diagnosed functioning pancreatic NETs for subsequent surgical removal.

In incidental lesions, imaging-guided FNA may be considered, depending on the possible influence on concomitant surgical management.

Computed Tomography

In Non-Enhanced CT (NECT) scanning functional tumors are depicted as lesions varying in size with cystic and necrotic areas. Additional calcifications may be obvious; whereas small tumors may not be identified. In Contrast-Enhanced CT (CECT) images relevant neoplasms are recognized as hyperdense lesions on the arterial phase due to their hypervascular appearance (Figure 33).

In case of functional insulinomas delayed scan presents a solid/ ring enhancement pattern. Enhancing metastases in the liver and lymph nodes are also detected in the same phase. Non-functional NETs are characterized with a similar depiction in NECT imaging.

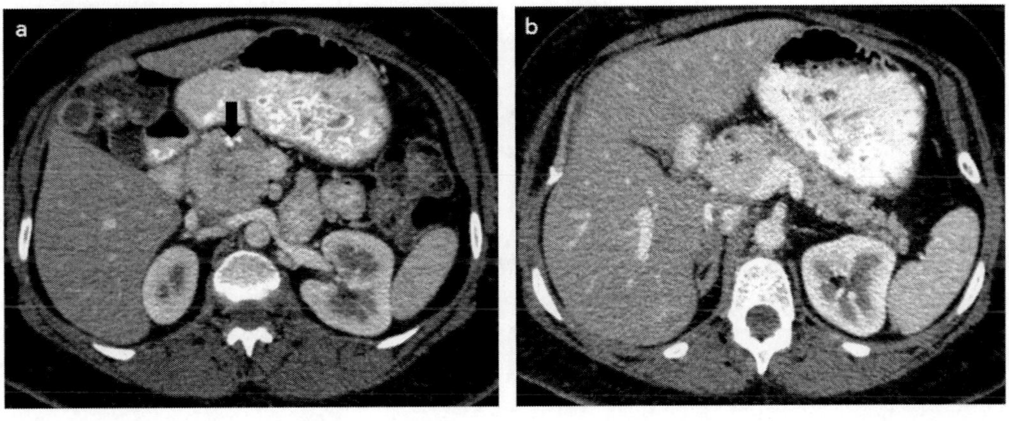

Figure 33. Abdominal CT of a non-functioning pancreatic neuroendocrine tumor: Pancreatic phase of enhancement: a, b) Hypervascular inhomogeneous pancreatic head lesion with calcifications (thick black arrow).

Nevertheless, in CECT depiction an enhancing hypervascular viable tumor as well as metastatic lesions is identified along with non-enhancing cystic or necrotic areas. Liver metastases are often extensive even in relatively healthy patients due to early invasion of PV. The presence of calcifications is indicative of local invasion and highly malignant behavior [109, 110].

Magnetic Resonance Imaging

Functional tumors behave as hypointense lesions on fat-saturated TlWI images with insulinomas presenting a solid or ring-enhancement pattern (Figure 34). Nevertheless, on delayed enhanced similar sequences NETs could be depicted as hyperintense solid enhancing lesions. On T2WI sequences both primary and secondary lesions are recognized as hyperintense areas. On the contrary, small non-functional NETs are usually isointense on T1WI images while large tumors appear heterogeneous with cystic and necrotic areas. On T2WI images increased size NETs often appear hyperintense. Finally, fat-saturated delayed enhanced TlWI sequences may reveal a small otherwise undetectable hyperintense NET [111, 112].

Endoscopic Ultrasonography

Another consistent indication for EUS is the localization of NETs, although specific limitations were recently analysed. The clinical scenario here is mostly quite different, since in functional endocrine tumors, the diagnosis is established on the basis of laboratory tests, and imaging is performed to identify the tumor for subsequent surgical removal. Problems can arise, if EUS is the only method to define the presence of the tumor, other preoperative tests are negative, palpation during surgery is doubtful and intraoperative imaging is inconclusive. Preoperative marking of the tumors has recently been suggested as a helpful adjunct but has not been extended beyond case report status [113].

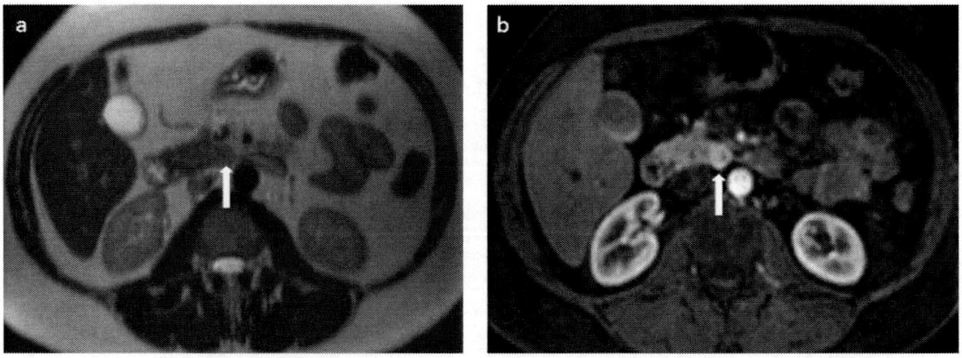

Figure 34. Abdominal MRI of an insulinoma: a) T2W image: Intermediate signal intensity lesion at the ucinate process of the pancreas (thick white arrow) b) 3D T1 Fat Suppression image: Arterial phase of enhancement: Homogeneously enhancing lesion at the ucinate process of the pancreas (thick white arrow).

The other setting are non-functional endocrine tumors which are mostly found incidentally even on transabdominal U/S [114]. They present as well demarcated, echo poor lesions in the pancreas (Figure 35, 36). FNA has been proposed to accomplish a tissue diagnosis, and further investigation from the specimens such as microsatellite loss analyses were recently performed and could be correlated to prognosis [115]. Therefore, EUS is still the diagnostic modality of choice in localizing NETs. In incidental lesions, FNA may be considered depending on the possible influcnce on subsequent management. Whether individual patients considered not being candidates for surgery can benefit from EUS-guided therapy using alcohol injection has to be evaluated [116].

Angiography

Conventional findings are indicative of hypervascular primary and secondary lesions. Subsequent hepatic venous sampling after intra-arterial stimulation of pancreas reveals elevated levels of hormones in case of functional NETs and decreased or absent elements for non-functional tumors.

Whole-Body Radionuclide Scanning

In contrast to pancreatic exocrine tumors, many of the NETs possess somatostatin receptors that allow them to be detected by a radiolabeled octreotide scan. A radioactive somatostatin analogue is injected intravenously, followed by whole-body radionuclide scanning.

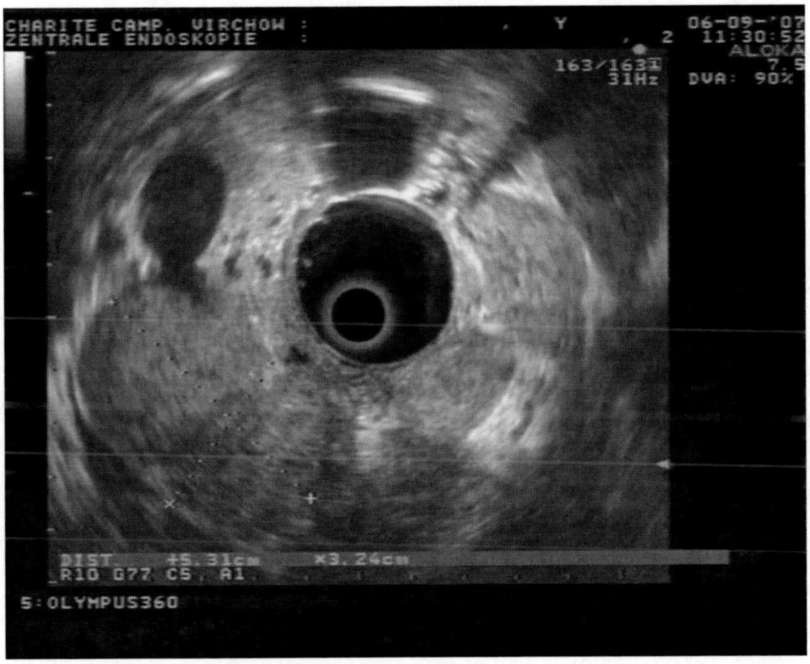

Figure 35. EUS depiction of an islet cell tumor of the tail of the pancreas.

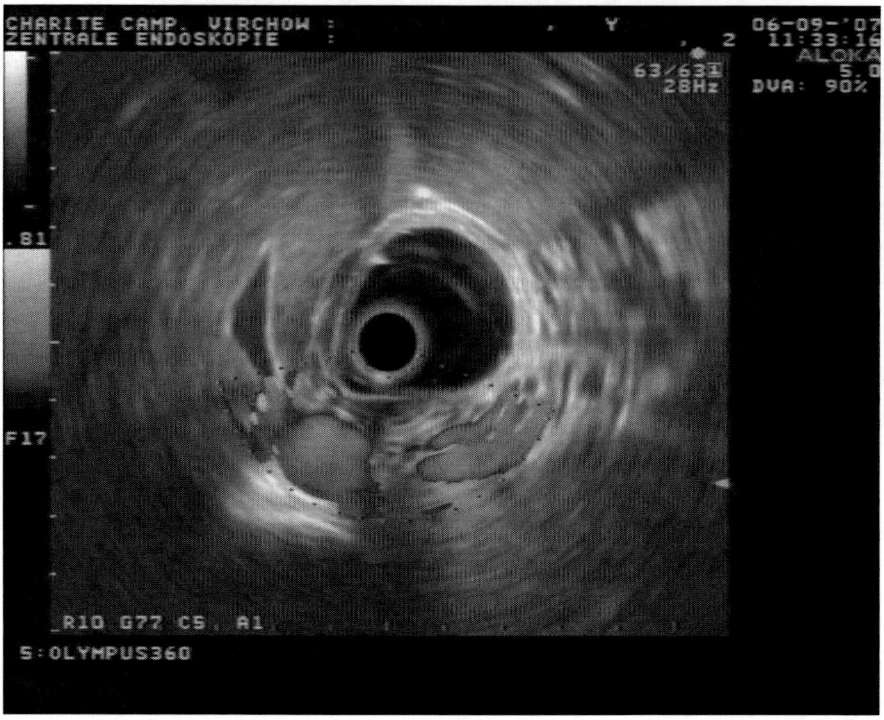

Figure 36. Power Doppler and contrast enhanced EUS findings indicative of advanced islet cell tumor of the pancreas and concomitant venous dilatation.

The success of this modality in localizing tumors and detecting metastases has decreased the use of older techniques such as angiography and selective venous sampling. Additional PET study with 68Ga (DFO)-octreotide may be complimentary in cases with disseminated disease.

Differential Diagnosis

- ✓ Pancreatic ductal adenocarcinoma
- ✓ Mucinous cystic tumor of the pancreas
- ✓ Metastases
- ✓ Serous cystadenoma of the pancreas

XI. Solid and Papillary Neoplasm

Definition

The term refers to a pancreatic mass of low malignant potential with solid and cystic features. Areas of central hemorrhage and necrosis are surrounded by solid and pseudopapillary structure [117].

Surgical Interventions

- ✓ Complete surgical excision

Imaging Modalities

The role of imaging modalities in case of solid and papillary neoplasm of the pancreas is to establish the diagnosis and assess whether surgical resection can be implemented.

Differential diagnosis of other cystic tumours categories and pseudocysts is only accomplished on the basis of specific imaging features as well as estimation of fluid aspirated with advanced imaging guided diagnostic procedures.

Ultrasound

Transabdominal U/S could only recognize fluid-debris levels with posterior enhancement.

Computed Tomography

NECT usually reveals an encapsulated, hypodense mass with limited calcification. Metastatic liver disease or lymph node involvement could rarely be encountered. In addition, on CECT images a well-defined heterogenous large mass is usually depicted.

Further low density areas of variable size within the lesion depend on the degree of concomitant hemorrhage and necrosis [118].

Magnetic Resonance Imaging

On TlWI images a large well-demarcated mass with central areas of mixed low and high signal intensity secondary to hemorrhage may be detected. The presence of capsule appears as rim of low intensity (Figure 37).

Angiography

Conventional angiography defines the presence of an avascular or hypovascular lesion depending on the degree of co-existing necrosis.

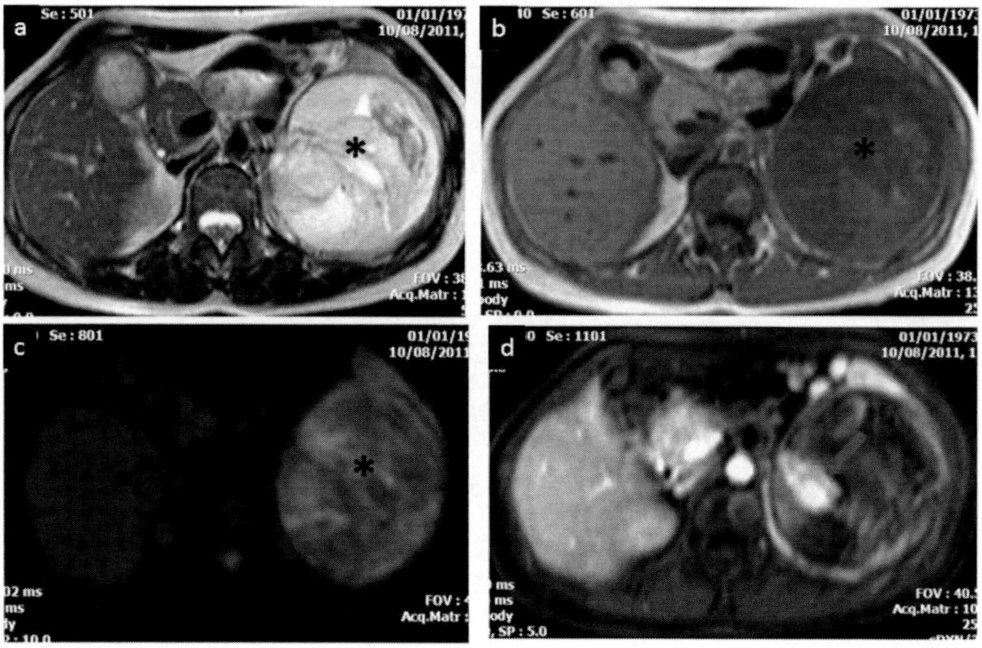

Figure 37. Abdominal MRI demonstrating a solitary pseudopapillary tumor of the pancreas: a) T2W image: Inhomogeneous predominantly high signal intensity lesion at the pancreatic tail (black asterisk), b) T1W image: Inhomogeneous predominantly low signal intensity, containing high intensity foci indicating hemorrhagic elements(black asterisk), c) Diffusion Weighted Image: Restricted diffusion pattern within the lesion (black asterisk), d) 3D T1 Fat Suppression image: Arterial phase of enhancement: Arterial enhancement of the solid portion of the lesion (thick red arrow).

Differential Diagnosis

- ✓ Pancreatic metastases
- ✓ Mucinous cystic tumor of the pancreas
- ✓ Exophytic gastric mass
- ✓ Serous cystadenoma of the pancreas
- ✓ Pseudocyst

XII. Pancreatic Lymphoma

Definition

Lymphoma can affect the pancreas. Primary involvement of the gland with no disease outside the pancreas also occurs. The clinical presentation often is similar to pancreatic adenocarcinoma, with vague abdominal pain and weight loss. Most common lymphoma is non-Hodgkin B cell subtype and is encountered usually in immunocompromised patients. Identification of a large mass often involving the head and body of the pancreas should raise suspicion. Percutaneous or EUS-guided biopsy will confirm the diagnosis in most cases.

If the diagnosis cannot be achieved preoperatively, laparoscopic exploration and biopsy are indicated [119].

Surgical Interventions

- ✓ There is no rolc for rcsection in the management of pancreatic lymphoma
- ✓ Endoscopic stenting to relieve jaundice followed by chemotherapy

Imaging Modalities

The role of imaging modalities in case of pancreatic lymphoma is to establish the diagnosis and achieve disease staging in order to avoid inadequate surgical interventions.

Differential diagnosis of other neoplastic disorders is only accomplished on the basis of specific imaging features as well as estimation of tissue aspirated with advanced imaging guided diagnostic procedures.

Computed Tomography

Pancreatic lymphoma is usually depicted as a homogeneous soft tissue mass with minimal enhancement. On occasion focal and circumscribed single or multiple masses may be encountered. Nevertheless, diffuse enlargement of pancreas with infiltrating tumor along with peri-pancreatic fat involvement could simulate acute pancreatitis (Figure 38).

Additional lymph node dissemination is often detected with lymphadenopathy below the level of renal veins consisting major determinant of the outcome. Dilatation of the pancreatic duct remains uncommon as well as encasement of the peri-pancreatic vessels [120, 121].

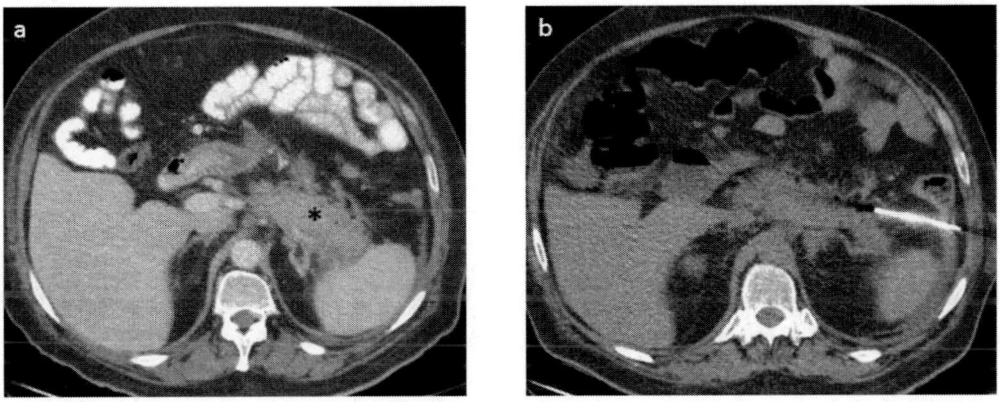

Figure 38. Abdominal CT in pancreatic lymphoma: Portal phase: a) Diffuse enlargement of the pancreatic tail in a patient with known Non Hodgkin lymphoma (black asterisk) b) Biopsy that revealed pancreatic involvement in lymphoma.

Differential Diagnosis

- ✓ Pancreatic ductal carcinoma
- ✓ Mucinous cystic tumor of the pancreas
- ✓ Pancreatic islet cell tumors

XIII. Pancreatic Metastases

Definition

The incidence of pancreatic metastases varies based on the primary malignant lesion. Solitary or multiple polypoid masses are usually recognized derived mainly from renal cell carcinoma (30%) and bronchogenic carcinoma (23%).

Cases of pancreatic secondary tumors due to advanced breast cancer, soft tissue sarcoma and primary tumors of the gastrointestinal track have also been described.

With regard to renal cell carcinoma it is common knowledge that may be isolated only to pancreas and detected occasionally several years or decades after initial diagnosis [122].

Surgical Interventions

- ✓ Surgical resection if metastasis is only isolated to the pancreas

Imaging Modalities

The role of imaging modalities in case of pancreatic metastases is to establish the diagnosis and achieve disease staging in order to avoid inadequate surgical interventions. Differential diagnosis of other neoplastic disorders is only accomplished on the basis of specific imaging features as well as estimation of tissue aspirated with advanced imaging guided diagnostic procedures.

Computed Tomography

Most common pancreatic metastases can be depicted as a discrete mass with variable enhancement pattern that usually mimics primary tumor.

Concomitant intra-abdominal metastases to the liver (36%), lymph nodes (30%) and adrenal glands (30%) may be recognized along with dilatation of the pancreatic duct or biliary tree and potential encasement of the major peri-pancreatic vascular structures [123].

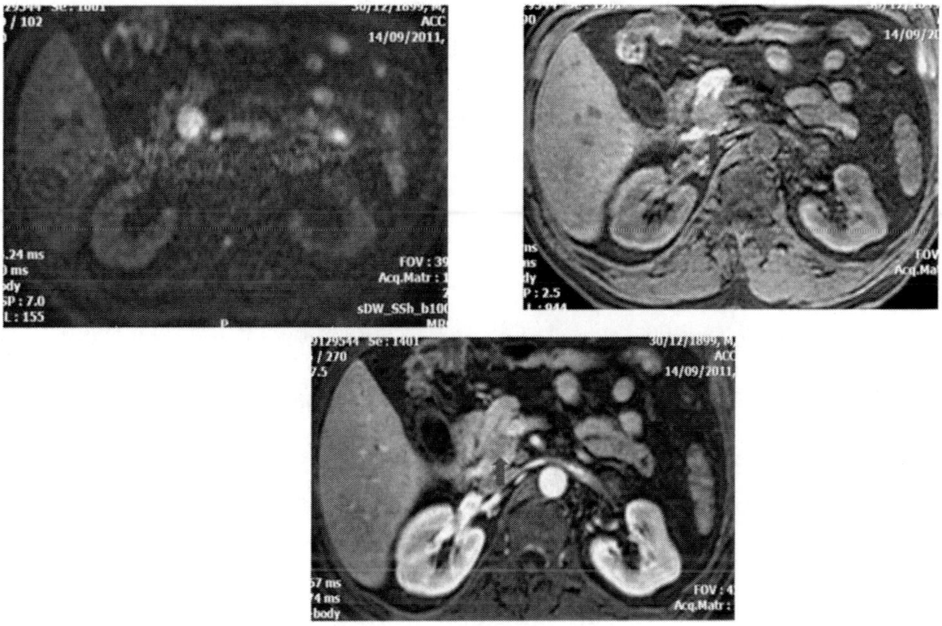

Figure 39. Abdominal MRI demonstrating metastasis to the pancreas from lung cancer. a) Diffusion Weighted image: Small hyperintense lesion (restricted diffusion pattern) at the pancreatic head (thick red arrow) b) T1 Fat Suppressed image: Hypointense lesion at the pancreatic head (thick red arrow) c) 3D T1 Fat Suppressed image after contrast medium administration: Hypovascular lesion at the pancreatic head (thick red arrow).

Magnetic Resonance Imaging

On TlWI images hypointense lesions with variable fat saturation are usually revealed. Smaller tumors present homogenous enhancement. On T2WI sequences slightly heterogenous and moderately hyperintense lesions as well as diffuse, enlarged metastases described as hypo-intense nodules may be recognized (Figure 39).

Differential Diagnosis

- ✓ Pancreatic ductal carcinoma
- ✓ Mucinous cystic tumor of the pancreas
- ✓ Pancreatic islet cell tumors

References

[1] Kamisawa, T., Yuyanq, T., Eqawa, N., et al., A new embryologic hypothesis of annular pancreas. *Hepatogastroenterology*. 2001;48(37):277-8.

[2] Harthun, N. L., Morse, J. H., Shaffer, H. A. Jr, et al., Duodenal obstruction caused by intraluminal duodenal diverticulum and annular pancreas in an adult. *Gastrointest. Endosc.* 2002;55(7):940-3.

[3] Shan, Y. S., Sy, E. D., Lin, P. W. Annular pancreas with obstructive jaundice: beware of underlying neoplasm. *Pancreas.* 2002;25(3):314-6.

[4] Lecesne, R., Stein, L., Reinhold, C., et al., MR cholangiopancreatography of annular pancreas. *J. Comput. Assist. Tomogr.* 1998;22(1):85-6.

[5] Balthazar, E. J. Acute pancreatitis: assessment of severity with clinical and CT evaluation. *Radiology.* 2002;223(3):603-13.

[6] Balthazar, E. J. Complications of acute pancreatitis: clinical and CT evaluation. *Radiol. Clin. North Am.* 2002;40(6):1211-27.

[7] Vitellas, K. M., Paulson, E. K., Enns, R. A., et al., Pancreatitis complicated by gland necrosis: evolution of findings on contrast-enhanced CT. *J. Comput. Assist. Tomogr.* 1999;23(6):898-905.

[8] Balthazar, E. J. Staging of acute pancreatitis. *Radiol. Clin. North Am.* 2002;40(6):1199-209.

[9] Zaheer, A., Singh, V. K., Qureshi, R. O., et al., The revised Atlanta classification for acute pancreatitis: updates in imaging terminology and guidelines. *Abdom. Imaging.* 2013;38(1):125-36.

[10] Aydin, H., Tatar, I. G., Hekimoglu, B. The role of diffusion weighted MR imaging in the diagnosis of acute pancreatitis. *Int. J. Emerg. Ment. Health.* 2014;16(2):308-14.

[11] Rana, S. S., Chaudhary, V., Sharma, R., et al., Comparison of abdominal ultrasound, endoscopic ultrasound and magnetic resonance imaging in detection of necrotic debris in walled-off pancreatic necrosis. *Gastroenterol. Rep.* (Oxf.). 2015 [Epub. ahead of print].

[12] Pocard, M., Soyer, P. CT of acute pancreatitis: A matter of time. *Diagn. Interv. Imaging.* 2015;96(2):129-31.

[13] Morgan, D. E., Baron, T. H., Smith, J. K., et al., Pancreatic fluid collections prior to intervention: Evaluation with MR imaging compared with CT and US. *Radiology.* 1997;203:773-8.

[14] Sriram, P. V., Kaffes, A. J., Rao, G. V., et al., Endoscopic ultrasound-guided drainage of pancreatic pseudocysts complicated by portal hypertension or by intervening vessels. *Endoscopy.* 2005;37(3):231-5.

[15] Cahen, D., Rauws, E., Fockens, P., et al., Endoscopic drainage of pancreatic pseudocysts: long-term outcome and procedural factors associated with safe and successful treatment. *Endoscopy.* 2005;37(10):977-83.

[16] Kahaleh, M., Shami, V. M., Conaway, M. R., et al., Endoscopic ultrasound drainage of pancreatic pseudocyst: a prospective comparison with conventional endoscopic drainage. *Endoscopy.* 2006;38(4):355-9.

[17] Remer, E. M., Baker, M. E. Imaging of chronic pancreatitis. *Radiol. Clin. North Am.* 2002;40(6):1229-42.

[18] D'Onofrio, M., De Robertis, R., Demozzi, E., et al., *World J. Gastroenterol.* 2014;20 (45):16881-90.

[19] Jenssen, C., Dietrich, C. F. Endoscopic ultrasound in chronic pancreatitis. *Z. Gastroenterol.* 2005;43(8):737-49.

[20] Thuler, F. P., Costa, P. P., Paulo, G. A., et al., Endoscopic ultrasonography and alcoholic patients: can one predict early pancreatic tissue abnormalities? *JOP*. 2005;6 (6):568-74.

[21] Ichikawa, T., Sou, H., Araki, T., et al., Duct-penetrating sign at MRCP: usefulness for differentiating inflammatory pancreatic mass from pancreatic carcinomas. *Radiology*. 2001;221(1):107-16.

[22] Kim, T., Murakami, T., Takamura, M., et al., Pancreatic mass due to chronic pancreatitis: correlation of CT and MR imaging features with pathologic findings. *AJR Am. J. Roentgenol*. 2001;177(2):367-71.

[23] Manfredi, R., Costamagna, G., Brizi, M. G., et al., Severe chronic pancreatitis versus suspected pancreatic disease: dynamic MR cholangiopancreatography after secretin stimulation. *Radiology*. 2000;214(3):849-55.

[24] Kahl, S., Glasbrenner, B., Leodolter, A., et al., EUS in the diagnosis of early chronic pancreatitis: a prospective follow-up study. *Gastrointest. Endosc*. 2002;55(4):507-11.

[25] Ardengh, J. C., Lopes, C. V., Campos, A. D., et al., Endoscopic ultrasound and fine needle aspiration in chronic pancreatitis: differential diagnosis between pseudotumoral masses and pancreatic cancer. *JOP*. 2007;8(4):413-21.

[26] Norton, I. D., Zheng, Y., Wiersema, M. S., et al., Neural network analysis of EUS images to differentiate between pancreatic malignancy and pancreatitis. *Gastrointest. Endosc*. 2001;54(5):625-9.

[27] Catalano, M. F., Lahoti, S., Geenen, J. E., et al., Prospective evaluation of endoscopic ultrasonography, endoscopic retrograde pancreatography, and secretin test in the diagnosis of chronic pancreatitis. *Gastrointest. Endosc*. 1998;48(1):11-7.

[28] Chowdhury, R., Bhutani, M. S., Mishra, G., et al., Comparative analysis of direct pancreatic function testing versus morphological assessment by endoscopic ultrasonography for the evaluation of chronic unexplained abdominal pain of presumed pancreatic origin. *Pancreas*. 2005;31(1):63-8.

[29] Kao, L. S., Bulger, E. M., Parks, D. L., et al., Predictors of morbidity after traumatic pancreatic injury. *J. Trauma*. 2003;55(5):898-905.

[30] Mayer, J. M., Tomczak, R., Rau, B., et al., Pancreatic injury in severe trauma: early diagnosis and therapy improve the outcome. *Dig. Surg*. 2002;19(4):291-7.

[31] Akhrass, R., Yaffe, M. B., Brandt, C. P., et al., Pancreatic trauma: a ten-year multi-institutional experience. *Am. Surg*. 1997;63(7):598-604.

[32] Brandwein, S., Farrell, J. J., Centeno, B. A., et al., Detection and tumor staging of malignancy in cystic, intraductal, and solid tumor of the pancreas by EUS. *Gastrointest. Endosc*. 2001;53:722-7.

[33] Yeh, H. C., Stancato-Pasik, A., Shapiro, R. S. Microcystic features at US: a nonspecific sign for microcystic adenomas of the pancreas. *Radiographies*. 2001;21(6):1455-61.

[34] Curry, C. A., Enq, J., Horton, K. M., et al., CT of primary cystic pancreatic neoplasms: Can CT be used for patient triage and treatment? AJR. *Am. J. Roentgenol*. 2000;175:99-103.

[35] Song, M. H., Lee, S. K., Kim, M. H., et al., EUS in the evaluation of pancreatic cystic lesions. *Gastrointest. Endosc*. 2003;57(7):891-6.

[36] Ahmad, N. A., Kochman, M. L., Brensinger, C., et al., Interobserver agreement among endosonographers for the diagnosis of neoplastic versus non-neoplastic pancreatic cystic lesions. *Gastrointest. Endosc*. 2003;58(1):59-64.

[37] Galanis, C., Zamani, A., Cameron, J. L., et al., Resected serous cystic neoplasms of the pancreas: a review of 158 patients with recommendations for treatment. *J. Gastrointest. Surg*. 2007;11(7):820-6.

[38] Hara, T., Kawashima, H., Ishigooka, M., et al., Mucinous cystic tumors of the pancreas. *Surg. Today*. 2002;32(11):965-9.

[39] Friedman, A. C., Clifford, P., Wynn, G., et al., CT of primary cystic pancreatic neoplasms: nihilism may be unwarranted. *AJR Am. J. Roentgenol*. 2001;177(2):469-70.

[40] Megibow, A. J., Lombardo, F. P., Guarise, A., et al., Cystic pancreatic masses: cross-sectional imaging observations and serial follow-up. *Abdom. Imaging*. 2001;26(6):640-7.

[41] Fernandez-del Castillo, C., Targarona, J., Thayer, S. P., et al., Incidental pancreatic cysts: clinicopathologic characteristics and comparison with symptomatic patients. *Arch. Surg*. 2003;138:427-34.

[42] Le Borgne, J., de Calan, L., Partensky, C. Cystadenomas and cystadenocarcinomas of the pancreas: a multi-institutional retrospective study of 398 cases. *Ann. Surg*. 1999; 230:152-61.

[43] Sedlack, R., Affi, A., Vazquez-Sequeiros, E., et al., Utility of EUS in the evaluation of cystic pancreatic lesions. *Gastrointest. Endosc*. 2002;56: 543-7.

[44] Brandwein, S., Farrell, J. J., Centeno, B. A., et al., Detection and tumor staging of malignancy in cystic, intraductal, and solid tumor of the pancreas by EUS. *Gastrointest. Endosc*. 2001;53:722-7.

[45] Sugiyama, M., Izumisato, Y., Abe, N., et al., Predictive factors for malignancy in intraductal papillary-mucinous tumors of the pancreas. *Br. J. Surg*. 2003;90(10):1244-9.

[46] Prasad, S. R., Sahani, D., Nasser, S., et al., Intraductal papillary mucinous tumors of the pancreas. *Abdom. Imaging*. 2003;28(3):357-65.

[47] Peters, H. E., Vitellas, K. M. Magnetic resonance cholangiopancreatography (MRCP) of intraductal papillary-mucinous neoplasm (IPMN) of the pancreas: case report. *Magn. Reson. Imaging*. 2001;19(8):1139-43.

[48] Aithal, G. P., Chen, R. Y. M., Cunningham, J. T., et al., Accuracy of EUS for detection of intraductal papillary mucinous tumor of the pancreas. *Gastrointest. Endosc*. 2002;56: 701-7.

[49] Cellier, C., Cuillerier, E., Palazzo, L., et al., Intraductal papillary and mucinous tumors of the pancreas: accuracy of preoperative computed tomography, endoscopic retrograde pancreatography, and endoscopic ultrasonography, and long-term outcome in a large surgical series. *Gastrointest. Endosc*. 1998;47:42-9.

[50] Frossard, J. L., Amouyal, P., Amouyal, G., et al., Performance of endosonography-guided fine needle aspiration and biopsy in the diagnosis of pancreatic cystic lesions. *Am. J. Gastroenterol*. 2003;98:1516-24.

[51] Jemal, A., Siegel, R., Ward, E., et al., Cancer statistics, 2008. *CA Cancer J. Clin*. 2008; 58(2):71-96.

[52] Katz, M. H., Hwang, R., Fleming, J. B., et al., Tumornode-metastasis staging of pancreatic adenocarcinoma. *CA Cancer J. Clin*. 2008;58(2):111-25.

[53] Agarwal, B., Abu-Hamda, E., Molke, K. L., et al., Endoscopic ultrasound-guided fine needle aspiration and multidetector spiral CT in the diagnosis of pancreatic cancer. *Am. J. Gastroenterol*. 2004;99(5):844-50.

[54] Delbek, D., Pinson, C. W. Pancreatic tumors: role of imaging in the diagnosis, staging, and treatment. *J. Hepatobiliary Pancreat. Surg*. 2004;11:4-10.
[55] Loyer, E. M., David, C. L., Dubrow, R. A., et al., Vascular involvement in pancreatic adenocarcinoma: reassessment by thin-section CT. *Abdom. Imaging*. 1996;21(3):202-06.
[56] Varadhachary, G. R., Tamm, E. P., Abbruzzese, J. L., et al., Borderline resectable pancreatic cancer: definitions, management, and role of preoperative therapy. *Ann. Surg. Oncol*. 2006;13(8):1035-46.
[57] Katz, M. H., Pisters, P. W., Evans, D. B., et al., Borderline resectable pancreatic cancer: the importance of this emerging stage of disease. *J. Am. Coll. Surg*. 2008;206(5):833-46.
[58] Nakagohri, T., Kinoshita, T., Konishi, M., et al., Nodal involvement is strongest predictor of poor survival in patients with invasive adenocarcinoma of the head of the pancreas. *Hepatogastroenterology*. 2006;53(69):447-51.
[59] Maithel, S. K., Khalili, K., Dixon, E., et al., Impact of regional lymph node evaluation in staging patients with periampullary tumors. *Ann. Surg. Oncol*. 2007;14(1):202-10.
[60] DeWitt, J., Devereaux, B., Chriswell, M., et al., Comparison of endoscopic ultrasonography and multidetector computed tomography for detecting and staging pancreatic cancer. *Ann. Intern. Med*. 2004;141(10):753-63.
[61] Kamisawa, T., Isawa, T., Koike, M., et al., Hematogenous metastases of pancreatic ductal carcinoma. *Pancreas*. 1995;11(4):345-9.
[62] Hess, K. R., Varadhachary, G. R., Taylor, S. H., et al., Metastatic patterns in adenocarcinoma. *Cancer*. 2006;106(7):1624-33.
[63] Bluemke, D. A., Cameron, J. L., Hruban, R. H., et al., Potentially resectable pancreatic adenocarcinoma: spiral CT assessment with surgical and pathologic correlation. *Radiology*. 1995;197(2):381-5.
[64] Fayad, L. M., Mitchell, D. G. Magnetic resonance imaging of pancreatic adenocarcinoma. *Int. J. Gastrointest. Cancer*. 2001;30(1-2):19-25.
[65] Takehara, Y. Fast MR imaging for evaluating the pancreaticobiliary system. *Eur. J. Radiol*. 1999;29(3):211-32.
[66] Pamuklar, E., Semelka, R. C. MR imaging of the pancreas. *Magn. Reson. Imaging Clin. N. Am*. 2005;13(2):313-30.
[67] Sheridan, M. B., Ward, J., Guthrie, J. A., et al., Dynamic contrast-enhanced MR imaging and dual-phase helical CT in the preoperative assessment of suspected pancreatic cancer: a comparative study with receiver operating characteristic analysis. *AJR Am. J. Roentgenol*. 1999;173(3):583-90.
[68] Bipat, S., Phoa, S. S., van Delden, O. M., et al., Ultrasonography, computed tomography and magnetic resonance imaging for diagnosis and determining resectability of pancreatic adenocarcinoma: a meta-analysis. *J. Comput. Assist. Tomogr*. 2005;29(4):438-45.
[69] Ahualli, J. The double duct sign. *Radiology*. 2007;244(1):314-5.
[70] Johnson, P. T., Outwater, E. K. Pancreatic carcinoma versus chronic pancreatitis: dynamic MR imaging. *Radiology*. 1999;212(1):213-8.
[71] Gangi, S., Fletcher, J. G., et al., Time interval between abnormalities seen on CT and the clinical diagnosis of pancreatic cancer: retrospective review of CT scans obtained before diagnosis. *AJR Am. J. Roentgenol*. 2004;182(4):897-903.

[72] Lall, C. G., Howard, T. J., Skandarajah, A., et al., New concepts in staging and treatment of locally advanced pancreatic head cancer. *AJR Am. J. Roentgenol.* 2007; 189(5):1044-50.

[73] Tsiotos, G. G., Farnell, M. B., Sarr, M. G. Are the results of pancreatectomy for pancreatic cancer improving? *World J. Surg.* 1999;23(9):913-9.

[74] Bluemke, D. A., Fishman, E. K. CT and MR evaluation of pancreatic cancer. *Surg. Oncol. Clin. N. Am.* 1998;7(1):103-24.

[75] Tamm, E. P., Silverman, P. M., Charnsangavej, C., et al., Diagnosis, staging, and surveillance of pancreatic cancer. *AJR Am. J. Roentgenol.* 2003;180(5):1311-23.

[76] Lu, D. S., Reber, H. A., Krasny, R. M., et al., Local staging of pancreatic cancer: criteria for unresectability of major vessels as revealed by pancreatic-phase, thin-section helical CT. *AJR Am. J. Roentgenol.* 1997;168(6):1439-43.

[77] O'Malley, M. E., Boland, G. W., Wood, B. J., et al., Adenocarcinoma of the head of the pancreas: determination of surgical unresectability with thin-section pancreatic-phase helical CT. *AJR Am. J. Roentgenol.* 1999;173(6):1513-8.

[78] Zeman, R. K., Cooper, C., Zeiberg, A. S., et al., TNM staging of pancreatic carcinoma using helical CT. *AJR Am. J. Roentgenol.* 1997;169(2):459-64.

[79] Low, R. N. MR imaging of the peritoneal spread of malignancy. *Abdom. Imaging* 2007; 32(3):267-83.

[80] Pakzad, F., Groves, A. M., Ell, P. J. The role of positron emission tomography in the management of pancreatic cancer. *Semin. Nucl. Med.* 2006;36:248-56.

[81] Quon, A., Chang, S. T., Chin, F., et al., Initial evaluation of (18)F-fluorothymidine (FLT) PET/CT scanning for primary pancreatic cancer. *Eur. J. Nucl. Med. Mol. Imaging.* 2008;35:527-31.

[82] Herlin, G., Persson, B., Bergstrom, M., et al., 11C-harmine as a potential PET tracer for ductal pancreas cancer: in vitro studies. *Eur. Radiol.* 2003;13:729-33.

[83] Warburg, O. On the origin of cancer cells. *Science.* 1956;123:309-14.

[84] Gambhir, S. S., Czernin, J., Schwimmer, J., et al., A tabulated summary of the FDG PET literature. *J. Nucl. Med.* 2001;42:1S-93S.

[85] Lytras, D., Connor, S., Bosonnet, L., et al., Positron Emission Tomography does not add to Computed Tomography for the diagnosis and staging of pancreatic cancer. *Dig. Surg.* 2005;22(1-2):55-61.

[86] Sperti, C., Pasquali, C., Decet, G., et al., F-18-fluorodeoxyglucose positron emission tomography in differentiating malignant from benign pancreatic cysts: a prospective study. *J. Gastrointest. Surg.* 2005;9:22-8.

[87] Bares, R., Klever, P., Hauptmann, S., et al., F-18 fluorodeoxyglucose PET in vivo evaluation of pancreatic glucose metabolism for detection of pancreatic cancer. *Radiology.* 1994;192:79-86.

[88] Bares, R., Dohmen, B. M., Cremerius, U., et al., Results of positron emission tomography with fluorine-18 labeled fluorodeoxyglucose in differential diagnosis and staging of pancreatic carcinoma. *Radiologe.* 1996;36:435-40.

[89] Frohlich, A., Diederichs, C. G., Staib, L., et al., Detection of liver metastases from pancreatic cancer using FDG PET. *J. Nucl. Med.* 1999;40:250-5.

[90] Nishiyama, Y., Yamamoto, Y., Yokoe, K., et al., Contribution of whole body FDG-PET to the detection of distant metastasis in pancreatic cancer. *Ann. Nucl. Med.* 2005;19: 491-7.

[91] Fujita, N., Noda, Y., Kobayashi, G., et al., Endoscopic approach to early diagnosis of pancreatic cancer. *Pancreas*. 2004;28:279-81.

[92] Brugge, W. R., Lee, M. J., Kelsey, P. B., et al., The use of EUS to diagnose malignant portal venous system invasion by pancreatic cancer. *Gastrointest. Endosc*. 1996;43: 561-7.

[93] Ahmad, N. A., Kochman, M. L., Lewis, J. D., et al., Endosonography is superior to angiography in the preoperative assessment of vascular involvement among patients with pancreatic carcinoma. *J. Clin. Gastroenterol*. 2001;32:54-8.

[94] Horwhat, J. D., Gerke, H., Acosta, R. D., et al., Focal or diffuse "fullness" of the pancreas on CT. Usually benign, but EUS plus/minus FNA is warranted to identify malignancy. *JOP* 2009;10:37-42.

[95] Yasuda, K., Mukai, H., Fujimoto, S., et al., The diagnosis of pancreatic cancer by endoscopic ultrasonography. *Gastrointest. Endosc*. 1988;34:1-8.

[96] Varadarajulu, S., Eloubeidi, M. A. The role of endoscopic ultrasonography in the evaluation of pancreaticobiliary cancer. *Gastrointest. Endosc. Clin. N. Am*. 2005;15: 497-511.

[97] Saftoiu, A., Popescu, C., Cazacu, S., et al., Power Doppler endoscopic ultrasonography for the differential diagnosis between pancreatic cancer and pseudotumoral chronic pancreatitis. *J. Ultrasound Med*. 2006;25:363-72.

[98] Klapman, J. B., Chang, K. J., Lee, J. G., et al., Negative predictive value of endoscopic ultrasound in a large series of patients with a clinical suspicion of pancreatic cancer. *Am. J. Gastroenterol*. 2005;100:2658-2661.

[99] Bhutani, M. S., Gress, F. G., Giovannini, M., et al., The No endosonographic detection of tumor (NEST) study: a case series of pancreatic cancers missed on endoscopic ultrasonography. *Endoscopy*. 2004;36(5):385-9.

[100] Agarwal, B., Abu-Hamda, E., Molke, K. L., et al., Endoscopic ultrasound-guided fine needle aspiration and multidetector spiral CT in the diagnosis of pancreatic cancer. Am. *J. Gastroenterol*. 2004;99:844-50.

[101] Hartwig, W., Schneider, L., Diener, M. K., et al., Preoperative tissue diagnosis for tumors of the pancreas. *Br. J. Surg*. 2009;96:5-20.

[102] Eloubeidi, M. A., Jhala, D., Chhieng, D. C., et al., Yield of endoscopic ultrasound guided fine-needle aspiration biopsy in patients with suspected pancreatic carcinoma. *Cancer*. 2003;99:285-92.

[103] Fritscher-Ravens, A., Brand, L., Knofel, W. T., et al., Comparison of endoscopic ultrasound-guided fine needle aspiration for focal pancreatic lesions in patients with normal parenchyma and chronic pancreatitis. *Am. J. Gastroenterol*. 2002;97:2768-75.

[104] Harewood, G. C., Wiersema, M. J. Endosonography-guided fine needle aspiration biopsy in the evaluation of pancreatic masses. *Am. J. Gastroenterol*. 2002;97:1386-91.

[105] Ahmad, N. A., Lewis, J. D., Ginsberg, G. G., et al., EUS in preoperative staging of pancreatic cancer. *Gastrointest. Endosc*. 2000;52:463-8.

[106] Kochman, M. L. EUS in pancreatic cancer. *Gastrointest. Endosc*. 2002; 56:S6-S12.

[107] McLean, A. M., Fairclough, P. D. Endoscopic ultrasound in the localisation of pancreatic islet cell tumours. *Best Pract. Res. Clin. Endocrinol. Metab*. 2005;19(2):177-93.

[108] Anderson, M. A., Carpenter, S., Thompson, N. W., et al., Endoscopic ultrasound is highly accurate and directs management in patients with neuroendocrine tumors of the pancreas. *Am. J. Gastroenterol.* 2000;95(9):2271-7.

[109] Stafford Johnson, D. B., Francis, I. R., Eckhauser, F. E., et al., Dual-phase helical CT of nonfunctioning islet cell tumors. *J. Comput. Assist. Tomogr.* 1998;22(1):59-63.

[110] Sohaib, S. A., Reznek, R. H., Healy, J. C., et al., Cystic islet cell tumors of the pancreas. *AJR Am. J. Roentgenol.* 1998;170(1):217.

[111] Ichikawa, T., Peterson, M. S., Federle, M. P., et al., Islet cell tumor of the pancreas: biphasic CT versus MR imaging in tumor detection. *Radiology.* 2000;216(1):163-71.

[112] Thoeni, R. F., Mueller-Lisse, U. G., Chan, R., et al., Detection of small, functional islet cell tumors in the pancreas: selection of MR imaging sequences for optimal sensitivity. *Radiology.* 2000;214(2):483-90.

[113] Ashida, R., Yamao, K., Okubo, K., et al., Indocyanine green is an ideal dye for endoscopic ultrasound-guided fine-needle tattooing of pancreatic tumors. *Endoscopy.* 2006;38(2):190-2.

[114] Gines, A., Vazquez-Sequeiros, E., Soria, M. T., et al., Usefulness of EUS-guided fine needle aspiration (EUS-FNA) in the diagnosis of functioning neuroendocrine tumors. *Gastrointest. Endosc.* 2002;56(2):291-6.

[115] Chang, F., Chandra, A., Culora, G., et al., Cytologic diagnosis of pancreatic endocrine tumors by endoscopic ultrasound-guided fine-needle aspiration: a review. *Diagn. Cytopathol.* 2006;34(9):649-58.

[116] Jurgensen, C., Schuppan, D., Neser, F., et al., EUS-guided alcohol ablation of an insulinoma. *Gastrointest. Endosc.* 2006;63(7):1059-62.

[117] Madan, A. K., Weldon, C. B., Long, W. P., et al., Solid and papillary epithelial neoplasm of the pancreas. *J. Surg. Oncol.* 2004;85(4):193-8.

[118] Buetow, P. C., Buck, J. L., Pantongrag-Brown, L., et al., Solid and papillary epithelial neoplasm of the pancreas: imaging-pathologic correlation on 56 cases. *Radiology.* 1996;199(3):707-11.

[119] Behrns, K. E., Sarr, M. G., Strickler, J. G. Pancreatic lymphoma: is it a surgical disease? *Pancreas.* 1994;9(5):662-7.

[120] Shah, S., Mortele, K. J. Uncommon solid pancreatic neoplasms: ultrasound, computed tomography, and magnetic resonance imaging features. *Semin. Ultrasound CT MR.* 2007;28(5):357-70.

[121] Merkle, E. M., Bender, G. N., Brambs, H. J. Imaging findings in pancreatic lymphoma: differential aspects. *AJR Am. J. Roentgenol.* 2000;174(3):671-5.

[122] Kassabian, A., Stein, J., Jabbour, N., et al., Renal cell carcinoma metastatic to the pancreas: a single-institution series and review of the literature. *Urology.* 2000;56(2): 211-5.

[123] Ng, C. S., Loyer, E. M., Iyer, R. B., et al., Metastases to the pancreas from renal cell carcinoma: findings on three-phase contrast-enhanced helical CT. *AJR Am. J. Roentgenol.* 1999;172(6):1555-9.

In: The Role of Imaging Technology …
Editor: Georgios Tsoulfas

ISBN: 978-1-63483-490-2

Chapter 9

The Role of Imaging in Esophageal Surgery

Efstathios Kotidis*[*], *Konstantinos Sapalidis* and *Manos-Georgios Pramateftakis

Department of Surgery, Aristotle University of Thessaloniki, Thessaloniki, Greece

Abstract

The esophagus is a muscular tube connecting the pharynx with the stomach and represents an integral part of the digestive system. There is a wide range of diseases (congenital, functional, structural, trauma and neoplasia) affecting the esophagus. These combined with the fact that it is located in both the thoracic and the abdominal cavity, make the diagnosis and management of esophageal problems a significant challenge, even for the more experienced practitioners. Knowledge of the most current imaging technology can play a critical role in forming a successful strategy.

Introduction

The esophagus is a muscular tube connecting the pharynx with the stomach. It is 23-37 cm long with a diameter of 1-2 cm and is divided into three parts:

a) cervical: the cervical esophagus is in continuity with the oropharynx, commences at the lower border of cricoid cartilage (at level of C5/6) or cricopharyngeus muscle and continuous until the level of the thoracic aperture.
b) thoracic: extents from the thoracic aperture (T1) to the oesophageal hiatus (T11)
c) abdominal: from oesophageal hiatus and is continuous with the cardia of the stomach at the gastro-oesophageal junction.

[*] Corresponding author: E. Kotidis. E-mail: skotidis@gmail.com.

It courses inferiorly to the left of the midline in the neck and superior mediastinum returning to the midline at T5 before coursing to the left again of the midline in the posterior mediastinum and in its inferior aspect curving anteriorly to pass through the diaphragm into the abdominal cavity. The esophagus has three normal constrictions, due to its compression against the adjacent structures that should not be confused for pathological constrictions: The *cervical constriction* due to the cricoid cartilage at the level of C5/6, the *thoracic constriction* due to the aortic arch at the level of T4/5 and the abdominal constriction at the oesophageal hiatus (T10/11).

Its arterial blood supply comes from the thyroid artery (upper third), esophageal branches of the thoracic aorta (middle third) and esophageal branches of the left gastric artery (lower third. Regarding the venous drainage, the upper third drains to the brachiocephalic veins, the middle to the azygos and the lower third to the left gastric vein. The lymphatic drainage follows the arterial supply. The nerve supply is from the sympathetic trunk and the vagal plexus. Histologically, the oesophagus is characterised by the luck of serosal layer. It consists of the outer muscularis propria, the inner muscularis propria, the submucosa, the muscularis mucosae and the mucosa. It is covered by stratified squamous epithelium that abruptly changes to columnar epithelium in the lower oesophagus [1, 2]. The commonest pathologies of the esophagus include oesophageal cancer, benign oesophageal neoplasms, hiatus hernias, achalasia and other motility disorders, gastroesophageal reflux disease (GORD), esophageal rupture (Boerhaave syndrome), esophageal strictures (Schatzki ring or oesophageal web) and esophageal diverticula [2]. The radiographic imaging modalities of the esophagus include barium swallow, CT, endoscopic ultrasonography, MRI, and PET/CT. Barium swallow is the main radiological method of assessing the oesophagus. Endoscopic ultrasonography is used for evaluation of the depth of the oesophageal cancer. CT or MRI are used to diagnose hiatal hernias, diverticuli and tumors of the esophagus and to stage esophageal cancer. PET/CT is only use in staging esophageal malignancies [2].

CONGENITAL DISORDERS

Oesophageal atresia is the commonest of the congenital anomalies of the esophagus. It refers to an absence in contiguity of the oesophagus due to an inappropriate division of the primitive foregut into the trachea and oesophagus. It may be suspected on antenatal ultrasound or in the neonate due to inability to swallow saliva or milk, aspiration during early feedings, or failure to successfully pass a catheter into the stomach.

It is frequently associated with a tracheo-oesophageal fistula. As such, the types of oesophageal atresia / tracheo-oesophageal fistula can be divided into proximal atresia with distal fistula (85%) isolated oesophageal atresia (8-9%), isolated fistula (H-type) (4-6%), double fistula with intervening atresia (1-2%), proximal fistula with distal atresia [3, 4] (1%).

Radiographic Features

A plain chest x ray may show a dilated pharyngeal pouch, or the presence of air in the stomach and bowel in the setting of oesophageal with a distal tracheo-oesophageal fistula.

If an oesophago-gastric (feeding) tube insertion has been attempted this may show the tube blind looping and turning back at the upper thoracic part of the oesophagus or heading into the trachea and/or bronchial tree.

A contrast swallow fluoroscopy may show contrast blindly ending and pooling in an oesophageal stump and/or may show evidence of the tracheo-oesophageal fistula (Images 1, 2). CT scan with 3D detailed visualisation of anatomy has also been trialed but is not part of routine investigation.

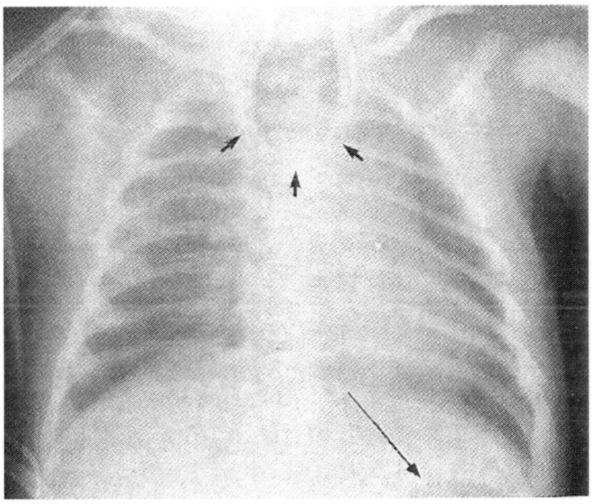

Image 1. Type I congenital atresia. The nasogastric tube folds at the level of the atresia.

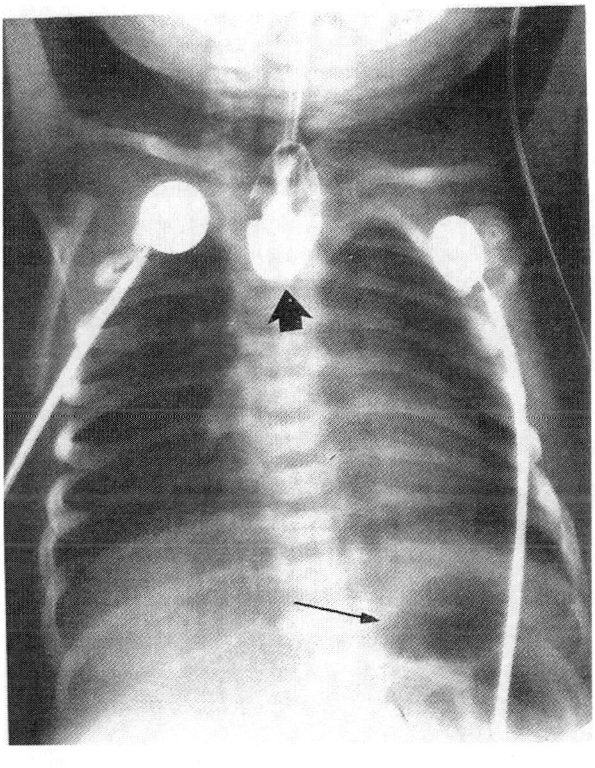

Image 2. The same patient after the administration of water soluble contrast.

Foreign Bodies

The presence of foreign bodies in the esophagus is more common in children. They are usually impacted in the first natural stricture of the esophagus at the level of the cricopharingeal muscle. In most cases the history along with a plain x ray are enough for the diagnosis [5, 6, 7] (Images 3, 4).

Esophageal Diverticula

Esophageal diverticulum is a pouch arising from the esophagus. It's lumen is in continuity with the esophageal lumen. They can occur in all ages but are more frequent in adults and elderly people. Based on their pathology, they are divided into *true* and *false* diverticula. True diverticula include all esophageal layers while false diverticula contain only mucosa and submucosa herniating through the muscular layer (e.g., Zenker's diverticulum).

Based on their pathophysiology they are divided into *traction diverticula* which occur secondary to pulling forces on the outer aspect of the oesophagus and *pulsion diverticula* which occur secondary to increased intraluminal pressure (e.g., Zenker diverticulum).

According to their location, they are divided into upper, middle and lower diverticula. Upper diverticula are generally pulsion diverticula and include Zenker's and Killian Jamieson diverticulum. Zenker's diverticulum is actually a pharyngeal pouch, located just proximal to the upper esophageal sphincter. Killian Jamieson diverticulum is infrequently encountered compared with the Zenker's and is located just below the cricopharyngeal muscle.

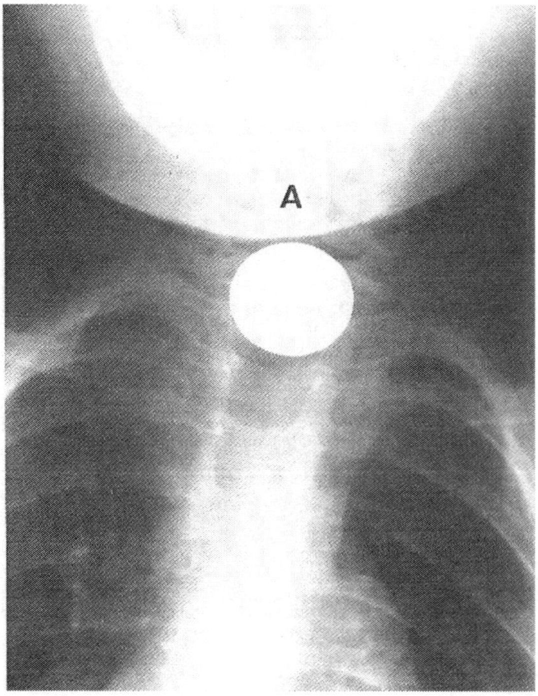

Image 3. Impacted foreign body (coin). Anteroposterior view.

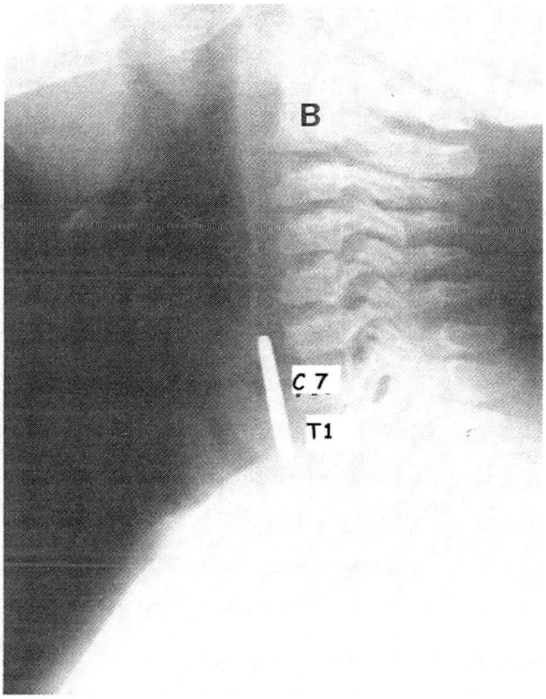

Image 4. Impacted foreign body (coin). Lateral view.

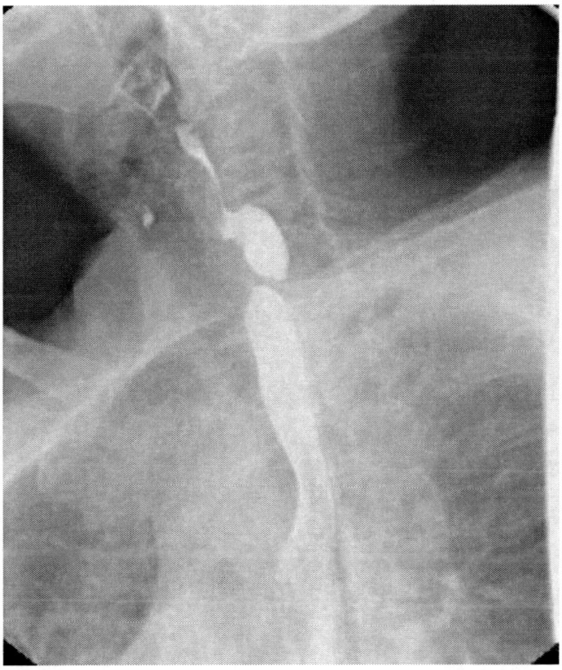

Image 5. Zenker's diverticulum.

The middle esophageal diverticula can be both traction and pulsion diverticula (Image 5). Traction diverticula may occur secondary to scarring, fibrosis and inflammatory processes in the mediastinum pulling on the oesophageal wall.

They are more frequently located close to the tracheal bifurcation. They are usually small, rarely exceeding 2cm in diameter and in most cases asymptomatic.

Pulsion diverticula are usually false diverticula and occur secondary to abnormally increased intraluminal pressure against a weak esophageal segment.

Finally, lower or epiphrenic oesophageal diverticula are pulsion diverticula that occur through weak or defective sites of the muscular layer of the lower esophagus, usually in combination with achalasia or hiatus hernias. They are usually larger than middle esophageal diverticula and may be complicated with infection or perforation.

A rare condition mimicking diverticula is esophageal pseudodiverticulosis. It may occur in all age groups, but more commonly in the 6th and 7th decades. They represent dilated excretory ducts of the deep oesophageal mucosal glands [8, 9].

Radiographic Features

A barium swallow is the study of choice. *Zenker's diverticula* present as an outpouching arising from the midline of the posterior wall of the distal pharynx near the pharyngoesophageal junction. The pouch is best identified during swallowing and is best seen on the lateral view, on which the diverticulum is typically noted at the C5-6 level (Image 6). *Epiphrenic diverticula* present as outpouching of the distal esophagus, best seen in prone oblique views (Image 7).

Pseudodiverticula are best seen with a single contrast, rather than a double contrast, thin barium examination (Image 8). The findings are numerous tiny flask-shaped outpouchings usually diffusely distributed or clustered. CT scan may also be used to confirm the diagnosis and to provide more anatomic information that may facilitate the surgical treatment [9].

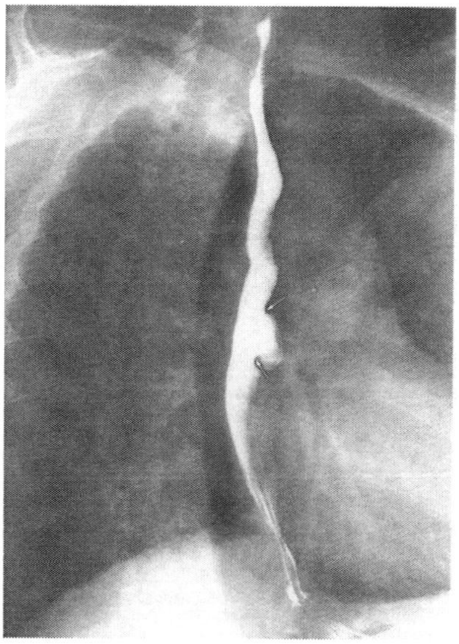

Image 6. Middle esophageal traction diverticulum.

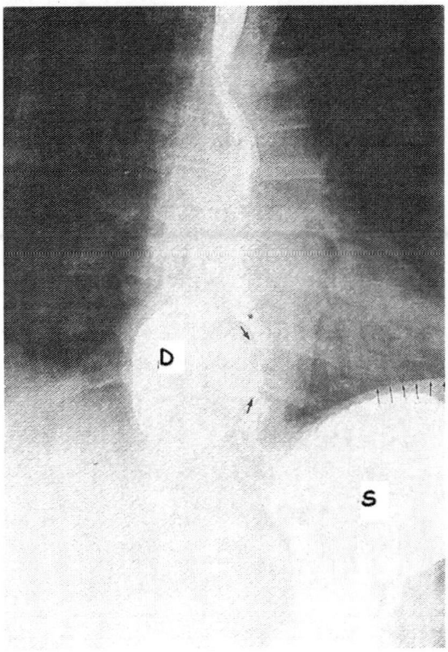

D = diverticulum, S = stomach.

Image 7. Epiphrenic diverticulum.

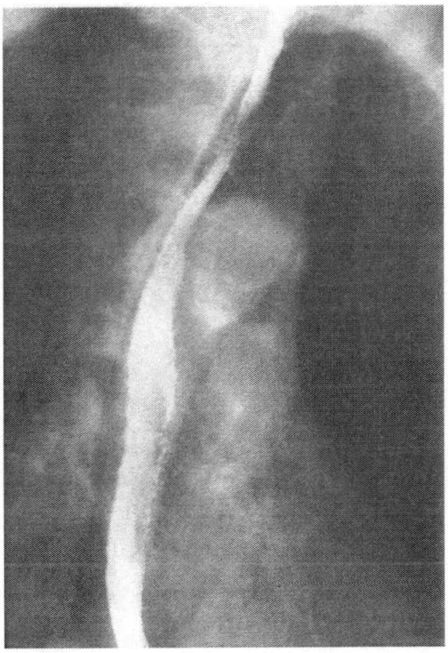

Image 8. Intramural pseudodiverticula.

ESOPHAGEAL VARICES

Esophageal varices are extremely dilated submucosal veins of the lower third of the esophagus. They are most often a consequence of portal hypertension, commonly due to cirrhosis; patients with esophageal varices have a strong tendency to develop bleeding.

The majority of blood from the esophagus is drained via the esophageal veins to the azygos vein, which in turn drains directly into the superior vena cava. These veins have no part in the development of esophageal varices. The remaining blood from the esophagus is drained into the superficial veins lining the esophageal mucosa, which drain into the left gastric vein (coronary vein), which in turn drains directly into the portal vein. These superficial veins (normally only approximately 1 mm in diameter) become distended up to 1-2 cm in diameter in case of portal hypertension. Normal portal pressure is approximately 9 mmHg compared to an inferior vena cava pressure of 2-6 mmHg.

This creates a normal pressure gradient of 3-7 mmHg. If the portal pressure rises above 12 mmHg, this gradient rises to 7-10 mmHg. A gradient greater than 5 mmHg is considered portal hypertension. At gradients greater than 10 mmHg, blood flow through the hepatic portal system is redirected from the liver into areas with lower venous pressures. This means that collateral circulation develops in the lower esophagus, abdominal wall, stomach, and rectum. The small blood vessels in these areas become distended, becoming more thin-walled, and appear as varicosities [10].

Radiographic Features

Lobulated masses in the posterior mediastinum or silhouetting of the aorta may be seen in plain x rays. Barium swallow with small amount of barium is the study of choice. Relaxation of the esophagus, in order not to compress the varices, is important.

Therefore, a sustained valsalva manoeuvre is important to preclude swallowing, since each swallow initiates a primary peristaltic wave that lasts for at least 10-30 seconds. The usual findings are thickened and interrupted mucosal folds, tortuous radiolucencies of variable size and location or "worm eaten" smooth lobulated filling defects (Images 9, 10).

A CT scan may also be useful to confirm the diagnosis. The commonest appearance is thickened esophageal wall with lobulatted outer contour, scalloped esophageal luminal masses and marked enhancement following dynamic CT. In case of paraesophageal varices right or left sided soft tissue masses may be seen [10, 11, 12] (Image 11).

Esophageal Strictures

Oesophageal strictures refer to any persistent intrinsic narrowing of the oesophagus.

They are usually caused by inflammatory or neoplastic processes such as caustic ingestion, mediastinal radiation, esophagitis, scleroderma or congenital stenosis.

Radiographic Features

Benign strictures typically show smooth concentric narrowing. Malignant strictures are characteristically abrupt, asymmetric, eccentric narrowings with irregular, nodular mucosa (Image 12).

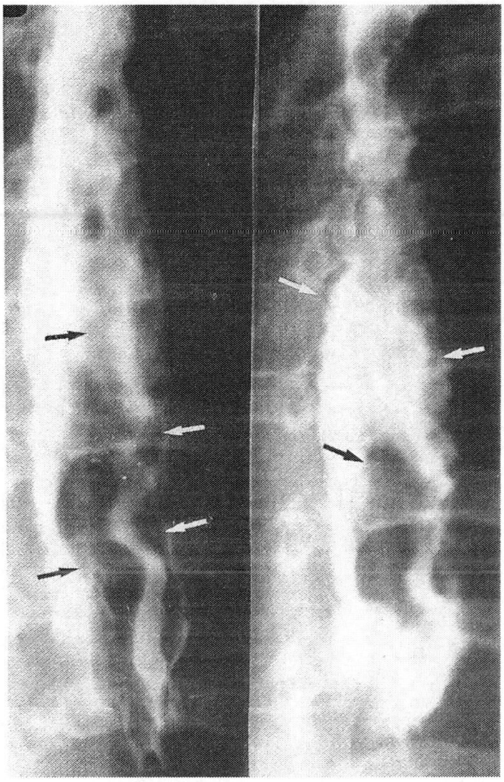

Image 9. Esophageal varices on barium swallow test.

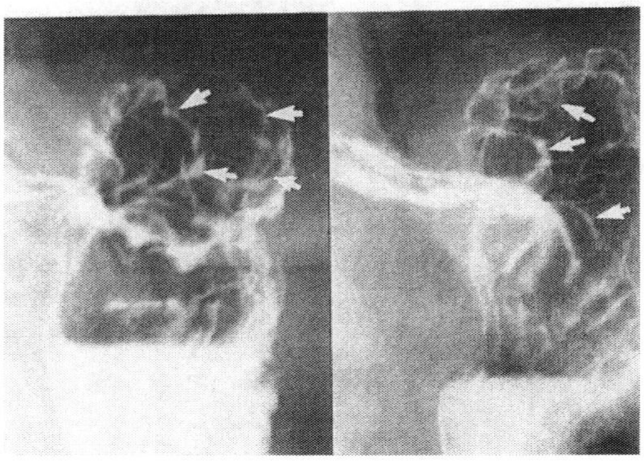

Image 10. Gastric varices.

Tapered margins may occur with malignant lesions because of the ease of submucosal spread of tumour. All esophageal strictures should be investigated with upper endoscopy to rule out malignancy [13, 14].

Esophageal Perforation

Esophageal perforation is a rare but serious medical emergency with very high mortality rate, especially if the diagnosis is delayed.

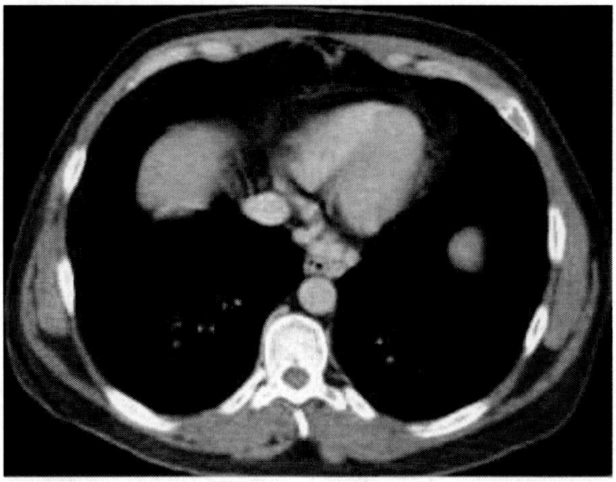

Image 11. CT scan demonstrating esophageal varices.

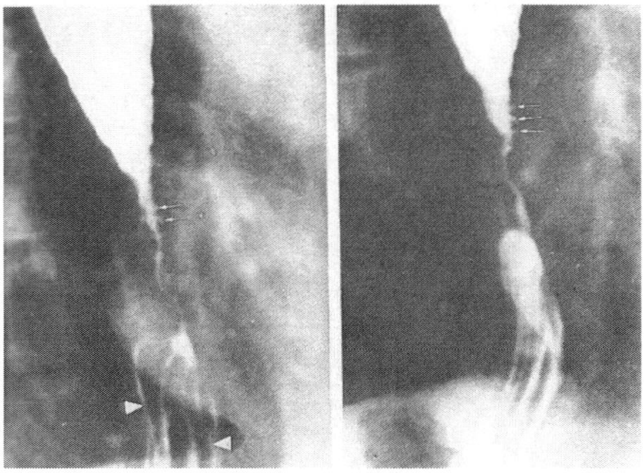

Image 12. Benign esophageal stricture secondary to esophagitis. A large sliding hiatus hernia is also seen.

Most perforations are iatrogenic, post dilatation or thoracic surgery. Other causes include trauma, foreign body ingestion, erosive material ingestion, esophageal cancer or spontaneous post vomiting rupture (Boerhaave syndrome). If perforation is not detected during the instrumentation, the patient will develop neck, chest or epigastric pain, dyspnoea, dysphagea and sepsis [15]. Subcutaneous emphysema may also be present.

Radiographic Features

Plain chest x-ray may show pneumomediastinum, pneumothorax and/or pleural effusion indicative of mediastinitis. Contrast swallow with water soluble agent is more sensitive, and should be done within 24 hours to confirm the diagnosis. CT scan may also be useful to evaluate the extent of pleural effusion and mediastinitis.

Once diagnosed, the esophageal perforation should immediately be treated either endoscopically or laparoscopically [15, 16].

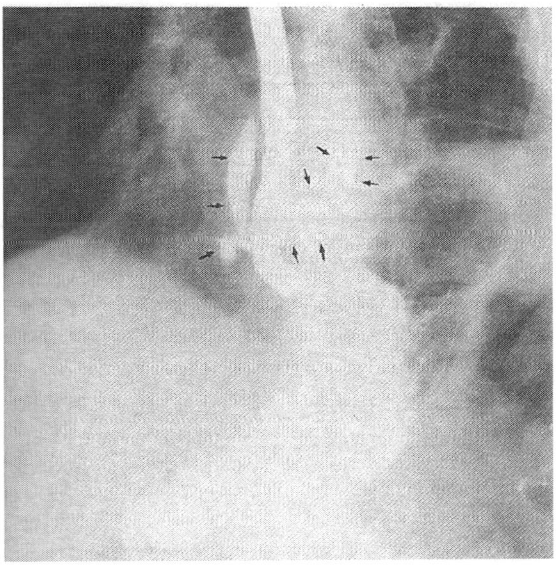

Image 13. Gastrographin swallow demonstrating iatrogenic perforation of the esopagus.

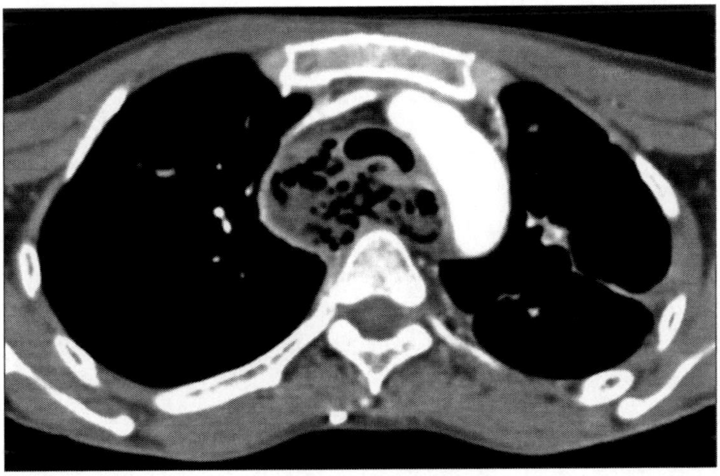

Image 14. CT scan after iatrogenic perforation of the esophagus. The scan shoes collection of fluid and air in the mediastinum.

SCHATZKI RING

Schatzki ring is a relatively common lower esophageal ring found in nearly 10% of barium swallows. It is located 2-3 cm above the hiatus and is thought to be a congenital anomaly formed by redundant pleats of mucosa. Its clinical presentation depends on its luminal diameter.

Most rings are asymptomatic unless the luminal diameter is < 13mm. In such cases they present with dysphagia especially to solid food. Interestingly, patients with Schatzki ring have lower incidence of Barret's esophagus. If they are symptomatic, boogie or balloon dilatation is the treatment of choice [17].

Radiographic Features

Single contrast barium swallow is the study of choice. Its sensitivity is even higher than endoscopy. A Valsalva manoeuvre may be useful to increase the sensitivity of the test.

A circumferential narrowing at the gastro-oesophageal junction, often a few centimeters above the diaphragmatic hiatus, is the commonest feature (15).

Hiatus Hernia

Hiatus hernia (HH) is the herniation of abdominal viscera through the esophageal hiatus into the posterior mediastinum or the thoracic cavity. Depending on the location of the gastroesophageal junction, hiatus hernias are divided into sliding, where the junction is displaced up in the posterior mediastinum and paraesophageal hernias, where the junction is not displaced. Many patients with HH are asymptomatic and it is an incidental finding. However, symptoms may include epigastric or chest pain, post prandial fullness, nausea and vomiting. Sometimes HH are considered synonymous with gastro-oesophageal reflux disease (GORD) but there is a poor correlation between the two conditions. The most common content of a HH is the stomach. Large HH containing stomach may result in gastric volvulus, which in turn presents as intestinal obstruction and may result in ischaemia or infarction [18].

There are two main types of hiatus hernia, although they may co-exist:

Sliding Hiatus Hernia

This is the most common type of hiatus hernia (95%). The gastro-oesophageal junction (GOJ) is usually displaced by more than 2 cm above the hiatus. The oesophageal hiatus is often abnormally widened to 3-4 cm (the upper limit of normal is 15 mm).

The gastric fundus may also be displaced above the diaphragm and present as aretrocardiac mass on a chest radiograph. The presence of an air-fluid level in the mass suggests the diagnosis. Small, sliding hiatus hernias commonly reduce in the upright position.

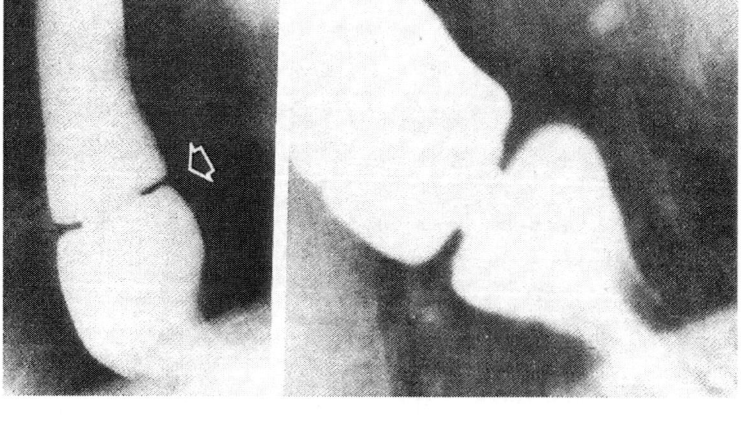

Image 15. Schatzki ring.

The mere presence of a sliding hiatus hernia is of limited clinical significance in most cases. The function of the lower oesophageal sphincter and the presence of gastro-esophageal reflux disease (GERD) are the crucial factors in producing symptoms and causing complications [18, 19].

Para-Oesophageal Hiatus Hernia

The para-oesophageal hiatus hernia is much less common than the sliding type (5%). The GOJ remains in its normal location while a portion of the stomach herniates above the diaphragm.

Mixed Hiatus Hernia

The two types of hiatus hernias may also coexist. The GOJ is displaced into the thorax with a large portion of the stomach, which is usually abnormally rotated.

Radiographic Features

A plain x ray may reveal retrocardiac opacity with air – fluid level. Single contrast barium swallow is diagnostic on most cases (Image 16, 17).

CT scan may be necessary to clarify in more detail the content and the relations of the hernia sack, especially in large paraesophageal hernias (Image 18). The differential diagnosis includes retrocardiac lung abscess or empyema and epiphrenic esophageal diverticulum [18].

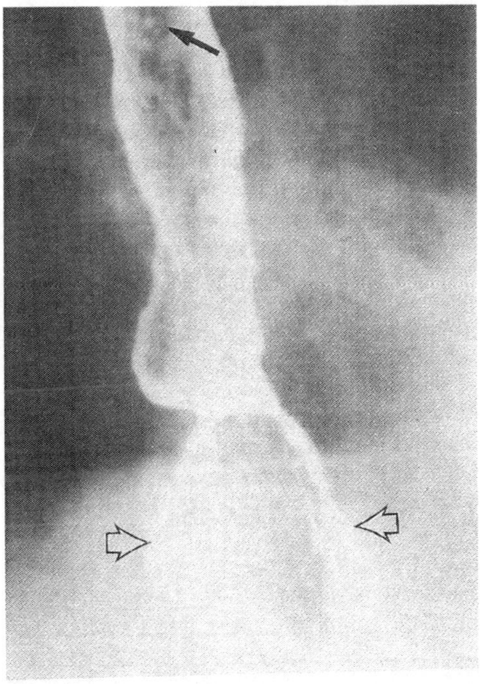

Image 16. Sliding hiatus hernia.

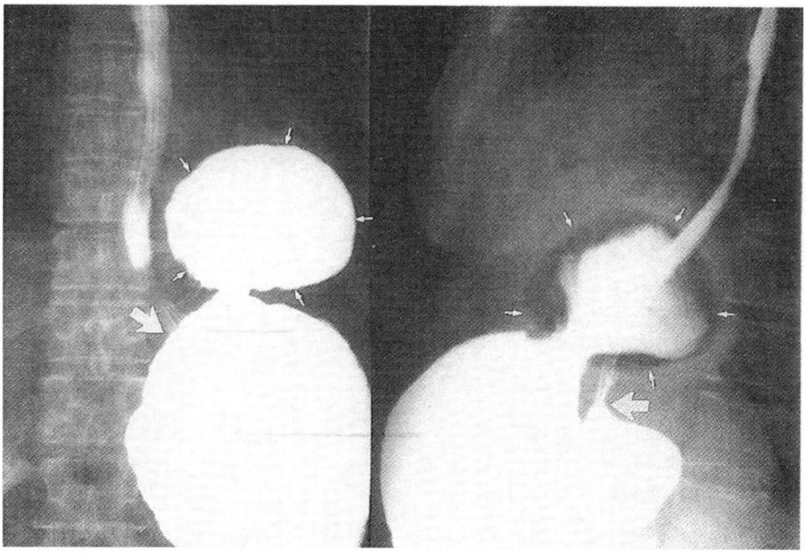

Image 17. Paraesophageal hiatus hernia.

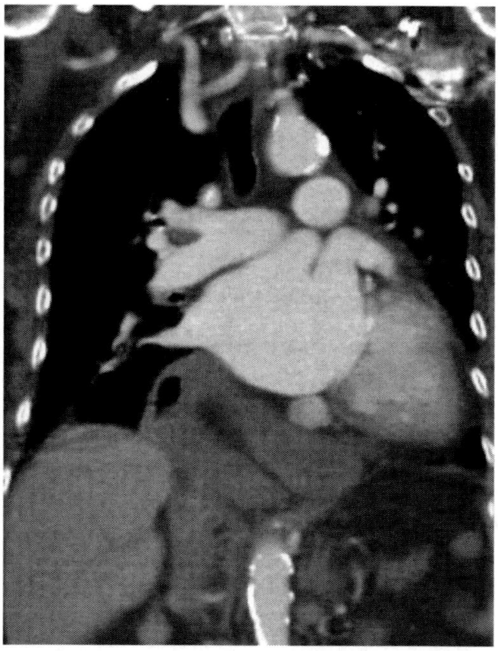

Image 18. CT scan demonstrating sliding hiatus hernia.

Gastroesophageal Reflux Disease (GERD)

Gastroesophageal reflux disease occurs when the amount of gastric juice that refluxes into the esophagus exceeds the normal limit, causing symptoms with or without associated esophageal mucosal injury. Typical esophageal symptoms include heartburn, regurgitation and dysphagia.

Abnormal reflux can also cause atypical (extraesophageal) symptoms, such as coughing and/or wheezing, hoarseness, sore throat, otitis media, noncardiac chest pain, enamel erosion or other dental manifestations. A history of nausea, vomiting, or regurgitation should alert the physician to evaluate for delayed gastric emptying. Patients with suspected gastroesophageal reflux disease should be investigated with upper gastrointestinal endoscopy, esophageal manometry and ambulatory 24-hour pH monitoring. Ambulatory 24-hour pH monitoring is the criterion standard in establishing a diagnosis of gastroesophageal reflux disease [19].

Radiographic Features

Upper gastrointestinal contrast-enhanced studies are the initial radiologic procedure of choice in the workup gastroesophageal reflux disease. Plain chest radiographic findings are not useful in evaluating of this condition, but they are helpful in assessing pulmonary status and basic anatomy. Chest images may also demonstrate a large hiatal hernia, but small hernias can be easily missed. Currently, no role exists for computed tomography scanning, magnetic resonance imaging, or ultrasonography in the routine evaluation of patients with reflux disease [20].

Achalasia

Achalasia is a primary esophageal motility disorder characterized by the absence of esophageal peristalsis and impaired relaxation of the lower esophageal sphincter (LES) in response to swallowing. The LES is hypertensive in about 50% of patients. These abnormalities cause a functional obstruction at the gastroesophageal junction (GEJ).

It is most frequently seen in middle and late adulthood (30-70 years of age) with no gender predilection. In most cases achalasia is idiopathic, however an identical appearance is seen in patients with Chagas disease.

Authors differ as to whether they reserve the term achalasia for idiopathic cases, or whether they include Chagas disease. Symptoms of achalasia include dysphagia (most common), regurgitation, chest pain, heartburn and weight loss. Initially symptoms are intermittent. Patients may also present with a complication of long standing achalasia:

- oesophageal carcinoma: is the most dreaded complication and is seen in approximately 5%, and most often in the mid oesophagus. It is thought to relate to the chronic irritation of the mucosa by stasis of food and secretions.
- aspiration pneumonia and eventually abscess formation
- candida oesophagitis
- acute airway obstruction: this is a rare complication requiring immediate esophageal decompression with nasogastric tube

Esophageal manometry is the criterion standard in the diagnosis of achalasia. Findings include incomplete LES relaxation in response to swallowing, high resting LES pressure, absent esophageal peristalsis.

Ambulatory esophageal pH monitoring to rule out gastroesophageal reflux disease and determine if abnormal reflux is being caused by treatment may also be necessary. Esophagogastroduodenoscopy to rule out cancer of the GEJ or fundus is usually done in most cases. Concomitant endoscopic ultrasonography is necessary if a tumor is suspected [21].

Radiographic Features

Chest x-ray findings include:

- right convex opacity behind right cardiac border; occasionally left convex opacity if thoracic aorta tortuous
- air-fluid level due to stasis in thoracic esophagus filled with retained secretions and food
- small or absent gastric air bubble
- anterior displacement and bowing of trachea on the lateral view

The chronic presence of fluid debris in the esophagus makes patients very prone to aspiration and thus patchy bilateral alveolar opacities representing acute or chronic aspiration pneumonia may be seen.

Barium Swallow

A barium swallow is able to not only confirm that the esophagus is dilated but is also able to assess for mucosal abnormalities (Image 19).

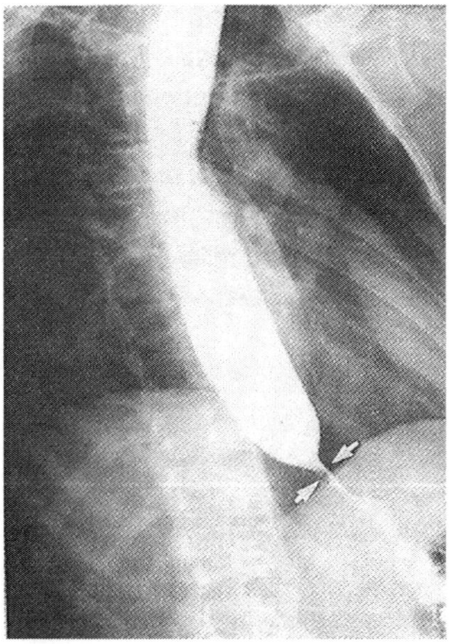

Image 19. Achalasia of the esophagus.

Findings include:

- failure of normal peristalsis to clear the esophagus of barium when the patient is in the recumbent position, with no primary waves identified
- uncoordinated, non-propulsive, tertiary contractions
- esophageal body dilatation, which is typically maximal in the distal esophagus
- pooling or stasis of barium in the esophagus when the esophagus has become atonic or non contractile (late feature in the disease)
- when barium column is high enough (patient standing) the hydrostatic pressure can overcome the LOS pressure allowing passage of esophageal content
- incomplete LOS relaxation that is not coordinated with esophageal contraction
- bird beak sign

CT

Patients with uncomplicated achalasia demonstrate a dilated thin walled esophagus filled with fluid/food debris. Overall CT has little role in directly assessing patients with achalasia, but is useful in assessing common complications. Careful assessment of the wall of the esophagus should be undertaken to identify any focal regions of thickening which may indicate malignancy. The lungs should be inspected for evidence of aspiration.

Differential Diagnosis

A number of entities may mimic achalasia, forming the so called 'achalasia pattern.' They include central and peripheral neuropathy, scleroderma, oesophageal malignancy or gastric carcinoma commonly referred as pseudoachalasia, oesophageal stricture, Chagas disease, non-specific oesophageal motility disorder and diffuse oesophageal spasm.

Treatment

The American College of Gastroenterology released new guidelines for the diagnosis and management of achalasia in July 2013. Treatment recommendations are as follows:

- Initial therapy should be either graded pneumatic dilation (PD) or laparoscopic surgical myotomy with a partial fundoplication in patients fit to undergo surgery
- Procedures should be performed in high-volume centers of excellence
- Initial therapy choice should be based on patient age, sex, preference, and local institutional expertise
- Botulinum toxin therapy is recommended for patients not suited to PD or surgery
- Pharmacologic therapy can be used for patients not undergoing PD or myotomy and who have failed botulinum toxin therapy (nitrates and calcium channel blockers most common) [20].

Esophageal Cysts

Esophageal cysts were initially described esophageal cysts as duplications. They can be divided into two categories. Simple epithelial-lined cysts and esophageal duplication, which is an embryologic duplication of a portion of the muscle and submucosa of the esophagus without epithelial duplication. Esophageal cysts are rare. Many patients with esophageal cysts are asymptomatic and never diagnosed. The true incidence of esophageal cysts is unknown, since no large study has defined it.

They are usually grouped with other benign lesions of the esophagus, comprising up to 20% of benign esophageal lesions. Up to 80% of them are diagnosed in childhood.

The diagnosis and treatment of esophageal cysts is still evolving. Diagnosis is aided by the relatively recent developments of CT scans and endoscopic ultrasonography. Treatment is currently moving from thoracotomy to less-invasive procedures, including video-assisted thoracoscopic surgery (VATS) and endoscopic treatment.

Symptoms are caused by compression of surrounding structures. Sixty percent of esophageal cysts occur in the lower third of the esophagus, where difficulty swallowing from compression is the most common symptom; 20% occur in the upper third of the esophagus, where respiratory difficulty from compression of the tracheobronchial tree is the most common symptom; and 20% occur in the middle third of the esophagus, where retrosternal chest pain and difficulty swallowing are the most common symptoms. Posterior cysts in the lower third of the esophagus can cause cardiac arrhythmias. The larger the cyst, the greater the chance of it causing symptoms [22].

Maldevelopment of the posterior division of the primitive foregut is the embryologic defect responsible for esophageal cysts. Esophageal cysts develop from aberrant elements of the esophageal wall. Simple cysts are duplication of the epithelium, whereas true esophageal duplications are duplications of the submucosa and the muscle wall without duplication of the epithelium. The lining of the cyst can vary and can include squamous columnar, cuboidal, pseudostratified, ciliated, and gastric mucosae. Hemorrhage can be the presenting symptom if gastric mucosa is present in the cyst. The other types of mucosa are not specifically associated with particular symptoms [22].

Radiographic Features

Plain chest radiographs can reveal a cyst within the mediastinum.

Barium swallow studies reveal compression of the esophagus without ulceration.

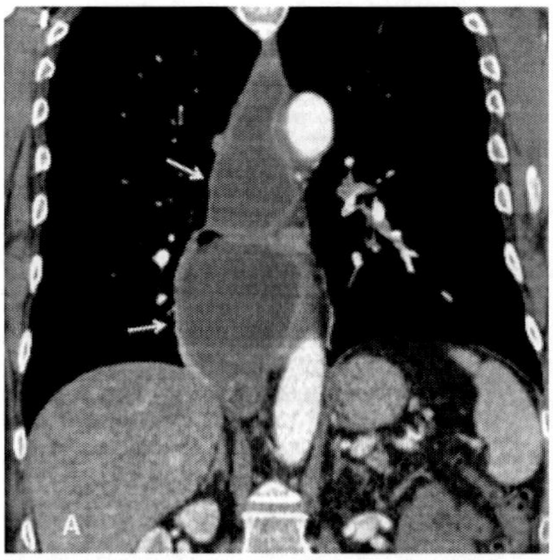

Image 20. CT scan. Achalasia of the esophagus.

CT scan reveals a fluid-filled cystic structure originating from the esophagus (Image 21).

Endoscopic ultrasonography reveals a cystic, filled structure in connection with the esophagus.

MRI scans can also help diagnose esophageal cysts.

All cysts should be resected unless the patient's other medical ailments prohibit operation.

Benign Esophageal Neoplasms – Leiomyoma

Benign neoplasms of the esophagus are extremely rare that constitute less than 1% of esophageal neoplasms. A number of benign esophageal tumors have been recognized. They include leiomyoma, fibrovascular polyp of the esophagus, papilloma, fibroma, haemangioma, hamartoma and neurofibroma. Esophageal leiomyoma is the most common, representing nearly two thirds of benign esophageal tumors.

Leiomyomas represent a hyperproliferation of bundles of smooth muscle cells that are well-demarcated by adjacent tissue or by a smooth connective tissue capsule. They usually arise as intramural growths, most commonly along the distal two thirds of the esophagus. They are multiple in approximately 5% of patients. The majority is discovered incidentally or during investigation for dysphagia. The clinical presentation would often depend on the size of tumour. Small tumours (< 5 cm) usually have no symptoms, while large tumours may cause dysphagia, regurgitation, oesophageal obstruction, chest pain, cough or bleeding. They typically involve the mid to distal oesophagus [23, 24].

Radiographic Features

Esophageal leiomyoma can be visualized using barium swallow. The classic appearance is a smooth concave mass underlying intact mucosa.

Distinct sharp angles are seen at the junction of the tumor and normal tissue. Encroachment onto the esophageal lumen usually is observed (Image 22).

Esophageal ultrasonography can be helpful in demonstrating a smooth, typically round, mass located in the muscularis without encroachment into the overlying mucosa or underlying adventitia.

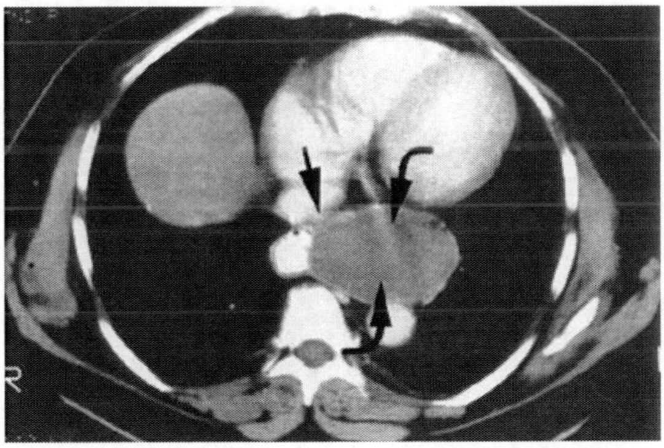

Image 21. Esophageal duplication cyst.

CT scan is even more accurate in diagnosing leiomyomas of the esophagus. Common findings include ovoid intramural solitary mass with a smooth surface, narrowing of oesophageal lumen, displacement of the esophagus, moderate diffuse contrast enhancement with no signs of invasion of adjacent tissues.

The presence of calcifications is almost pathognomonic. Imaging differential considerations include oesophageal carcinoma, leiomyosarcoma of the oesphagus, oesophageal hamartoma and other mediastinal tumours arising close to the oesophagus. The overall prognosis is excellent. If tumour is small (< 5 cm) and asymtomatic treatment is non necessary. Otherwise surgical enucleation is recommended [23].

Esophageal Carcinoma

Carcinoma of the esophagus remains a devastating disease because it is usually not detected until it has progressed to an advanced incurable stage. Oesophageal cancer is responsible for < 1% of all cancers and 4-10% of all gastrointestinal malignancies.

It represents a disease in epidemiologic transition. Until the 1970s, the most common type of esophageal cancer in the United States was squamous cell carcinoma, which has smoking and alcohol consumption as risk factors; since then, there has been a progressive increase in the incidence of esophageal adenocarcinoma, for which the most common predisposing factor is gastroesophageal reflux disease (GERD) [25].

Presenting signs and symptoms of esophageal cancer include dysphagia, initially for solids and eventually progressing to include liquids, weight loss, bleeding epigastric or retrosternal pain, bone pain with metastatic disease, hoarseness, persistent cough. Clinical examination is typically normal unless the cancer has metastasized. In metastatic disease the commonest findings are hepatomegaly and lymphadenopathy in the laterocervical or supraclavicular areas. Diagnosis is based on esophagogastroduodenoscopy which allows direct visualisation and biopsy of the tumor [25, 26].

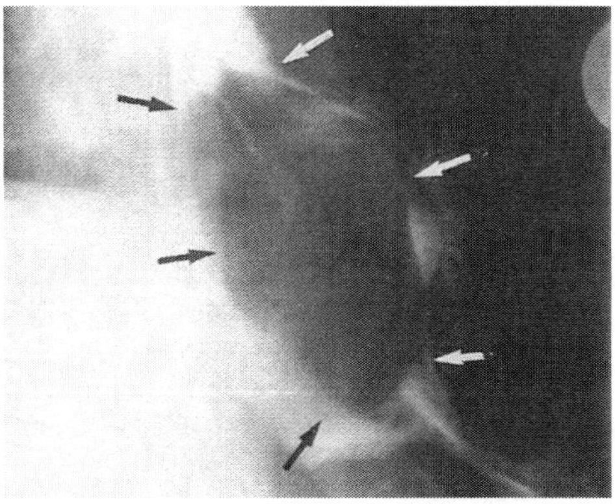

Image 22. Esophageal leiomyoma.

Radiographic Features

Barium esophagography is a useful initial examination in the evaluation of a patient with esophageal complaints. It is unique among esophageal studies for assessing both morphology and motility and therefore remains the study of choice for characterization of esophageal strictures. Esophageal carcinoma may demonstrate a variety of appearances on barium esophagram such as irregular stricture, pre-stricture dilatation with 'hold up' and shouldering of the stricture (Image 24, 25, 26).

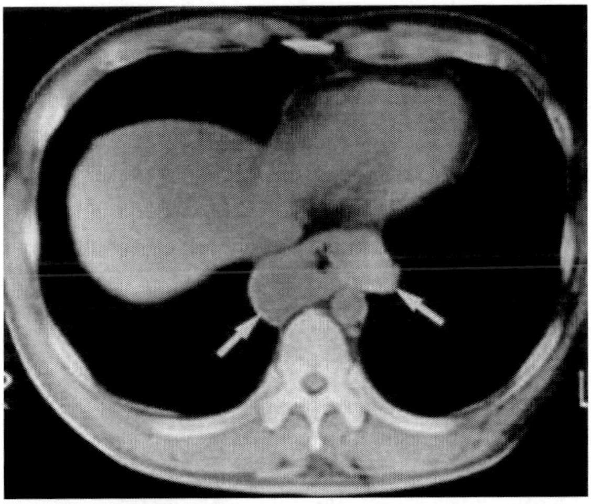

Image 23. CT scan. Esophageal leiomyoma.

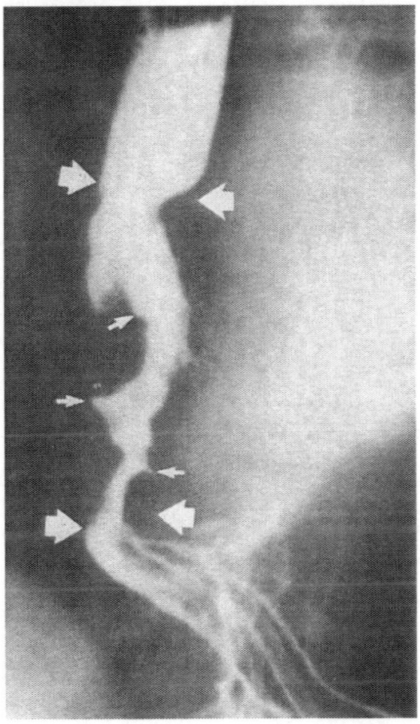

Image 24. Barium swallow illustrating carcinoma of the lower third of the esophagus in a patient with sliding hiatus hernia.

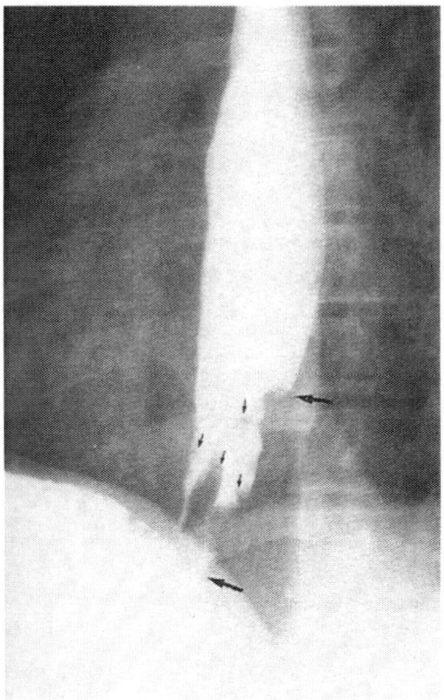

Image 25. Barium swallow illustrating esophageal carcinoma.

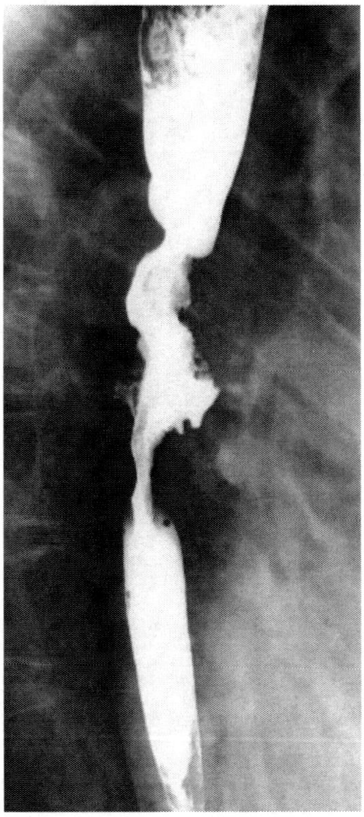

Image 26. Barium swallow illustrating carcinoma of the middle third of the esophagus.

Esophageal endoscopy permits direct inspection and biopsy of the esophageal mucosa for histologic diagnosis. For the purpose of staging esophageal carcinoma, EUS (Image 27), contrast-enhanced CT (Images 28, 29), and PET (Image 30) each offer unique information [26].

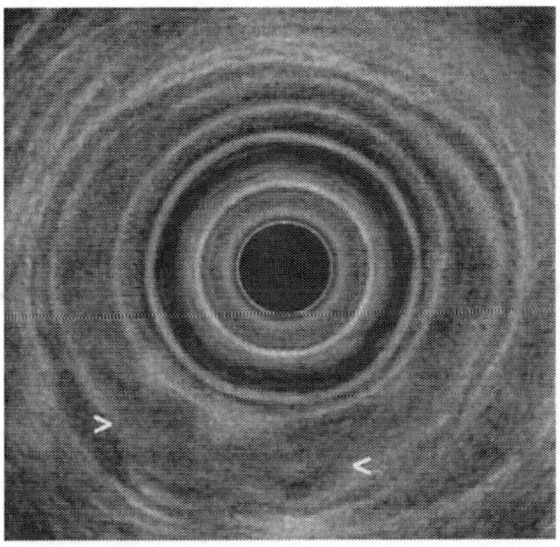

Image 27. EUS showing adenocarcinoma of the esophagus.

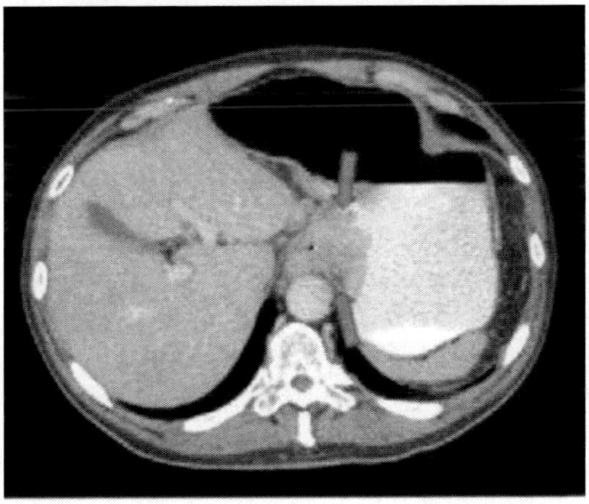

Image 28. CT scan in a patient with adenocarcinoma of the gastroesophageal junction.

Each of the diagnostic modalities has its limitations. Barium esophagography has optimal sensitivity for the detection of lesions when a double-contrast technique is used. Such technique requires that the patient be able to stand upright, which may not be possible with all patients. For bulkier obstructive lesions, an air-contrast technique may not be possible, and a detailed mucosal examination may not be achieved distal to the obstruction.

A notable limitation of CT in diagnosis involves the characterization of lymph nodes. With CT scans, size criteria are used to determine possible metastatic involvement; however, lymph nodes may be enlarged because of infectious or inflammatory aetiologies. Conversely, subcentimeter lymph nodes may harbour metastatic tumor.

Endoscopic ultrasonography (EUS) is highly operator dependent. Another limitation of EUS is its inability to pass the malignant stricture with the transducer. This limitation may result in an incomplete examination.

However, the use of a dedicated 8-mm-diameter esophagoprobe for EUS allows complete examination in most patients [25-27].

With PET, the resolution and cost remain the primary limitations. Subcentimeter foci of tumor metabolism may not be detected.

Staging of Esophageal Carcinima

Contrast-enhanced CT plays an important role in the staging of esophageal carcinoma. Attention is directed to determining the extent of the local tumor, invasion of mediastinal structures, involvement of supraclavicular mediastinal or upper abdominal lymph nodes and distant metastases. These observations are useful in distinguishing between T3 and T4 lesions and in determining the N and M status.

CT examination should extend from the thoracic inlet through the liver. Routine oral contrast material should be administered. It should be obtained during full inspiration when patients are evaluated for esophageal carcinoma since inward bowing or the trachea and mainstem bronchi during expiration may produce the false impression of tracheobronchial invasion. Common CT findings include eccentric or circumferential wall thickening > 5 mm, perioesophageal soft tissue and fat stranding, dilated fluid- and debris-filled oesophageal lumen proximal to an obstructing lesion.

Tracheobronchial invasion appears as displacement of the airway (usually the trachea or left mainstem bronchus) as a result of mass effect by the oesophageal tumour. A careful search for lymph nodes is an essential component of the interpretation.

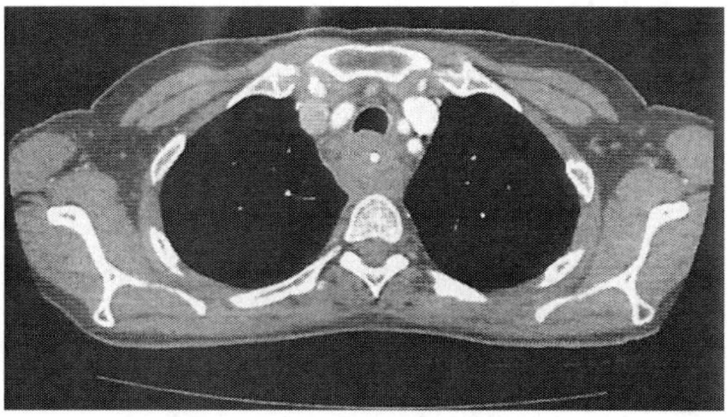

Image 29. CT scan illustrating scuamous cell carcinoma of the middle esohagus.

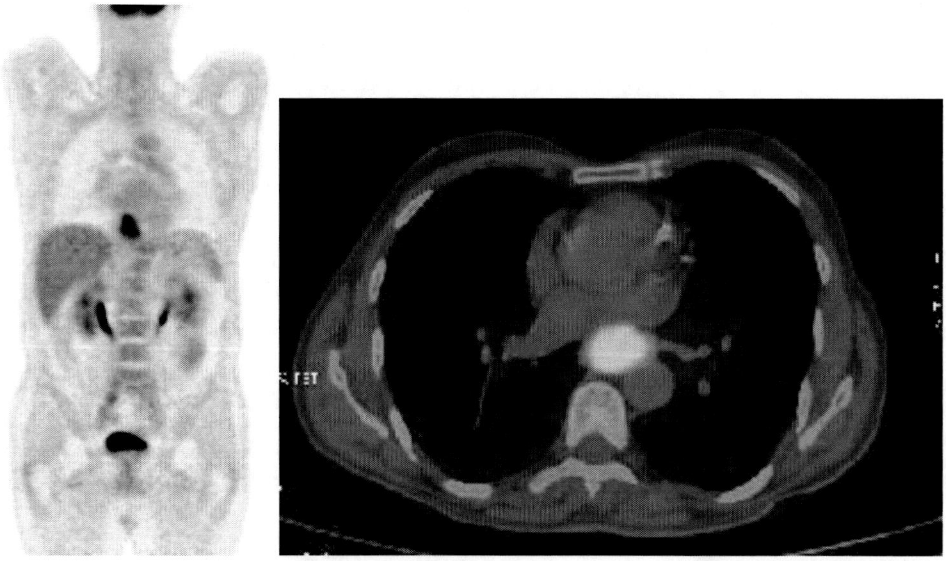

Image 30. PET scan and PET/CT in a patient with adenocarcinoma of the lower third of the esophagus.

A short-axis diameter exceeding 1 cm is considered abnormal for lymph nodes in all mediastinal locations except those in the subcarinal region, in which 1.4 cm is the upper limit of normal. Because lymph nodes may harbor metastases without being enlarged, noting the location of any identified lymph nodes is important. In addition, remembering that lymph nodes may be enlarged because of inflammatory or infectious aetiologies is important. Its sensitivity for the detection of lymph node metastases is in the range of 60-80%. Its specificity is higher, approximatcly 90%.

Magnetic resonance imaging (MRI) has the advantage of direct multiplanar imaging capabilities, which may be of particular use in assessing tracheobronchial, aortic, and pericardial invasion. Currently, MRI has not yielded other significant advantages compared with CT in the staging of esophageal carcinoma. The sensitivity and specificity of MRI for the determination of tumor invasion are equivalent to those of CT.

EUS, unlike CT, allows visualization of the distinct layers within the esophageal wall. Alternating circumferential layers define the mucosal interface (hyperechoic), the mucosa (hypoechoic), the submucosa (hyperechoic), the muscularis propria (hypoechoic), and the adventitial interface (hyperechoic). Such resolution permits the distinction of T1, T2, T3, and T4 tumors. Esophageal carcinoma appears as a hypoechoic lesion disrupting the normal circumferential layers.

However, with standard EUS equipment, often only 3 layers are seen in the esophageal wall: the mucosa and submucosa (hyperechoic), the muscularis propria (hypoechoic), and the adventitial interface (hyperechoic). Local lymph nodes are also demonstrated by using EUS. Nodes are considered malignant if they are round, if they are hypoechoic, and if they have well-defined borders. Usually, benign nodes are hyperechoic and less well defined [27, 28].

T-stage accuracy with EUS is in the range of 79-94%. At this time, only EUS is useful in distinguishing T1 and T2 lesions. N-stage accuracy is in the range of 69-90%. Distant metastases cannot be reliably identified with EUS because of the limited field of view.

PET is quickly becoming a standard oncologic imaging modality. The technique is useful not only for the primary detection of tumor and metastases, but also for the further characterization of abnormalities discovered by using other imaging modalities.

The sensitivity of PET in assessing nodal metastasis is reportedly 33-83%, but studies have shown the superiority of PET to CT and EUS for determining the N status while PET is more sensitive than CT for the detection of distant metastases.

REFERENCES

[1] Buttler, P. *Applied radiological anatomy*. Cambridge University Press. (1999) ISBN: 0521481104.

[2] Ryan, S. *Anatomy for Diagnostic Imaging*. Saunders Ltd. ISBN:0702029718.

[3] Berrocal, T., Madrid, C., Novo, S., et al., Congenital anomalies of the tracheobronchial tree, lung, and mediastinum: embryology, radiology, and pathology. *Radiographics*. 24 (1): e17.

[4] Lam, W. W., Tam, P. K., Chan, F. L., et al., Esophageal atresia and tracheal stenosis: use of three-dimensional CT and virtual bronchoscopy in neonates, infants, and children. *AJR. Am. J. Roentgenol*. 2000;174(4): 1009-12.

[5] Emslander, H. C., Bonadio, W., Klatzo, M. Efficacy of esophageal bougienage by emergency physicians in pediatric coin ingestion. *Ann. Emerg. Med*. Jun. 1996;27(6): 726-9.

[6] Gilchrist, B. F., Valerie, E. P., Nguyen, M. Pearls and perils in the management of prolonged, peculiar, penetrating esophageal foreign bodies in children. *J. Pediatr. Surg*. Oct. 1997;32(10):1429-31.

[7] Jaramillo, D., Cleveland, R. N., Blickman, J. G. Radiologic management of esophageal foreign bodies. *Semin. Intervent. Radiol*. 8:198-203.

[8] Palanivelu, C., Rangarajan, M., Maheshkumaar, G. S., et al., Minimally invasive surgery combined with peroperative endoscopy for symptomatic middle and lower esophageal diverticula: a single institute's experience. *Surg. Laparosc. Endosc. Percutan. Tech*. 2008;18(2): 133-8.

[9] Baker, M. E., Zuccaro, G., Achkar, E., et al., Esophageal diverticula: patient assessment. *Semin. Thorac. Cardiovasc. Surg*. 1999;11(4): 326-36.

[10] D'Journo, X. B., Ferraro, P., Martin, J., et al., Lower oesophageal sphincter dysfunction is part of the functional abnormality in epiphrenic diverticulum. *Br. J. Surg*. 2009;96 (8): 892-900.

[11] Luketic, V. A., Sanyal, A. J. Esophageal varices. I. Clinical presentation, medical therapy, and endoscopic therapy. *Gastroenterol. Clin. North Am*. Jun. 2000;29(2):337-85.

[12] Pieters, P. C., Miller, W. J., DeMeo, J. H. Evaluation of the portal venous system: complementary roles of invasive and noninvasive imaging strategies. *Radiographics*. Jul.-Aug. 1997;17(4):879-95.

[13] Kim, S. H., Kim, Y. J., Lee, J. M., Choi, K. D., Chung, Y. J., Han, J. K., et al., Esophageal varices in patients with cirrhosis: multidetector CT esophagography--comparison with endoscopy. *Radiology*. Mar. 2007; 242(3):759-68.

[14] Karasick, S., Lev-toaff, A. S. Esophageal strictures: findings on barium radiographs. *AJR Am. J. Roentgenol*. 1995;165(3): 561-5. *AJR Am. J. Roentgenol*.

[15] Hasimoto, C. N., Cataneo, C., Eldib, R., et al., Efficacy of surgical versus conservative treatment in esophageal perforation: a systematic review of case series studies. *Acta Cir. Bras*. 2013;28(4): 266-71.

[16] Søreide, J. A., Viste, A. Esophageal perforation: diagnostic work-up and clinical decision-making in the first 24 hours. *Scand. J. Trauma Resusc. Emerg. Med*. 2011;19 (1): 66.

[17] Müller, M., Gockel, I., Hedwig, P., et al., Is the Schatzki ring a unique esophageal entity?. *World J. Gastroenterol*. 2011;17(23): 2838-43.

[18] Kahrilas, P. J., Kim, H. C., Pandolfino, J. E. Approaches to the diagnosis and grading of hiatal hernia. *Best Pract. Res. Clin. Gastroenterol*. 2008; 22(4):601-16.

[19] Huang, X., Zhu, H. M., Deng, C. Z., et al., Gastroesophageal reflux: the features in elderly patients. *World J. Gastroenterol*. Oct. 1999;5(5):421-423.

[20] Lacy, B. E., Weiser, K. Esophageal motility disorders: medical therapy. *J. Clin. Gastroenterol*. May-Jun. 2008;42(5):652-8.

[21] Gonlachanvit, S., Fisher, R. S., Parkman, H. P. Diagnostic modalities for achalasia. *Gastrointest. Endosc. Clin. N. Am*. Apr. 2001;11(2):293-310.

[22] Jeung, M. Y., Gasser, B., Gangi, A., et al., Imaging of cystic masses of the mediastinum. *Radiographics*. 2002;22 Spec. No (suppl. 1): S79-93.

[23] Weissleder, R., Wittenberg, J., Harisinghani, M. G. *Primer of diagnostic imaging*. Mosby Inc. (2007) ISBN:0323040683.

[24] Gupta, V., Lal, A, Sinha, S. K., Nada, R., Gupta, N. M. Leiomyomatosis of the esophagus: experience over a decade. *J. Gastrointest. Surg*. Feb. 2009;13(2):206-11.

[25] Takashima, S., Takeuchi, N., Shiozaki, H., et al., Carcinoma of the esophagus: CT vs MR imaging in determining resectability. *AJR Am. J. Roentgenol.* Feb. 1991;156(2): 297-302.

[26] Levine, M. S., Chu, P., Furth, E. E., et al., Carcinoma of the esophagus and esophagogastric junction: sensitivity of radiographic diagnosis. *AJR Am. J. Roentgenol.* Jun. 1997;168(6):1423-6.

[27] Rankin, S. C., Taylor, H., Cook, G. J., Mason, R. Computed tomography and positron emission tomography in the pre- operative staging of oesophageal carcinoma. *Clin. Radiol*. Sep. 1998;53(9):659-65.

[28] Levine, M. S., Halvorsen, R. A. Esophageal carcinoma. In: Gore, R. M., Levine, M. S., Laufer, I., eds. *Textbook of Gastrointestinal Radiology*. Philadelphia: WB Saunders Co; 1994:446-78.

In: The Role of Imaging Technology …
Editor: Georgios Tsoulfas

ISBN: 978-1-63483-490-2

Chapter 10

The Role of Imaging in Gastric Surgery

Efstathios Kotidis*[*], *Manos-Georgios Pramateftakis* and *Nikolaos Michalopoulos
Department of Surgery, Aristotle University of Thessaloniki, Thessaloniki, Greece

Abstract

The esophagus is an integral part of the digestive system. There is a wide range of diseases (congenital, functional, structural, trauma and neoplasia) affecting the stomach, and as a result knowledge of the most current imaging technology is critical for accurate diagnosis and a successful management. This chapter will present the various imaging modalities and discuss their advantages and disadvantages.

Introduction

The stomach lies between the oesophagus and the duodenum in the upper abdomen. It is divided into four distinct regions. The cardia, which is the area that receives the oesophagus (gastro-oesophageal junction); the fundus, which is formed by the upper curvature; the body, the main central region of the organ; and the pylorus (antrum), which represents the lower section of the stomach that facilitates emptying into the small intestine (Image 1).

Entry of food into the stomach is controlled by the lower esophageal sphincter and exit from the stomach by the pyloric sphincter. These are under the control of several mechanisms including stimulant (parasympathetic) and inhibitory (orthosympathetic) control from the anterior gastric, posterior, superior and inferior coeliac and myenteric nerve plexuses.

The inner mucosal surface has many rugal folds that act to increase the surface area of the stomach lining and increase its efficiency.

---

[*] Corresponding author: E. Kotidis. E-mail: skotidis@gmail.com.

Its arterial supply is provided by the right gastric artery (inferior lesser curvature), the left gastric artery (superior lesser curvature and cardia), the right gastroepiploic artery (inferior greater curvature), the left gastroepiploic artery (superior greater curvature) and the short gastric vessels (fundus). Regarding the venous drainage, the left and right gastric veins drain to portal vein, the short gastric vein and left gastroepiploic vein drain to splenic vein and the right gastroepiploic vein drain to superior mesenteric artery. Lymphatics drain with arteries to the coeliac lymph nodes.

The gastric wall is composed of four layers: the mucosa includes the internal layer of epithelium the lamina propria and the muscularis mucosae; the submucosa which is a fibrous layer of connective tissue under the mucosa; the muscularis externa which is composed of three muscular layers (inner oblique, middle circular and outer longitudinal); and the serosa, the outermost layer of the stomach wall consisting of connective tissue which is continuous with the peritoneum.

The stomach wall contains several different types of glandular tissue. The cardia, fundus and pylorus all have different types of glands and are composed of a variety of different cells:

- Mucous cells: secrete a mucus gell layer and are found throughout the stomach [1, 2]
- Parietal (oxyntic) cells: secrete gastric acid and intrinsic factor throughout the stomach
- Chief (zymogenic) cells: secrete pepsinogen and rennin in the fundus only
- Enteroendocrine (APUD) cells: secrete a variety of products and are found throughout the stomach

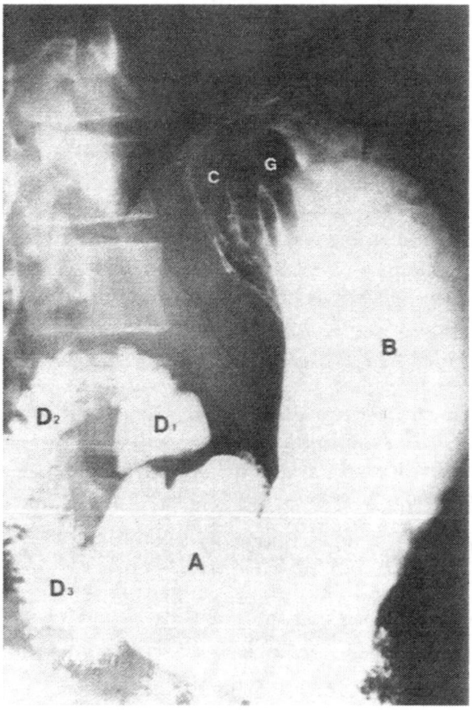

C = cardia, G = fundus, B = body, A = antrum, D = duodenum.

Image 1. Double contrast swallow.

Gastric Diverticulum

The gastric diverticulum is a sac-like projection usually originated from the gastric fundus, located usually 1-2cm below the gastroesophageal junction.

It is the least common among gastrointestinal diverticula. The incidence varies from 0.01% to 0.11% at endoscopy studies. It is usually asymptomatic and, in some cases, could presents as a vague sensation of fullness immediately after meals or as gastric discomfort. Complications like ulceration, perforation, torsion, hemorrhage and malignancy are rare and an indication for surgical treatment [3].

Gastric diverticulum may be congenital (true diverticula that have all layers of the gastric wall) or acquired (false diverticula) and arise virtually anywhere along the stomach.

In imaging studies gastric diverticulum could mimic an adrenal mass. Surgical resection is recommended when the diverticulum is large, symptomatic or complicated [4].

Radiographic Features

A well defined saccular collection of barium protracting from the gastric wall is seen in barium swallow test (Image 2). CT scan may be needed and it shows a well defined saccular collection of fluid or gas, being filled by the iodinated oral contrast, demonstrating communication with the gastric cavity.

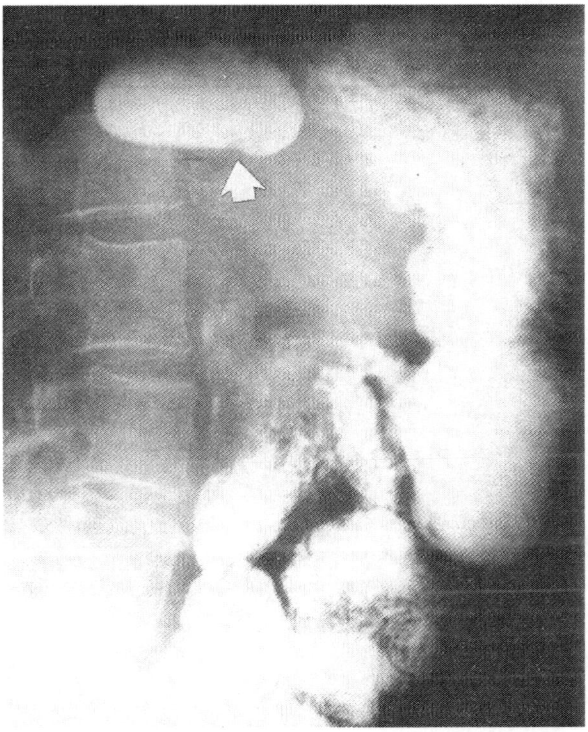

Image 2. Gastric diverticulum in the posterior wall of the cardia.

Gastric Volvulus

Gastric volvulus is a rare clinical entity defined as an abnormal rotation of the stomach of more than 180°, creating a closed-loop obstruction that can result in incarceration and strangulation. Borchardt described the classic triad associated with gastric volvulus: severe epigastric pain, retching without vomiting, and inability to pass a nasogastric tube [5].

Classification

The most frequently used classification system of gastric volvulus relates to the axis around which the stomach rotates, including organoaxial, mesentericoaxial, and combined.

Organoaxial type: In an organoaxial gastric volvulus, the stomach rotates around an axis that connects the gastroesophageal junction and the pylorus. The antrum rotates in opposite direction to the fundus of the stomach. This is the most common type of gastric volvulus and it is usually associated with diaphragmatic defects. Strangulation and necrosis commonly occur with organoaxial gastric volvulus.

Mesentericoaxial type: The mesentericoaxial axis bisects the lesser and greater curvatures. The antrum rotates anteriorly and superiorly so that the posterior surface of the stomach lies anteriorly. The rotation is usually incomplete and occurs intermittently. Vascular compromise is uncommon. Patients with mesentericoaxial gastric volvulus usually present without diaphragmatic defects and usually have chronic symptoms.

Combined type: The combined type of gastric volvulus is a rare form in which the stomach twists mesentericoaxially and organoaxially. This type of gastric volvulus makes up the remainder of cases and is usually observed in patients with chronic volvulus.

According to etiology, gastric volvulus can be classified as either type 1 (idiopathic) or type 2 (congenital or acquired).

Type 1: Idiopathic gastric volvulus comprises two thirds of cases and is presumably due to abnormal laxity of the gastrosplenic, gastroduodenal, gastrophrenic, and gastrohepatic ligaments. This allows approximation of the cardia and pylorus when the stomach is full, predisposing to volvulus. Type 1 gastric volvulus is more common in adults but has been reported in children.

Type 2: Type 2 gastric volvulus is found in one third of patients and is usually associated with congenital or acquired abnormalities that result in abnormal mobility of the stomach. The most common causes of gastric volvulus in adults are diaphragmatic defects.

Symptoms

Symptoms of gastric volvulus may range from mild abdominal pain and vomiting, when no or partial outlet obstruction is present, to severe pain and retching, when there is complete obstruction and ischemia.

Fiberoptic endoscopy has a limited role in the diagnosis of gastric volvulus because the twist precludes passage of the endoscope [6].

Radiographic Features

Typically, the first examination to be performed in the patient with symptoms referable to the chest and/or abdomen is a plain radiograph. Plain radiography may demonstrate findings that are indistinguishable from those that are produced by other causes of gastric atony or obstruction. In mesenteroaxial volvulus, the distended stomach appears spherical on supine images. Two air-fluid levels are visible on the upright film: 1 in the fundus, which is inferior, and 1 in the antrum, which is superior. Organoaxial volvulus is difficult to diagnose on plain images. The stomach lies horizontally and contains a single air-fluid level on upright views. No characteristic beak is observed. However, the modality is useful for excluding other causes of the patient's symptoms, such as pneumoperitoneum or pneumothorax.

Although this is a good examination to start with, the most definitive study is the upper GI barium study. Barium study is highly sensitive and specific. It is generally considered to be the criterion standard for diagnosis (Image 3). However, the diagnosis may be missed in cases of intermittent torsion. The upper GI series may show only a paraesophageal hernia during a symptom-free interval, leading to a false-negative diagnosis.

CT scanning and MRI are not typically considered to be the diagnostic examinations of choice in patients who are evaluated for gastric volvulus. However, the multiaxial reconstructions that are afforded by helical CT in particular may be preferred to the images obtained with conventional barium study, particularly in the acutely ill patient who is unable to tolerate a fluoroscopic examination. In addition, chronic gastric volvulus is often discovered incidentally in patients undergoing CT scanning for an unrelated condition.

Ultrasonography as a technique for the detection of gastric disease (and of gastric volvulus in particular) is still in its infancy. Angiography is often used in the evaluation of massive or refractory GI hemorrhage. Although it is a rare cause of such hemorrhage, gastric volvulus should be considered. The angiographic appearance is sensitive and specific during an acute episode.

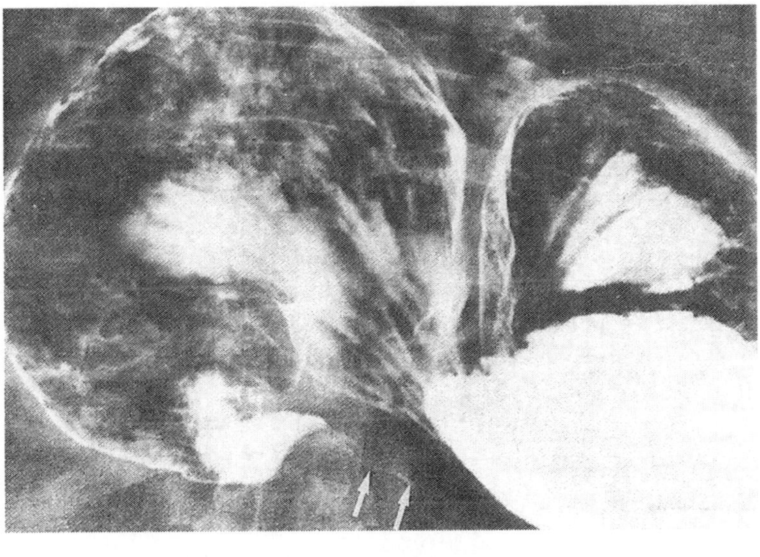

Image 3. Double contrast swallow test illustrating mesentericoaxial gastric volvulus.

MENETRIER DISEASE

Ménétrier disease (MD) is a form of rare idiopathic hypertrophic gastropathy. The exact aetiology is not well known. The juvenile form has been linked to cytomegaloviral infection and usually resolves spontaneously. The adult form tends to progress with time and TGF-A activation of the EGFR receptor has been implicated. The characteristic of the disease is gastric mucosal hypertrophy, which may cause the rugae to resemble convolutions of the brain. Rugal thickening is predominantly caused by the expansion of the epithelial cell compartment of the gastric mucosa.

It most commonly affects the gastric fundal region also any part of the stomach may be involved. Achlorhydria, hypoproteinaemia and oedema comprise the classic triad. It is thought to be caused by protein-loss in the digestive system, protein-losing enteropathy. Acid production may be compromised. Hypoproteinaemia may lead to ascites and pleural effusions. Imaging differential considerations for diffuse rugal thickening include gastric lymphoma, which may also occur as part of post transplant lymphoproliferative disorder affecting the stomach and other forms of gastritis (infective gastritis, radiation gastritis, eosinophilic gastritis). Treatment includes high protein diet to correct hypoproteinaemia, PPI to treat attendant gastritis, EGFR monocloncal antibody (Cetuximab) or gastrectomy.

Radiographic Features

On fluoroscopy MD is usually characterised by giant rugal folds (Images 3, 4). On contrast-enhanced CT images, the thickened rugae appear as areas of thickened mucosa that project into the gastric lumen to a degree that may resemble convolution of brain [7].

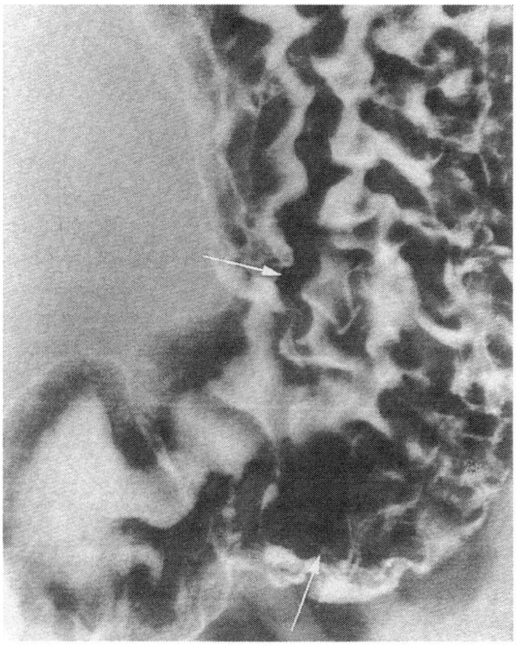

Image 4. Menetrier's disease. The arrows indicate the hypertrophic mucosal folds.

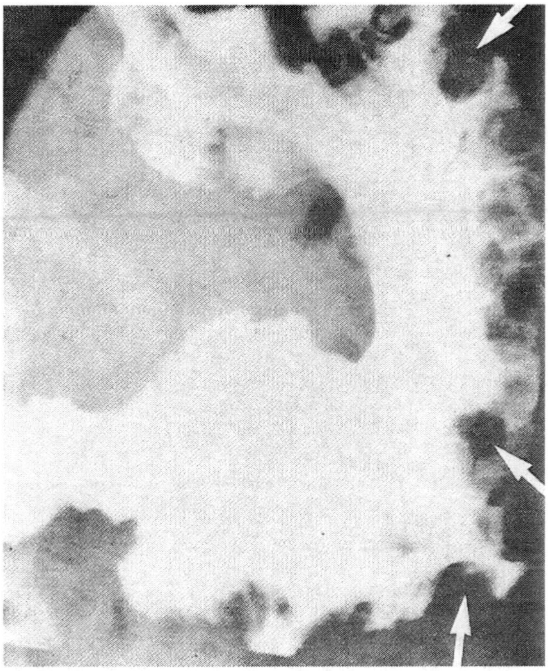

Image 5. Barium swallow test in a patient with Menetrier's disease.

Peptic Ulcer Disease

Peptic ulcer disease (PUD) encompasses a number of entities, united by the presence of mucosal ulceration secondary to the effects of gastric acid. Since the recognition of *Helicobacter pylori* as a common causative agent, and the development of powerful anti-acid medications, peptic ulcer disease has become comparatively rare in western populations.

Generally peptic ulcer disease is encountered more frequently in males (M:F 3:1) and usually in the older population.

Risk factors include *Helicobacter pylori* infection, NSAIDs, corticosteroids, severe physiological stress/illness (e.g., admission to intensive care) and Zollinger-Ellison syndrome. The majority of cases are due to infection with *Helicobacter pylori.*

This can be confirmed with biopsies obtained at endoscopy and urea breath test, the combination of the two resulting in a detection rate of close to 100% [8]. Gastric and duodenal ulcers usually cannot be differentiated based on history alone, although some findings may be suggestive.

Epigastric pain is the most common symptom of both gastric and duodenal ulcers. It is characterized by a gnawing or burning sensation and occurs after meals—classically, shortly after meals with gastric ulcer and 2-3 hours afterward with duodenal ulcer. A peptic ulcer may present acutely as upper gastrointestinal bleeding (14%), perforation (6%) or gastric outlet obstruction (1%). Upper GI endoscopy is the preferred diagnostic test in the evaluation of patients with suspected PUD. Endoscopy provides an opportunity to visualize the ulcer, to determine the presence and degree of active bleeding, and to attempt hemostasis by direct measures, if required.

Endoscopy should be performed early in patients older than 45-50 years and in patients with associated so-called alarm features. When dyspeptic symptoms lead to identification of upper gastrointestinal ulceration (usually via endoscopy) patients are typically treated with acid lowering medications and tested for *Helicobacter pylori*, which if found is then eradicated.

This is important not only to prevent recurrence of peptic ulceration and reflux oesophagitis but also because it is associated with a number of malignancies including B-cell lymphoma and gastric adenocarcinoma [8].

Radiographic Features

Although historically barium studies were the mainstay of investigation for suspect peptic ulceration, endoscopy has in most centres largely replaced the barium meal. Many current younger radiologists have rarely if ever performed a full diagnostic barium meal, and the 'art' of this examination is gradually being lost. Barium meals are performed with liquid barium and an effervescent to distend the stomach with gas and allow a 'double contrast' image (Images 6, 7). Features of ulceration include pocket of barium filling the ulcer crater (85% round; 15% linear) and radiating folds of mucosa away from the ulcer. 10-15% of ulcers are multiple while postbulbar ulcers should raise the possibility of Zollinger-Ellison syndrome especially if ulcers are multiple and gastric folds are thickened.

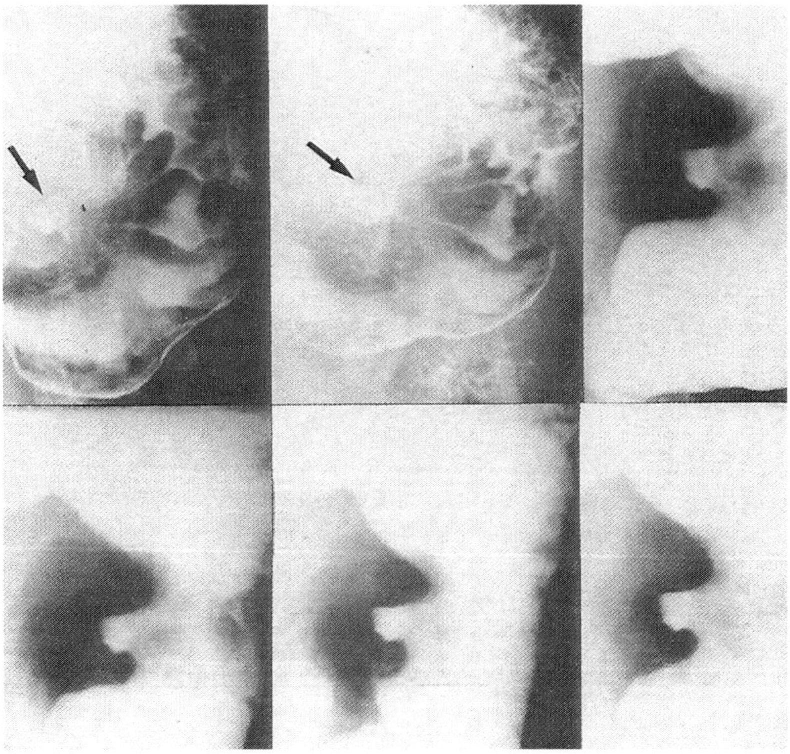

Image 6. Benign gastric ulcer.

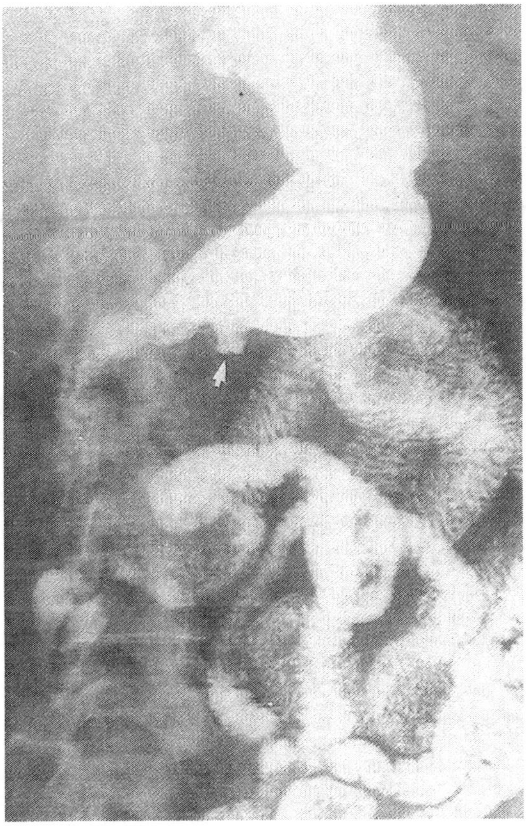

Image 7. Benign gastric ulcer.

In patients presenting acutely, a chest radiograph may be useful to detect free abdominal air when perforation is suspected (Image 8). However, even in the acute setting CT is the modality of choice for assessing a patient with acute abdominal pain, especially in cases where plain chest x ray fails to demonstrate the presence of free intra-abdominal air. In some settings, CT scan may be able to identify the site of bleeding prior to endoscopy. Haemorrhage, though, is challenging to identify and requires a multi-phase scan without positive oral contrast (typically non-contrast, arterial and delayed phase scans are obtained) and the presence of active bleeding. Extravasation and pooling/accumulation of contrast into the lumen of the bowel may be seen. Angiography may be necessary in patients with a massive GI bleed in whom endoscopy cannot be performed. An ongoing bleeding rate of 0.5 mL/min or more is needed for the angiography to be able to accurately identify the bleeding source. Angiography can depict the source of the bleeding and can help provide needed therapy in the form of a direct injection of vasoconstrictive agents [6, 8].

Benign Gastric Tumors

With the advent of modern techniques and the widespread use of gastric endoscopy, benign gastric wall lesions are now diagnosed more frequently and can be studied using the tissue obtained by biopsy or polypectomy.

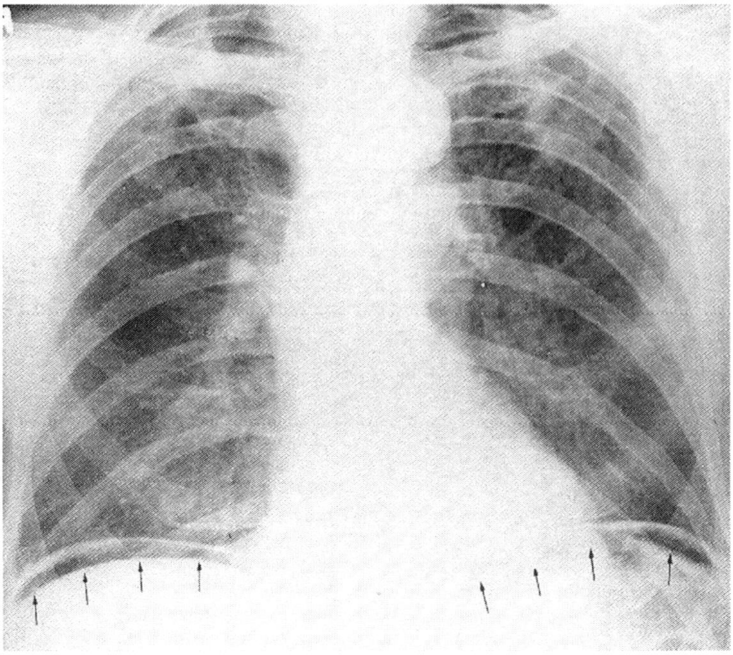

Image 8. Chest x-ray demonstrating free subphrenic air collection secondary to perforation of peptic ulcer.

All layers of the stomach wall have the potential to produce tumorous growths. In 40% of patients with benign gastric tumors, the lesions are mucosal tumors. Another 60% are nonmucosal based. Gastric polyps are defined as luminal lesions projecting above the plane of the mucosal surface and are relatively frequent in routine pathology practice.

Various subtypes of gastric polyps are recognized and divided into nonneoplastic and neoplastic and are also further classified by their association with polyposis syndromes [9].

Mucosal tumors are divided into nonneoplastic and neoplastic polyps.

Not neoplastic polyps include could either associated with polyposis syndrome (Peutz-Jeghers, juvenile polyps, Cowden disease, Cronkhite Canada syndrome, Gardner syndrome) or not associated with polyposis syndromes (hyperplastic polyps, inflammatory polyps, ectopic pancreas). Neoplastic polyps include fundic gland polyps, adenomatous polyps and gastric carcinoids [9, 10].

Nonmucosal tumors could be mesenchymal (GIST, lipoma, fibroma, glomus tumor) or vascular (hemangioma or lymphangioma). Many tumors are found incidentally on gastroscopy. Small tumors are usually asymptomatic, but larger tumors can ulcerate and cause occult bleeding and anemia. Large antral tumors cause intermittent gastric outlet obstruction. If ulcerated, these tumors may cause epigastric pain similar to a peptic ulcer.

Radiographic Features

Air-contrast studies of the stomach are sensitive in delineating mucosal details and lesions (Image 9). Lesions are often found incidentally by computerized tomography scan or other radiological evaluations of the upper gastrointestinal tract (Image 10).

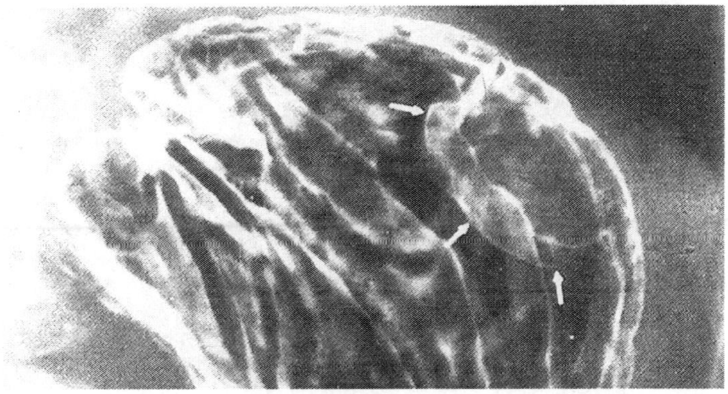

Image 9. Double contrasts swallow illustrating a leiomyoma of the stomach.

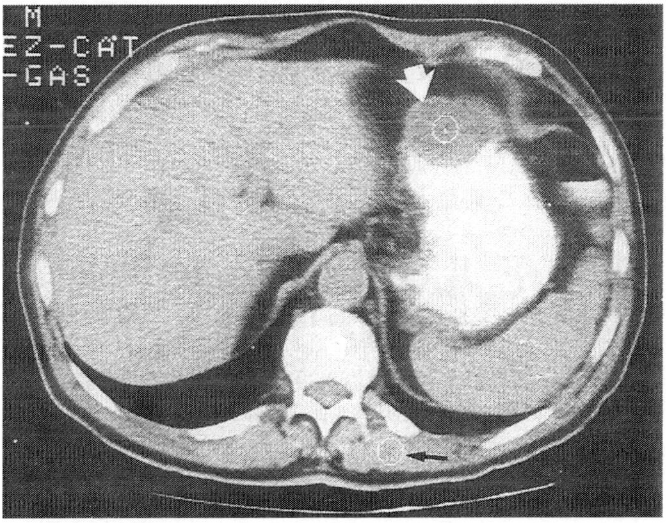

Image 10. CT scan in the same patient as in image 9.

Endoscopy however is the procedure of choice for both diagnostic and therapeutic purposes. If small superficial lesions are removed endoscopically, follow-up should include a regular annual endoscopy. Endoscopic biopsies are difficult to interpret and may be misleading because deep layers of the stomach wall or the tumor are not sampled. Snare biopsies that retrieve the whole specimen are preferred whenever technically possible. Endoscopic ultrasound (EUS) is helpful in broad-based lesions, where the relationship of the tumor to the layers of the stomach is important (Image 11). Disruption of the normal sonographic appearance of 5 layers on EUS may signify invasion [11].

Gastric Carcinoma

Gastric cancer is the second most common cause of cancer-related death in the world, and it remains difficult to cure, primarily because most patients present with advanced disease. In most developed countries, however, rates of stomach cancer have declined dramatically over the past half century.

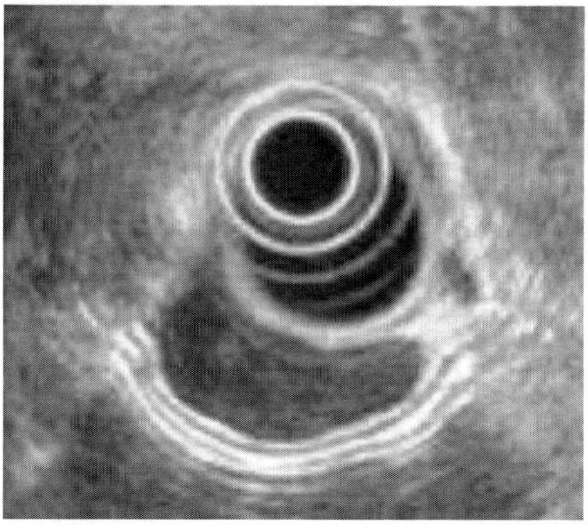

Image 11. EUS in a patient with gastric GIST.

Decreases in gastric cancer have been attributed in part to widespread use of refrigeration and therefore decreased contamination of food by carcinogenic compounds arising from the decay of unrefrigerated meat products as well as decreased intake of salt. Another reason is the lower rates of chronic *Helicobacter pylori* infection, thanks to improved sanitation and use of antibiotics, and increased screening in some countries [12].

Adenocarcinomas account for approximately 95% of all malignant gastric neoplasms. The remaining 5% of tumors are lymphomas, leiomyosarcomas, carcinoids, or sarcomas.

Early disease has no associated symptoms; however, some patients with incidental complaints are diagnosed with early gastric cancer. Most symptoms of gastric cancer reflect advanced disease. Patients may complain of indigestion, nausea or vomiting, dysphagia, postprandial fullness, loss of appetite, melena, hematemesis, and weight loss [13].

Late complications include pathologic peritoneal and pleural effusions; obstruction of the gastric outlet or the gastroesophageal junction. Other symptoms may include intrahepatic jaundice caused by hepatomegaly; extrahepatic jaundice; and inanition resulting from starvation or cachexia of tumor origin. The differential diagnosis can be broad and includes gastric lymphoma, gastric metastasis, gastric stromal tumour (GIST), gastritis, benign gastric (peptic) ulcer, Menetrier disease, secondary changes from pancreatitis (from extrinsic inflammatory change). Endoscopy and biopsy (at least 6 samples) of any gastric lesion is the cornerstone in the diagnosis of gastric gancer. Esophagogastroduodenoscopy has a diagnostic accuracy of 95%. In selected cases, endoscopic ultrasound may be helpful in assessing depth of penetration of the tumor or involvement of adjacent structures. Depending on the depth of tumor invasion into the gastric wall, gastric adenocarcinoma is divided into early, if the tumor invades no more deeply than the submucosa, irrespective of lymph node metastasis and advanced if the tumor invades deeper than the submucosa [14].

Radiographic Features

Radiological methods are often the initial examination that raises suspicion for gastric carcinoma, besides being used in the staging of the disease.

Single-contrast barium studies have an overall sensitivity of 75% in the detection of gastric cancer, but double-contrast barium examinations have a sensitivity of 90-95% in gastric cancer detection, comparable to that of endoscopy (Images 12, 13). Double-contrast upper GI series and barium swallows may be helpful in delineating the extent of disease when obstructive symptoms are present or when bulky proximal tumors prevent passage of the endoscope to examine the stomach distal to an obstruction.

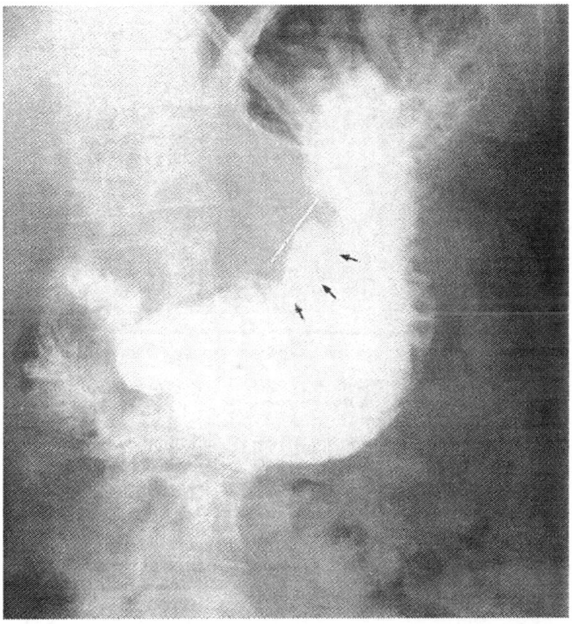

Image 12. Fluoroscopy test demonstrating gastric carcinoma.

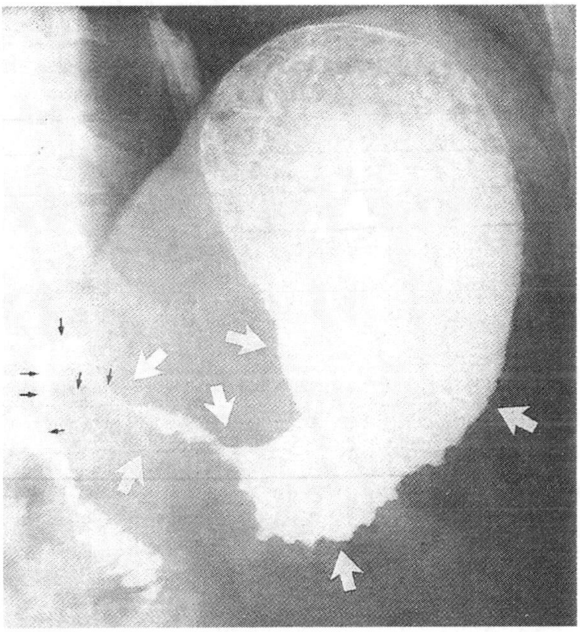

Image 13. Fluoroscopy test demonstrating linitis plastic.

Depending on the fluoroscopy findings, early gastric cancer is divided into three types.

type I: elevated lesion, protrudes > 5 mm into lumen (polypoid)

type II: superficial lesion (plaque-like, mucosal nodularity, ulceration)

type III: shallow, irregular ulcer crater with adjacent nodular mucosa and fusion or amputation of radiation folds.

Likewise, advanced gastric cancer may be polypoidal, ulcerative, or infiltrating lesions on barium studies.

With ulcerated carcinomas, an irregular crater is located in a rind of malignant tissue. Infiltrating carcinomas result in irregular narrowing of the stomach, with nodularity or spiculation of the mucosa Submucosal spread of tumors may result in pseudoachalasia or secondary achalasia with tapered, beaklike narrowing of the distal esophagus and infiltration of the gastric cardia. Ultrasound is not useful, unless a large epigastric mass is present or on endoscopic ultrasound study.

CT is currently the staging modality of choice because it can help identify the primary tumor, assess for local spread, and detect nodal involvement and distant metastases.

Additionally, CT is used to monitor a patient's response to treatment. Detection of gastric carcinoma is improved by using thin-section sequences and helical CT (14, 15). The early arterial phase is used to assess enhancement of the gastric wall; the later portal venous phase is used to assess the liver parenchyma for metastases. CT scans may show polypoidal mass with or without ulceration, focal wall thickening with mucosal irregularity or ulceration, wall thickening with the absence of normal mucosal folds (infiltrative lesions), focal infiltration of the gastric wall, variable thickening of the wall and marked contrast enhancement (typical of scirrhous lesions). Finally, mucinous carcinomas have low attenuation due to their high mucin content and which may contain calcification.

The depth of tumor invasion is not accurately assessed with CT. Tumor invasion of the perigastric fat is seen as soft-tissue stranding. Tiny 4- to 8-mm nodules may be observed. These may coalesce into sheets of tumor in advanced cases. Overall, the accuracy of determining the T-stage with CT is approximately 66%. CT depicts 75% of nodes larger than 5 mm in diameter, but it does not depict tumor in normal-sized nodes. CT is not useful in distinguishing between enlarged nodes due to reactive changes and those due to tumor. Because the portal vein drains the stomach, the liver is the most common site for hematogenous metastases (see the first image below).

Less common sites are the lungs (see the second image below), adrenal glands, and kidneys. Bony and cerebral metastases are uncommon. ntraperitoneal and omental metastases are common in advanced gastric cancer. They consist of nodules, localized fluid collections, and irregular thickening and stranding of the mesentery and omentum. Ascites and small-bowel obstruction may occur. Gastric carcinoma is the most common primary tumor to metastasize to the ovaries. These ovarian metastases are usually bilateral and are known as Krukenberg tumors. CT may fail to depict tiny omental and peritoneal deposits; small pelvic deposits may be overlooked as well [11-13].

MRI studies in which a breath-hold, fast-imaging technique and water were used showed accuracy rates comparable to those of helical, biphasic CT scanning. In T staging, the accuracy of MRI is 73%, compared with 67% for CT. In N staging, the accuracy of MRI is 55%, compared with 59% for CT. EUS has improved the accuracy of local staging of gastric carcinomas. Unlike CT and MRI, EUS can depict individual layers of the gastric wall, with a rotating high-frequency probe inserted via an endoscope.

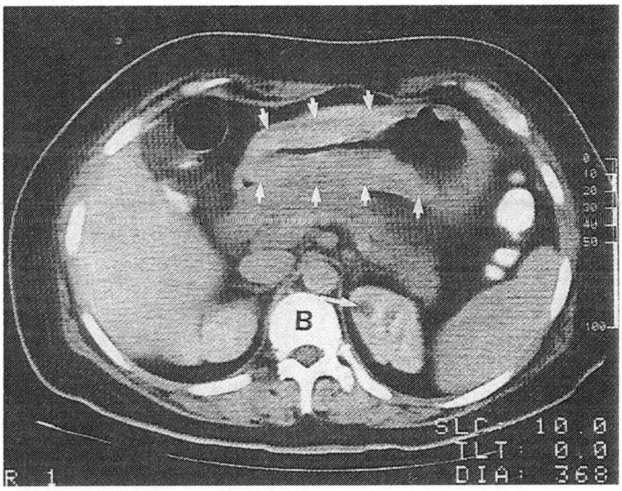

Image 14. CT scan illustrating thickening of the gastric wall because of adenocarcinoma of the antrum.

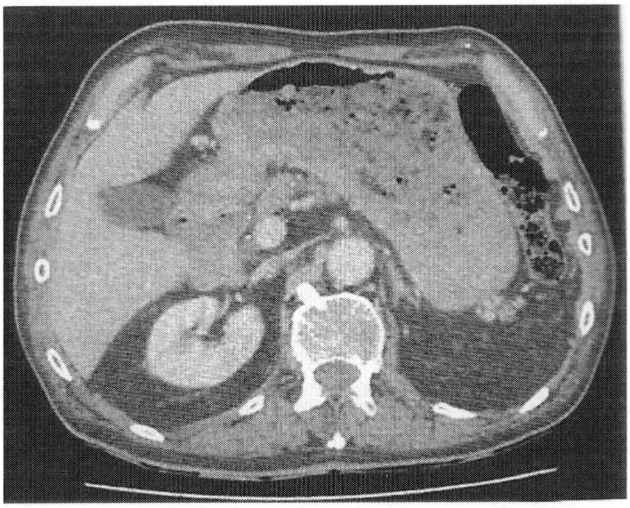

Image 15. CT scan in a patient with gastric outlet obstruction secondary to gastric cancer.

The gastric wall is visualized as 5 concentric bands: Mucosa – Echogenic, Muscularis mucosa – Hypoechoic, Submucosa – Echogenic, Muscularis propria – Hypoechoic andSerosa – Echogenic.

A gastric tumor is demonstrated as a hypoechoic mass with varying mural invasion. Regarding N staging, involved nodes are rounder and more hypoechoic than normal nodes. However, EUS is limited to an area 5 cm from the probe. It cannot be used to assess distant metastases or nodes more than 5 cm away from the probe. Intraoperative US and laparoscopy have an accuracy of 81% in T staging and an accuracy of 93% in N staging; however, the necessary equipment and expertise are not widely available.

PET scanning may be useful in the staging and postoperative assessment of gastric carcinomas. The only limitation of PET is that involved local lymph nodes cannot be separated from the primary tumor. Thus, its role in N staging is limited [15].

GASTRIC LYMPHOMA

Gastric lymphoma may either represent secondary involvement by systemic disease or primary malignancy confined to the stomach. Primary gastric lymphoma is an uncommon condition accounting for about 2% of all lymphomas. It is the most common source of lymphomas in the gastrointestinal tract. Typically primary gastric lymphoma occurs in adults in the 6th decade of life, without gender predilection. Secondary gastric lymphoma matches the demographics of the underlying lymphoma [16]. Patients usually present with long standing epigastric pain and/or dyspepsia which is attributable to *Helicobacter pylori* rather than the lymphoma *per se*. Three distinct types of gastric lymphoma are recognised:

- low-grade MALT lymphoma, accounting for 60% of all primary gastric lymphomas
- primary sporadic lymphoma, the vast majority of which are B-cell non-Hodgkins lymphoma
- secondary involvement of the stomach by systemic lymphoma

Mucosa-associated lymphoid tissue (MALT) lymphoma are strongly associated withHelicobacter pylori (85-98% of cases). These are low-grade lymphomas and may regress following treatment of Helicobacter infection. It is very important to differentiate gastric lymphoma from gastric adenocarcinoma and GIST since the treatment of lymphoma is primarily chemotherapy.

Subtotal gastrectomy, with post-operative chemotherapy is undertaken in refractory cases, or in the setting of complications, including gastric outlet obstruction [17].

Radiographic Features

Appearances in barium swallow vary from normal, to grossly abnormal. Possible appearances include bull's eye appearance due to central ulceration, filling defects, thickened gastric rugae or linitis plastica. On CT scan, gastric lymphomas typically present with marked thickening of the gastric wall with extensive lateral extension of the tumour representing its submucosal spread.

In some instances the submucosal spread involves nearly all the stomach, mimicking linitis plastica. In such cases, mural involvement may even extend across the pylorus into the duodenum or superiorly into the oesophagus. The mass is usually homogeneous in attenuation, but may contain focal areas of low density representing necrosis. Extensive retroperitoneal and local nodal enlargement is often seen.

Endoscopic ultrasound with EUS needle biopsy may be necessary to diagnose and to stage the disease. Hematological parameters are usually checked to assist with staging and to exclude concomitant leukemia [16, 17].

REFERENCES

[1] *Gray's Anatomy* 39th Edition, Elsevier.

[2] Butler, P., Mitchell, A., Healy, J. C. *Applied Radiological Anatomy.* Cambridge University Press. (2012) ISBN:0521766664.

[3] Mohan, P., Ananthavadivelu, M., Venkataraman, J. Gastric diverticulum. *CMAJ.* 2010; 182(5):E226.

[4] DuBois, B., Powell, B., Voeller, G. Gastric diverticulum: "a wayside house of ill fame" with a laparoscopic solution. *JSLS.* 2012;16(3): 473-7.

[5] Abbara, S., Kalan, M. M., Lewicki, A. M. Intrathoracic stomach revisited. *AJR Am. J. Roentgenol.* 2003;181(2): 403-14. AJR *Am. J. Roentgenol.*

[6] Underman, R. B. Essential radiology, clinical presentation, pathophysiology, imaging. *Thieme Medical Pub.* (2006) ISBN: 1588900827.

[7] De Sousa, L. C., Piza, M. R., Da Costa, S. S. Diagnosis of Meniere's disease: routine and extended tests. *Otolaryngol. Clin. North Am.* 2003; 35(3):547-64.

[8] Chey, W. D., Wong, B. C. American College of Gastroenterology guideline on the management of Helicobacter pylori infection. *Am. J. Gastroenterol.* Aug. 2007;102(8): 1808-25.

[9] Do Youn Park, MD; Gregory Y. Lauwers, MD. Gastric Polyps: Classification and Management. *Archives of Pathology and Laboratory Medicne.* Accepted October 2007; 132.

[10] Marcial, M. A., Villafana, M., Hernandez-Denton, J., et al., Fundic gland polyps: prevalence and clinicopathologic features. *Am. J. Gastroenterol.* Oct. 1993;88(10): 1711-3.

[11] Morais, D. J., Yamanaka, A., Zeitune, J. M., et al., Gastric polyps: a retrospective analysis of 26,000 digestive endoscopies. *Arq. Gastroenterol.* Jan-Mar 2007;44(1):14-7.

[12] Hallinan, J. T., Venkatesh, S. K. Gastric carcinoma: imaging diagnosis, staging and assessment of treatment response. *Cancer Imaging.* May 30 2013;13:212-27.

[13] Ge, M. Y., Yin, H. B., Wan, K. M., Ge, J. F., Jin, H. Computed tomography of gastrohepatic ligament involvement by gastric carcinoma. *Abdom. Imaging.* Aug. 2013; 38(4):697-704.

[14] Park, J. M., Jang, Y. J., Kim, J. H., Park, S. S., Park, S. H., Kim, S. J., et al., Gastric cancer histology: clinicopathologic characteristics and prognostic value. *J. Surg. Oncol.* Dec. 1 2008;98(7):520-5.

[15] Suzuki, H., Hasegawa, Y., Terada, A., Ogawa, T., Hyodo, I., Suzuki, M., et al., Limitations of FDG-PET and FDG-PET with computed tomography for detecting synchronous cancer in pharyngeal cancer. *Arch. Otolaryngol. Head Neck Surg.* Nov. 2008;134(11):1191-5.

[16] Buy, J. N., Moss, A. A. Computed tomography of gastric lymphoma. *AJR Am. J. Roentgenol.* 1982;138(5):859-65. *AJR Am. J. Roentgenol.*

[17] Yoo, C. C., Levine, M. S., Furth, E. E., et al., Gastric mucosa-associated lymphoid tissue lymphoma: radiographic findings in six patients. *Radiology.* 1998;208(1):239-43.

ISBN: 978-1-63483-490-2

Chapter 11

THE ROLE OF IMAGING IN UROLOGY

Michelle Kim,[1,*] MD, PhD,
Douglas A. Mata,[2] MD, MPH
and Dicken S. C. Ko,[1] MD, FRCSC
[1]Department of Urology, Massachusetts General Hospital,
Harvard Medical School, Boston, MA, US
[2]Department of Pathology, Brigham and Women's Hospital,
Harvard Medical School, Boston, MA, US

ABSTRACT

In this chapter, we examine the various imaging modalities used to evaluate the genitourinary (GU) tract. Advances in imaging technology have improved the clinical practice of urology and continue to be an active area of growth. Imaging modalities used by urologists include plain film radiography, ultrasonography (US), computed tomography (CT), magnetic resonance imaging (MRI), radionuclide studies, and positron emission tomography (PET). Each modality plays an important role in the diagnosis and management of urologic diseases and when used appropriately, provides cost-effective care. This chapter explores indications for these modalities and their optimal use.

Keywords: Imaging, urology, uroradiology

PLAIN FILM RADIOGRAPHY

1. The Kidneys, Ureters, and Bladder (KUB) Film

Summary: Plain film abdominal radiographs are frontal, supine radiographs of the abdomen that capture the kidneys, ureters, and bladder and are often called KUBs. The KUB

* Corresponding author: Michelle M. Kim, MD, PhD. Department of Urology, Massachusetts General Hospital, 55 Fruit Street, GRB 1102, Boston, MA 02114. Tel: 617-726-2797, fax: 617-726-6131, e-mail: mkim27@partners.org.

may be used as a primary study or as a scout film in anticipation of the use of contrast media [1].

In urology, KUBs are often used in the diagnosis of renal calculus disease and to assess the positioning of indwelling devices such as ureteral stents [1]. They are more commonly used to investigate the etiologies of non-GU processes such as bowel obstructions or bony fractures that may indicate the presence of urologic injuries. Because of the advent of the CT scan, use of the KUB has become limited. Nonetheless, it remains a cost-effective tool for monitoring residual stone burden after therapy for urolithiasis.

Technique: Placement of the patient is in the supine position [1]. The radiograph is obtained using an anterior-to-posterior (AP) exposure and should include the diaphragm superiorly and the pubic symphysis inferiorly. Oblique films may be used to aid in visualization and to clarify the location of peritoneal structures relative to the GU tract.

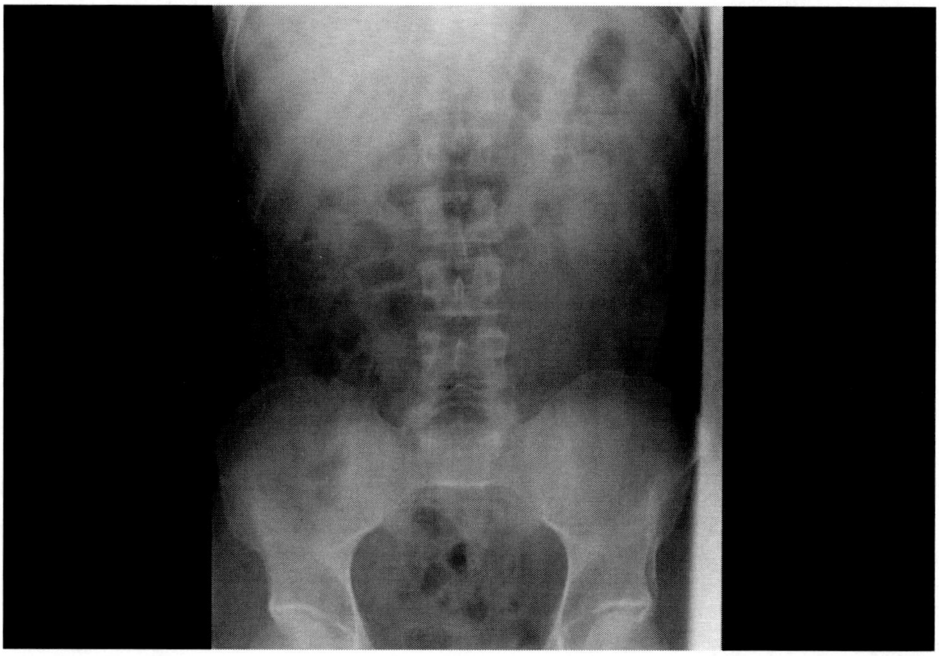

Figure 1. Kidneys, ureters, and bladder (KUB) film.

Limitations: The sensitivity of the KUB for the detection of uroliths can be adversely affected by overlying stool, bowel gas, or bony structures [1]. Non-GU calcifications in the pelvic veins or other vascular structures may also be confused with ureteral calculi. Poorly calcified, uric acid, or indinavir stones may be radiolucent and therefore not visualized. The KUB is also of limited use for evaluating soft tissue abnormalities.

2. Intravenous Urography (IVU)

Summary: IVU is used to demonstrate abnormalities of the renal collecting system, ureters, and bladder. IVU is widely considered obsolete and has now been replaced by US, CT, and MRI in most developed countries.

In resource poor healthcare systems, an important indication for IVU is the investigation of renal and ureteral anatomy in the setting of suspected obstruction (i.e., secondary to nephrolithiasis or following surgery).

IVU is also indicated for patients with unexplained hematuria to diagnose the presence of tumors or other anatomical abnormalities. IVU can also be used in the operating room to opacify the collecting system during extracorporeal shock wave lithotripsy (ESWL), to facilitate access during percutaneous nephrolithotomy (PCNL), or to assess renal trauma burden intraoperatively in trauma patients with suspected renal injuries who did not undergo preoperative imaging.

Technique: A bowel prep may be needed to facilitate the visualization of the ureters and upper collecting system [1]. Placement of the patient is in the supine position. A scout KUB is taken to confirm correct positioning and exposure. A 50 to 100 mL bolus of contrast is injected. The nephrogenic phase radiograph is captured almost immediately after injection as the contrast is excreted from the bloodstream. Additional films are taken at five-minute intervals based on the clinical scenario. Abdominal compression and oblique views may be used to better visualize the ureters and to precisely differentiate ureteral stones from pelvic calcifications. Post-void films are obtained to evaluate for the presence of bladder outlet obstruction, or bladder-filling defects such as stones or malignancies.

Limitations: IVU has been largely replaced by CT and MRI for other diagnostic purposes given that they provide greater anatomic detail and three-dimensional reconstructions.

3. Retrograde Pyelography

Summary: Retrograde pyelography is a procedure in which contrast in injected into the upper urinary tract in a retrograde fashion to opacify the ureters and collecting system [1]. Retrograde pyelograms help identify filling defects (e.g., stones, tumors) and delineate renal anatomy in preparation for surgery. It is commonly used intraoperatively to opacify or to distend the collecting system to assist in percutaneous access of the kidney, ureteroscopy, or stent placement.

Similar to an IVU, the retrograde pyelogram can also play a role in the workup of hematuria, in the surveillance of urothelial carcinoma, and in the evaluation of traumatic or iatrogenic injury to the ureter or collecting system. In children, retrograde pyelograms are indicated for evaluation of congenital or acquired ureteral obstruction and for elucidation of deformities of the ureters or intrarenal collecting system.

Technique: Retrograde pyelograms are performed with the patient under regional or general anesthesia [2]. The patient is placed in the dorsal lithotomy position. An abdominal plain film is initially obtained to ensure appropriate positioning. Cystoscopy is performed to visualize the ureteral orifice.

A ureteral catheter or a cone tip catheter is inserted and contrast is injected into the upper urinary tract [1]. Contrast may be diluted to 50% with sterile saline to prevent subtle filling defects from being obscured.

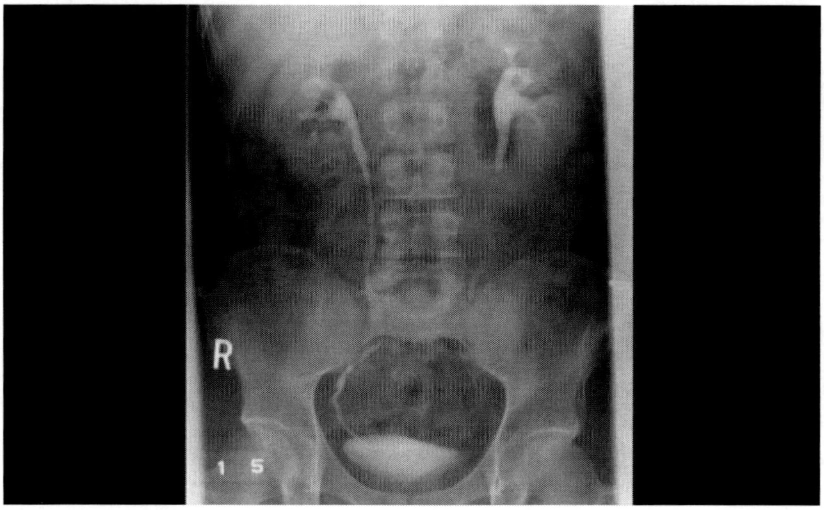

Figure 2. Retrograde pyelogram.

Care should be taken to prevent over-distension of the collecting system and contrast backflow, which can introduce infected urine into the vascular system (by pyelolymphatic drainage) as well as systemic absorption of contrast media with resultant adverse systemic reactions. Retrograde pyelograms evaluate the upper urinary tract in real time and can be immediately interpreted as they are performed.

Limitations: Retrograde pyelography is difficult when the ureteral orifices cannot be properly identified or accessed [1]. Intravenous injection of methylene blue or indigo carmine (indigotindisulfonate sodium) can be used to identify the orifices. If trauma and extravasation of contrast occurs extraluminally, it is generally without serious complication. However, if large quantities of urine continue to extravasate, a stent may be indicated [2]. Retrograde pyelography should not be done in the setting of a urinary tract infection to avoid the risk of pyelonephritis and bacteremia.

4. Retrograde Urethrography

Summary: A retrograde urethrogram (RUG) is used to evaluate the integrity and anatomy of the anterior and posterior urethra [3]. It is essential for the diagnosis of urethral injury or stricture. RUGs are beneficial for demonstrating the length of a stricture when it cannot be determined by direct visualization. They can also show anatomy distal to a stricture that may not be readily visualized by voiding cystourethrogram.

RUGs are also commonly used if there is suspicion of a foreign body or urethral trauma with additional clinical findings such as blood at the meatus, gross hematuria, scrotal hematoma, or high-riding prostate by digital rectal examination. If urethral injury is suspected, a RUG should be performed before placing a Foley catheter. If urethral disruption is observed, a suprapubic tube (SPT) would be preferred.

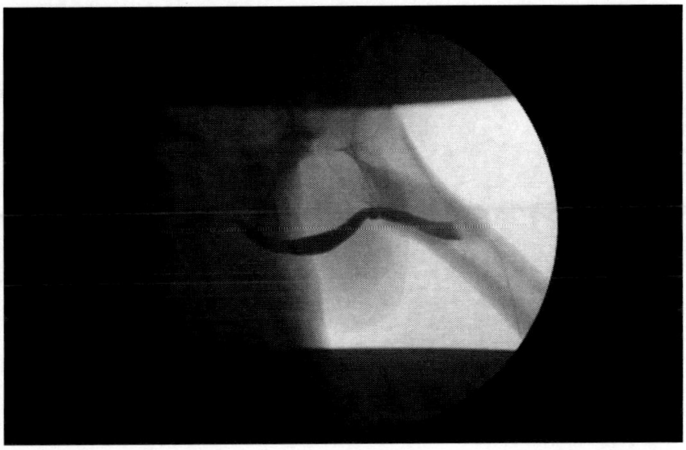

Figure 3. Retrograde urethrogram.

Technique: The patient is supine in a slightly oblique position with the penis on stretch [1]. A small Foley catheter is placed in the fossa navicularis, just past the urethral meatus, and inflated with 2 mL of sterile water. Thirty mL of contrast is injected into the catheter and a plain radiograph is obtained. A penile clamp can be used to keep the contrast in the urethra if desired. If contrast leakage is present, it suggests urethral injury and may help to determine whether surgery is indicated.

Limitations: RUGs provide limited information about surrounding soft tissue injury.

5. Cystogram

Summary: A cystogram evaluates the anatomy of the bladder and provides information about its size, shape, and contour [3]. Cystograms aid in the evaluation of intravesical pathology such as diverticula, fistulas, and trauma. Filling defects may provide information about stones or tumors. They are also indicated for evaluating inguinal hernias involving the bladder, colovesical or colovaginal fistulas, anastomotic integrity after surgery, and blunt or penetrating bladder trauma. Last, cystograms with contrast can be useful for studies of urodynamics.

Technique: The patient is placed in the supine position. A catheter is placed in the bladder and filled with 200 to 400 mL of contrast under gravity at 30-cm height. Adequate filling is necessary to ensure visualization of bladder extravasation or intravesical pathology [1]. AP and oblique films are taken to assess for lesions, including posterior lesions, which may be obscured.

The patient is instructed to void three times, after which post-void images are taken to evaluate the quantity of urine left behind. A final radiograph of the kidneys may be performed to evaluate for occult vesicoureteral reflux not seen during the procedure itself.

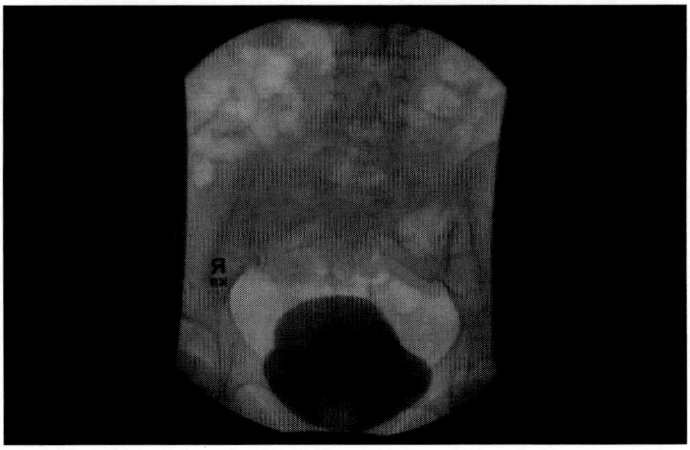

Figure 4. Cystogram.

Limitations: While the cystogram uses less radiation than a pelvic CT scan, it is less sensitive and specific for the diagnosis of most intravesical pathologies except the detection of bladder rupture [1].

6. Voiding Cystourethrogram (VCUG)

Summary: A VCUG is used to visualize the anatomy of the urethra and bladder during micturition [2]. The exam is most commonly used in children with UTIs to assess for the presence of vesicoureteral reflux. VCUG is indicated for all boys with recurrent UTIs, boys with abnormalities on US after their first UTI, girls less than three years of age with their first UTI, girls less than five years of age with their first febrile UTI, older girls and women with pyelonephritis or recurrent UTIs, and in the setting of suspected bladder obstruction, trauma, or rupture. VCUGs should be avoided in patients with untreated UTIs, contrast media hypersensitivity, or fevers within the past day.

Technique: The patient is placed in the supine or semi-upright position using a table capable of reaching the full upright position [2]. A pelvic plain film is obtained. In children, a 5 to 8 French (F) feeding tube is used to fill the bladder with contrast using patient comfort as a guide to determine the appropriate volume [1]. In adults, a standard catheter is placed and the bladder is filled with 200 to 400 mL of contrast. The catheter is removed and an AP film is obtained. The patient is instructed to void while additional AP and oblique films are taken.

The bladder neck and urethra may be evaluated by fluoroscopy during voiding. Oblique views may demonstrate low grade reflux that cannot be captured on an AP film. The exam ends when the patient voids while the radiologist is watching under fluoroscopy. Consumption of fluid promotes excretion of contrast media after the procedure. It is important to watch the contrast during voiding, as this is when the bladder has the most pressure and when reflux will most likely occur.

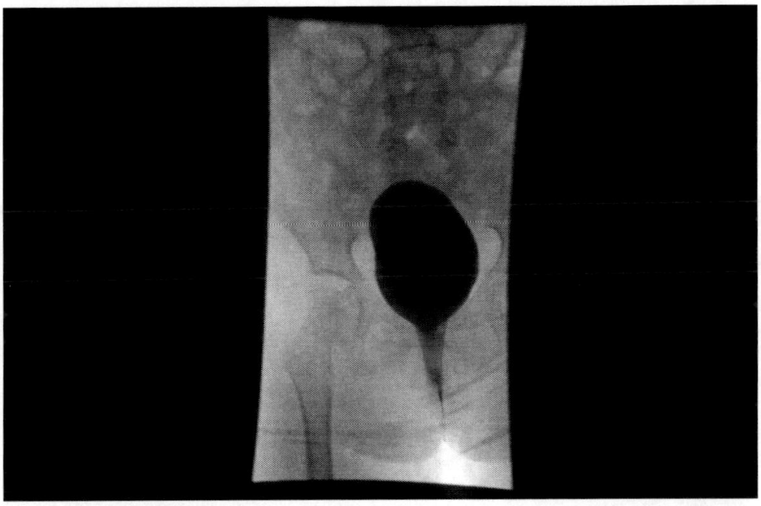

Figure 5. Voiding cystourethrogram.

Limitations: A VCUG requires filling the bladder with a catheter, which is difficult in children and in patients with anatomic abnormalities of the urethra or bladder neck [1]. Bladder filling may lead to autonomic dysreflexia in patients with spinal cord injuries and stimulate bladder spasms in some patients.

ULTRASONOGRAPHY

US uses the mechanical properties of sound to provide real-time images and is commonly used in urology for diagnosis, interventional management, and longitudinal follow up [3]. US is inexpensive, portable, and radiation-free. However, its specificity depends on the skill level of the operator and the body habitus of the patient.

1. Renal US

Summary: Renal US provides a cost-effective method of investigating renal lesions. A curved array transducer of 3.5 to 5.0 MHz is used in adults; higher frequencies can be used in children [1]. Intraoperative renal US during open or laparoscopic cases typically employs a linear transducer of 6 to 10 MHz given the physical proximity of the organ.

Renal US is indicated for the assessment of renal and perirenal masses; upper GU tract dilation; flank pain during pregnancy; hematuria in patients who are not candidates for other imaging modalities; or impaired renal function. Renal US may also be used for interventional procedures such as renal biopsies, renal mass ablation, or nephrostomy tube placement. Vascular abnormalities including renal artery stenosis, renal vein thrombosis, arteriovenous fistulas, and pseudoaneurysms can also be detected by renal US with Doppler concurrent imaging.

Technique: US of the right kidney is performed with the patient supine. The kidney is located in the mid-clavicular line in the right upper quadrant [1]. The transducer is moved laterally until the mid-sagittal plane of the kidney to visualize the anterior and posterior kidney. The, probe is rotated 90 degrees counter clockwise and the kidney is imaged in the transverse plane which includes visualization of the renal hilum. Imaging of the left kidney is similar except that it is slightly more cephalad due to the absence of the liver. It is more difficult to image due to interference from bowel gas from the splenic flexure and because the liver does not provide an acoustic window. Echogenic renal lesions include renal stones, angiomyolipomas (AMLs), renal cortical neoplasms, abscesses, and hematomas.

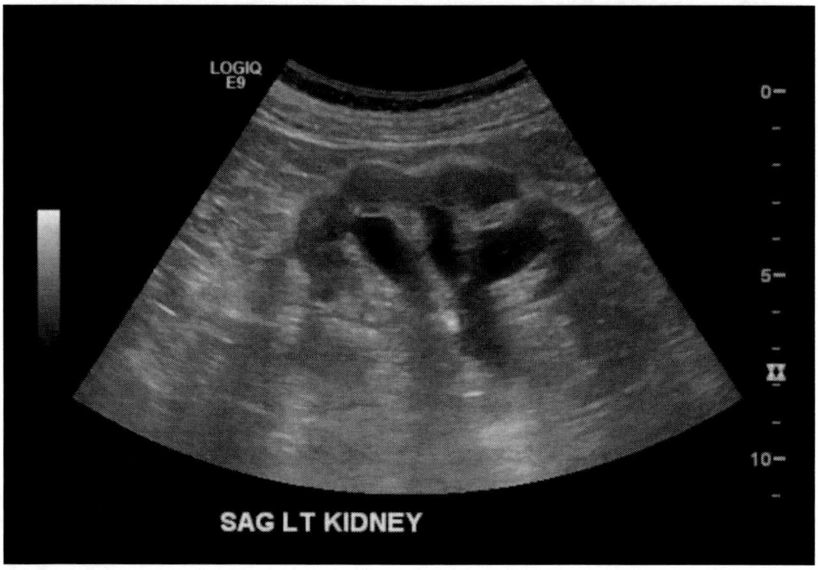

Figure 6. Renal ultrasound.

Limitations: Obesity, intestinal gas, and physical deformity are limitations to adequate US imaging studies [1]. Renal US is excellent for diagnosing benign renal lesions such as cysts, but has poor sensitivity for renal masses less than 2 cm as well as for masses other than angiomyolipomas (AML). More complicated lesions require correlation with another imaging modality, most commonly a CT scan.

2. Transabdominal Pelvic US

Summary: Transabdominal pelvic US, commonly referred to as bladder US, is used to image the lower GU tract in men and women [3]. Common indications for transabdominal pelvic US include assessment of bladder volume, post-void residual, bladder wall configuration and thickness, prostate size and morphology, and catheter placement. A curved array transducer is used. Of note, handheld BladderScan™ devices used in the clinic and wards for measuring bladder volumes and post-void residuals are based on US technology.

Technique: The patient is positioned supine. The bladder is moderately distended to ensure appropriate visualization. The bladder is scanned in the sagittal and transverse planes angling the probe into the pelvis to visualize the bladder beneath the pubic bone [1]. To visualize the prostate, the transducer is fanned inferiorly until the largest transverse diameter of the prostate is identified. Measurements of the width and height are obtained. The transducer is rotated 90 degrees clockwise to produce a true sagittal image of the prostate, which is again measured. Detection of hypertrophy or an enlarged median lobe should be noted to provide additional information regarding the length, size, and configuration of the prostatic urethra and median lobe. These data may provide secondary information about the etiology of bladder outlet obstruction.

Limitations: An under-distended or empty bladder will interfere with the identification of distal ureteral or bladder obstructions, stones, or tumors, and with the assessment of prostatic morphology.

3. Scrotal US

Summary: Scrotal US is an excellent tool for investigating intratesticular and extratesticular disease including testicular neoplasms, torsion, infection, and inguinal hernias [3]. It is commonly used with Doppler sonography to evaluate blood flow to provide detailed anatomic and physiologic information. Indications include assessment of scrotal or testicular mass, pain, or trauma. It may also be used in the infertility workup.

Technique: The patient is placed in the supine position with the scrotum supported on a towel. A high frequency linear array 6 to 12 MHz and 4 to 7.5 cm in width is used [1]. The sonographer starts with a sagittal view of testes from the midline medially and then laterally from the mid-transverse section to the upper and lower poles. The epididymis and scrotal contents are evaluated.

Limitations: The pathognomonic sign of torsion is the absence of intratesticular blood flow. Collateral blood flow may be preserved and it is important for the sonographer not to confuse its presence with that of intratesticular blood flow [1]. Imaging of the contralateral testis can be performed to confirm that the study is able to adequately detect intratesticular blood flow.

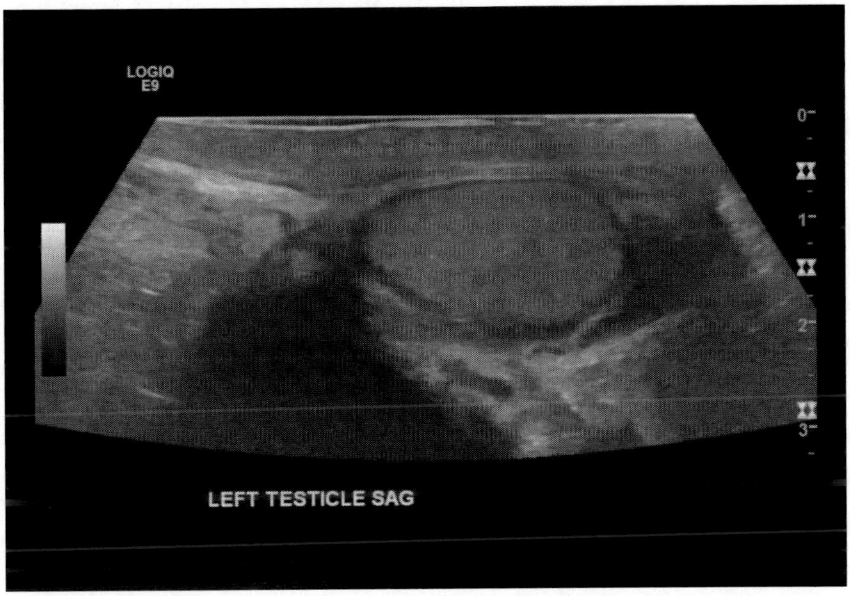

Figure 7. Scrotal ultrasound.

4. Penile US

Summary: Penile US is commonly used to assess the vascular supply of the penis for the diagnosis of erectile dysfunction secondary to arterial insufficiency and veno-occlusion etiologies. Moreover, penile US remains a mainstay for the diagnosis of traumatic injuries [1]. Penile US is also indicated for the evaluation corpora cavernosa fibrosis, urethral stricture or diverticulum, foreign body, priapism, and Peyronie's disease.

Technique: The patient is placed in the supine position. A 6 to 12 MHz linear array transducer is used to image the phallus in the longitudinal and transverse planes in a systematic fashion beginning at the base of the penis and proceeding distally to the glans [1]. Scanning the scrotum and perineum also allows for imaging of the proximal urethra and corporal bodies. Lubricating gels or intracavernosal injection of vasoactive substances may be useful for evaluating anatomy and vascular flow.

Limitations: Penile US has a limited sensitivity and specificity for the detection of penile arterial dysfunction. Pudendal arteriography may be needed to collect more definitive data prior to surgical intervention.

5. Transrectal US of the Prostate

Summary: Transrectal ultrasound (TRUS) allows for the visualization and evaluation of the prostate gland [3]. TRUS is used to guide prostate biopsy, to determine prostate volumes for brachytherapy and cryotherapy (e.g., by planimetry), and to evaluate benign prostatic hypertrophy (BPH). TRUS provides enough resolution to differentiate between the peripheral and transitional zones of the prostate so that the peripheral zone, in which cancers are more commonly located, can be targeted with the biopsy needle [1].

Technique: The patient is placed in left lateral decubitus position with the legs drawn inward [2]. A 6 to 10 MHz endorectal US probe is inserted into the rectum until it reaches the base of the prostate [1]. The probe is moved caudad to visualize the seminal vesicles, bladder neck, prostatic apex and proximal urethra. Complete evaluation of the prostate includes scanning in the sagittal and transverse planes, thoroughly inspecting the prostate for echogenic lesions, cysts, contour, and calcifications. The seminal vesicles and vas deferens should be fully visualized.

Limitations: The sensitivity and specificity of gray-scale TRUS is limited for the reliable detection of all cancers. Color and power Doppler imaging modes improve detection but biopsy remains the gold standard for diagnosis.

Tomography and Magnetic Resonance Imaging Modalities

1. X-Ray Computed Tomography

Summary: CT is often the imaging modality of choice for the diagnosis and management of urologic diseases and has largely replaced other types of imaging as the first-line imaging for nephrolithiasis, hematuria, and workup of renal or urothelial masses [1]. CT scans have advantages over plain film radiographs in that they eliminate superimposition of images of structures that obscure the organ of interest. CT scans of traumatic injuries of the bladder can be complemented by cystogram to better assess the location of the rupture.

Technique: The patient is placed in the supine position on a gantry that passes through the center of CT scanner [5]. The length of study depends on the indication.

Limitations: Although CT scans are generally associated with greater radiation exposure than IVUs, a low-dose CT stone protocol with minimal radiation exposure can be used to detect renal calculi. CT scans sometimes require radiocontrast agents, which often are not without side effects, for improved visualization. Contrast induced nephropathy, which is more prevalent in patients with preexisting renal insufficiency, diabetes, or hypovolemia, should be avoided. Metal implants may create radiographic artifacts.

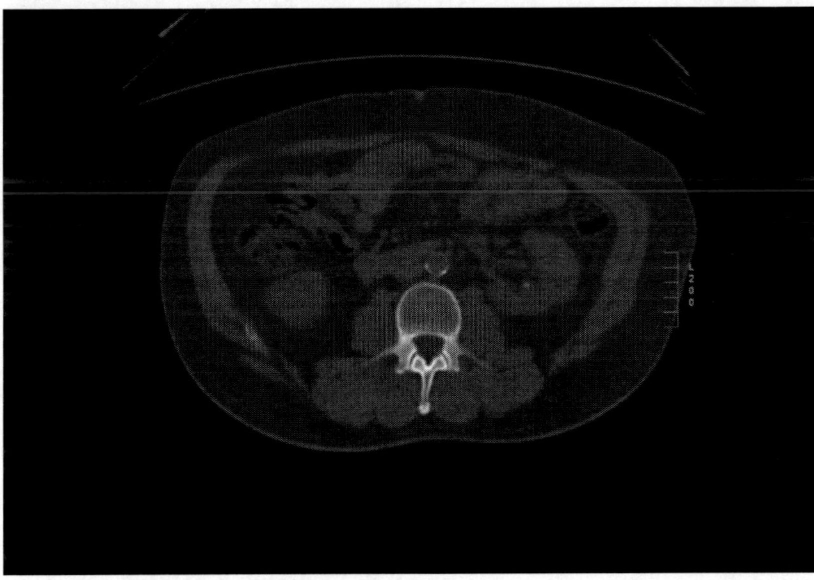

Figure 8. X-ray computed tomographic scan.

2. CT Urography

Summary: CT urography evaluates the entire GU tract using different phases of contrast enhancement [1, 3, 5]. Patients with hematuria and those presenting with flank or abdominal pain are often evaluated by CT urography.

1. The non-contrast phase scan provides an optimal set of images for detecting calcifications, and acts as a baseline for assessing the changes noted following contrast injection [5].
2. The arteriographic or early arterial phase scan is taken 20 seconds after contrast injection and evaluates arterial pathologies such as fibromuscular dysplasia or renal artery stenosis [3, 5].
3. The late arterial or corticomedullary phase is taken 40 seconds after contrast injection and allows for the detection of hypervascular renal masses [5]. This study should always be obtained when information about the renal vasculature is desired or if there may be an aneurysm, arteriovenous malformation, or fistula.

4. The nephrographic phase occurs 80 to 100 seconds after contrast injection and assesses the abdominal and pelvic viscera [5]. Non-hypervascular renal masses are best evaluated during this phase.
5. The excretory phase occurs two minutes after contrast injection and evaluates the collecting system [1, 5]. It is useful for evaluating hematuria and is more sensitive than retrograde pyelogram for detecting upper tract urothelial cancers.

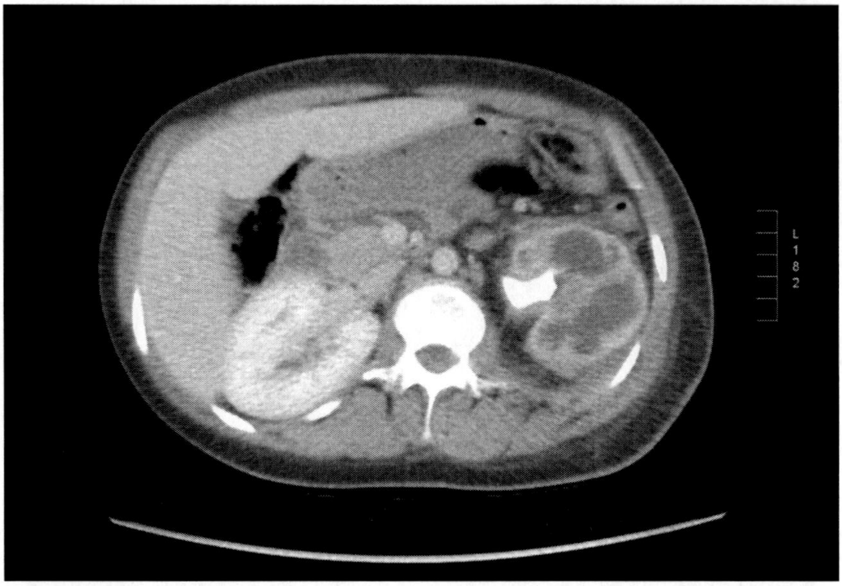

Figure 9. Computed tomographic urogram.

Technique: CT urography may be performed supine or prone [5]. Prone images help to precisely identify the locations of distal ureteral-vesical junction stones. If there is concern that the stone is in the distal ureter, other signs of obstruction helpfully differentiate it from pelvic calcifications. Non-contrast and excretory phase images should span the diaphragm to the pubic symphysis to visualize the entire GU tract.

Limitations: CT urography is not as sensitive as cystoscopy for the detection of intravesical tumors and should not be a substitute in the evaluation of hematuria. However, it can identify filling defects in the bladder caused by larger tumors. In patients with recurrent need for radiation exposure, low-dose CT protocols may be used with minimal sacrifice of diagnostic capabilities.

3. Magnetic Resonance Imaging

Summary: MRI uses magnetic fields and radio waves to provide excellent soft tissue resolution and can be used in patients who cannot be given iodinated contrast [1, 3, 5]. MRI images may be weighted to show different anatomical structures. Fluids such as urine have low signal and appear dark in T1-weighted images. Intravenous gadolinium contrast can be used to augment the relaxation of protons in T1-weighted images, making the kidneys brighter and increasing the chance of detecting renal masses. Fluids in T2-weighted images have higher signal and appear bright. In the kidney, this causes the cortex to appear brighter than the medulla. Urine in the bladder is also bright on T2-weighted images. MRI can differentiate among complex renal cysts, which may be filled with heterogeneous material, in ways that CT or US cannot. Blood breakdown products due to hemorrhage result in high signal on T1-weighted images, whereas they result in black rings around cyst walls on T2-weighted images.

MRI is often used to evaluate renal masses, staging of renal malignancies, as well as aid in the planning of surgery for RCC, particularly in the setting of renal vein or inferior vena cava (IVC) invasion [1, 3, 5].Detectable lesions are assessed for increases in signal intensity by comparing non-enhanced to gadolinium-enhanced T1-weighted images. Adrenal evaluation by MRI is useful because of variations in tissue density among the various adrenal lesions.

Technique: The patient is placed in the supine position on a gantry that passes through the bore of the magnet [3]. More than 30 minutes are needed for the scanner and patients will need to hold their breath for 20 to 30 seconds during each imaging sequence. If the patient is noncompliant, the image will be compromised.

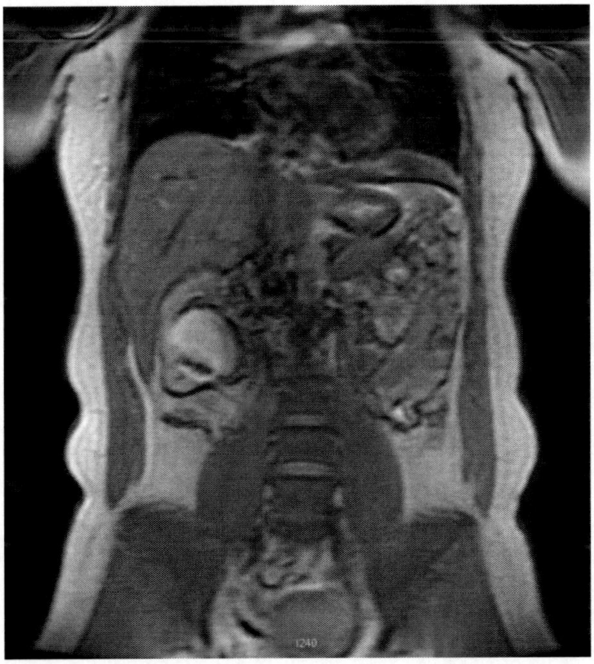

Figure 10. Magnetic resonance imaging scan.

Limitations: An important disadvantage of MRI is that patients must stay still for extended periods of time in enclosed environments [1]. If patients have difficulty with breath-holding, severe claustrophobia, pacemakers, sterile magnetic implants, retained magnetic foreign bodies, cochlear implants, neurovascular aneurysm clips, or cardiac defibrillators other imaging modalities are preferred. Gadolinium contrast agents should not be used in patients with renal insufficiency as it may lead to development of debilitating fibrosing dermopathy.

NUCLEAR MEDICINE

1. Positron Emission Tomography

Summary: PET allows for the detection of primary and metastatic cancers and for the determination of disease extent [4, 5]. PET is combined with high resolution CT to increase the detection of recurrent or metastatic cancers. For seminomas and nonseminomatous germ cell testicular tumors, PET/CT is more accurate than CT for staging of residual masses after chemotherapy [1].

PET/CT also has a promising role in clear cell RCC. The antibody cG250 recognizes carbonic anhydrase IX, which is related to unrestrained cancer growth, and positron-emitting radionuclide, iodine 124, has been successfully attached to it and injected into RCC patients. Other tracers are being developed for the detection of metastatic prostate cancer. Fewer studies have addressed the role of PET in bladder cancer.

Technique: Prior to the scan, a radioactive tracer isotope is injected into the blood [2]. After a waiting period during which the tracer becomes concentrated in the tissue of interest, the patient is scanned. Tissue concentrations are recorded as the tracer decays.

Limitations: The accuracy of PET can be compromised if it is performed within two weeks of completing chemotherapy due to decreased metabolism and increased macrophage activity.It is recommended that PET/CT be delayed for four to 12 weeks following chemotherapy [1].

2. Radioisotope Renography

Summary: Radioisotope renography plays an important role in providing information about kidney function[1, 5]. There are several commonly used agents in nuclear scintigraphy.

1. ^{99m}Tc-DTPA is used to evaluate obstruction and renal function. It is excreted through the kidney and requires a normal glomerular filtration rate (GFR) to provide accurate results.
2. ^{99m}Tc-DMSA, is cleared by filtration and secretion and localizes to the renal cortex. It is the standard test used to identify cortical defects and ectopic or aberrant kidneys, and can also differentiate between benign and malignant lesions.
3. ^{99m}Tc-MAG3, is cleared mainly through tubular secretion with approximately 10% cleared extra-renally. It is limited in its ability to measure GFR because it binds to plasma proteins. It is the study of choice to evaluate renal function and plasma flow in individuals with impaired renal function and urinary obstruction and to evaluate anatomical abnormalities.

Technique: The radioisotope is injected intravenously [1]. Gamma scintillation cameras measure radiation emitted from the radioisotope and digital workstations process and display the information. Of note, ^{99m}Tc-MAG3 works with diuretic scintigraphy to provide a differential of renal function and clearance time comparing the two kidneys. A diuretic, usually 0.5 mg/kg furosemide, is administered when maximum collecting system activity is visualized. The initial phase of the study is called the flow phase. Images are taken at 2-second intervals for two minutes. Images are taken at 1-second intervals for one minute. This phase demonstrates renal uptake, background clearance, and abnormal vascular lesions that may be due to AVM, tumors, or active bleeding. The second phase is called the renal phase. It is most useful for evaluating renal function. The time to peak uptake is typically between 2 and 4 minutes. During this phase, images are taken at 1-minute intervals for half an hour. In the last phase, the excretory phase, images are again taken at 1-minute intervals for half an hour. The half-life ($T_{1/2}$) is the time it takes for the collecting system activity to decrease by 50% from the time of diuretic administration.

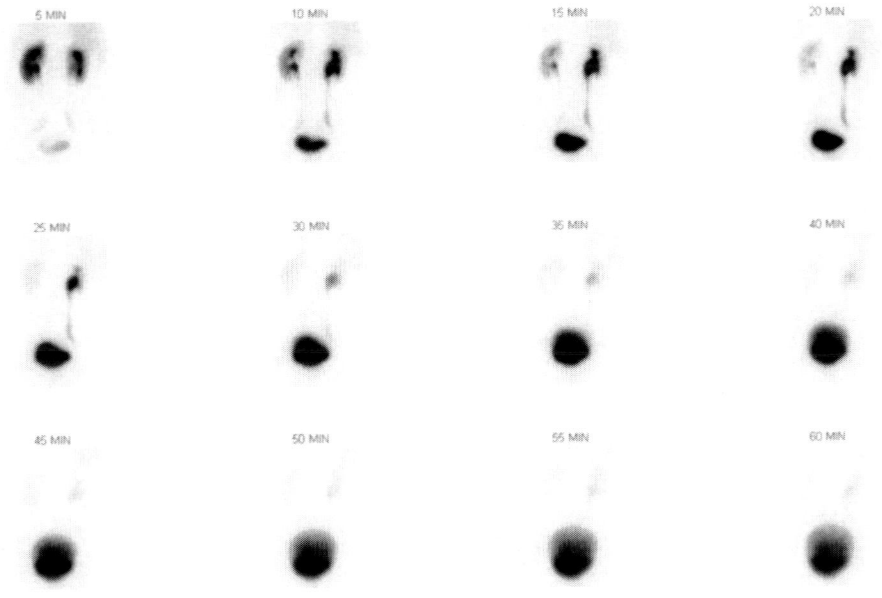

Figure 11. Radioisotope renogram.

Transit time through the collecting system of less than 10 minutes is consistent with a normal, non-obstructed system [1]. A $T_{1/2}$ of 10 to 20 minutes represents a mild to moderate delay and may indicate the presence of a mechanical obstruction. A $T_{1/2}$ greater than 20 minutes is consistent with a high grade obstruction. If ureteral stents are in place, the patient should have an unclamped bladder catheter.

Limitations: For diuretic scintigraphy, the $T_{1/2}$ is highly technician dependent because the diuretic must be given when the collecting system displays maximum activity.

3. Whole-Body Bone Scintigraphy

Summary: Whole-body bone scans are the most sensitive method for detecting bone metastases from primary prostate and renal cancers [5].

Technique: The patient is injected with a radioactive tracer and then scanned with a gamma camera, a device that detects the radiation emitted [3].

Limitations: A positive bone scan is not specific for cancer and may prompt the use of other imaging modalities (e.g., plain film radiography, CT, or MRI) to confirm the findings and correlate them with any prior history of fracture, trauma, surgery, or arthritis. Bone scans can be mistaken as normal if there is uniformly increased uptake in the bony structures due to diffuse metastatic bony disease.

REFERENCES

[1] Wein, A. J., Kavoussi, L. R., Novick, A. C., Partin, A. W., Peters, C. A. *Campbell-Walsh Urology: Expert Consult Premium Edition: Enhanced Online Features and Print*, 4-Volume Set, 10e. 10 edition. Philadelphia, PA: Saunders; 2011.

[2] Hanno, P. M., Guzzo, T. J., Malkowicz, S. B., Wein, A. J. *Penn Clinical Manual of Urology: Expert Consult - Online and Print*, 2e. 2 edition. Philadelphia, PA: Saunders; 2014.

[3] McAninch, J., Lue, T. F. *Smith and Tanagho's General Urology, Eighteenth Edition*. 18th edition. New York: McGraw-Hill Professional; 2012. Dunnick, R., Sandler, C., Newhouse, J. *Textbook of Uroradiology*. Fifth edition. Philadelphia: LWW; 2012.

[4] Kim, S. H., editor. *Radiology Illustrated: Uroradiology*. 2nd ed. 2012 edition. New York: Springer; 2012.

[5] Shoskes, D. A., Uzzo, R. G. *The American Urological Association Educational Review Manual in Urology*. 4th Ed. 2012. 4th edition. Castle Connolly Graduate Medical Publishing; 2012.

[6] Wang, L. J. *Key Diagnostic Features in Uroradiology: A Case-Based Guide*. 2015 edition. New York, NY: Springer; 2014.

In: The Role of Imaging Technology …
Editor: Georgios Tsoulfas
ISBN: 978-1-63483-490-2

Chapter 12

THE ROLE OF IMAGING IN PLASTIC SURGERY

Alexandros Mekras[1,*], MD, MSc, PhD, FICS and Vasileios Kalles[2], MD, MSc, PhD

[1]Verbundkrankenhaus Bernkastel/Wittlich, Germany
[2]Naval and Veterans Hospital of Athens, Athens, Greece

ABSTRACT

From the era that Röntgen discovered X-rays, imaging studies have been a significant adjunct in the clinicians' armamentarium. The rapid development of modern imaging techniques, as well as the increased accessibility to sophisticated imaging techniques, has allowed physicians to have access to detailed anatomical and functional information. Plastic surgery, being one of the surgical specialties that uses the most up-to-date technologies in both diagnosis and treatment, is a field that modern imaging techniques have had a significant impact on. Current applications of imaging in plastic surgery range from staging of melanoma patients to preoperative submillimeter-scale planning of perforator flaps. Nearly all currently available imaging techniques, including X-rays, Ultrasound, Computed Tomography, Magnetic Resonance Imaging, and Positron Emission Tomography, are being used as adjuncts in the diagnosis and/or staging of plastic surgical conditions and diseases. Furthermore, as accurate preoperative planning of plastic and reconstructive surgical procedures has been shown to be of high importance for both the patient as well as the health system by improving the surgical outcomes, imaging techniques, and more specifically CT – and MRI – based studies, have emerged as the outstanding gold standard techniques.

* Corresponding author: A. Mekras. Surgeon, Verbundkrankenhaus Bernkastel/Wittlich, Germany. E-mail: almekras @yahoo.gr.

INTRODUCTION

Over the past years, the field of imaging has seen continuous and increasingly rapid developments, regarding both the availability and the accessibility of imaging techniques. Imaging procedures nowadays integrate information strictly anatomical with high resolution images, and, in the case of molecular imaging, information on the functional nature of the tissue. All this detailed information allows plastic surgeons to have precise preoperative data that correlate with the clinical status of the patient.

As a result, imaging has become an essential part of preoperative planning for the patient undergoing a plastic surgical procedure, whether this should be reconstructive or aesthetic.

Apart from the classical applications of imaging in disease diagnosis and staging (such as skin melanoma), particular applications of preoperative imaging include perforator flap surgery and facial reconstruction, among others. It is now well established that accurate preoperative analysis can reduce the length of operations, enhancing the surgical design and minimizing unneeded dissections.

The modern imaging modalities that are now available can offer high–resolution, three–dimensional analysis of the vascular anatomy, and perfusion. Computed Tomography (CT) and magnetic resonance imaging (MRI) are the modalities that have lately been established as outstanding non–invasive techniques for the depiction of vascular and non–vascular systems.

This chapter will elaborate on the use and the importance of imaging techniques in plastic surgery, including the role of both CT and MR angiography, the techniques that are currently the state of the art in preoperative exploration of the vascular system.

1. DIAGNOSTIC IMAGING IN PLASTIC SURGERY

1.1. Skin Melanoma

Although skin melanoma accounts for only 5% of skin cancers, it represents nearly half of skin related deaths and globally, in 2012, melanoma occurred in 232,000 people and resulted in 55,000 deaths. Its prognosis is directly related to the clinical stage at presentation, and patients with metastatic disease survive for a median of 6-10 months (Table 2.1) [1, 2].

Melanoma can disseminate to virtually any organ of the human body, but has a predilection for the regional lymph nodes, liver, lung and brain [3]. Surgery remains the cornerstone of melanoma treatment, while imaging plays a key role in preoperative staging and postoperative follow – up. Although most imaging studies have a limited ability to diagnose melanoma, a variety of traditional or advanced imaging techniques are employed, in an attempt to detect occult metastases.

1.1.1. X – Rays

X – rays, the most classical imaging study, is a quick, inexpensive, and easy to perform technique, and can be applied in melanoma staging, especially since the lung is one of the most common metastatic sites. However, only a few lesions produce an appearance that can be correlated to a specific diagnosis. Investigating the use of chest X – ray in patients with localized melanoma, Terhune et al., [4] found that only 0.1% of the patients staged by this method were found to have occult metastatic lesions. In a more recent study, Hofmann et al., [5] reported that chest X - ray showed a yield of 0.2% and a false positive rate of 4.4%.

Still, a chest X – ray in a symptomatic patient remains of some use, and will also be useful as a routine preoperative screening exam.

1.1.2. Ultrasound

In melanoma, ultrasound has been used for both the diagnosis of skin lesions, and staging of regional nodes and abdominal organs. The ability of ultrasound to distinguish between basal cell papilloma and malignant melanoma has been investigated, and ultrasound has been reported to have sensitivity of up to 100%, but with low specificity rates [6, 7]. The addition of color Doppler in the investigation might also further improve accuracy [8].

Ultrasound has also been widely used in the evaluation of lymph node basins in melanoma staging. Compared to clinical examination, ultrasound has shown superior sensitivity rates, with comparable specificity, despite the fact that it is an operator – dependent technique [9-11]. However, in the era of the Sentinel Lymph Node Biopsy technique for lymph node staging of melanoma, ultrasound has limited utility, as its false negative rates remain high, especially in case of small metastatic deposits (2-4mm), and SLNB remains the golden standard for lymph node staging in clinically node – negative patients [12]. Finally, in distant metastases staging, ultrasound is not routinely used, but may be useful in the differential diagnosis of e.g., suspicious liver lesions.

1.1.3. Computed Tomography

Computed Tomography is the preferred imaging technique for the evaluation of abdominal metastases in melanoma patients. Liver metastases from melanoma are typically hypervascular lesions, and therefore the correct phase post contrast infusion is needed to be acquired. On the other hand, chest CT is also superior to chest radiography, more sensitive in detecting subcentimeter lesions and more capable to distinguish solitary from multiple pulmonary lesions [13]. In patients with normal chest radiography, the possibility of discovering additional metastasis in chest CT raises up to 19% in high – risk patients [14]. However, when the CT results in indeterminate findings, patients should undergo further imaging or diagnostic surgery.

1.1.4. Magnetic Resonance Imaging

Magnetic Resonance Imaging (MRI) is an excellent technique to delineate soft tissues, due to its high contrast resolution and multiplanar images.

Table 2.1. Expected survival of patients with melanoma

Stage	5 – year survival (%)
I	91 – 95
IIA	80
IIB	65
IIC	45
IIIA	65 – 70
IIIB	45 – 55
IIIC	25 – 30
IV	5 - 20

However, it still carries a lot of limitations, due to its high – cost, long examination times, and its patient – related contraindications (claustrophobia, pacemakers, certain surgical clips or metal prosthetic devices).

In melanoma patients, T1 – weighed images give a high signal density for melanoma deposits, consistent with the paramagnetic effect of melanin.

As a result of its increased soft – tissue contrast, MRI is more sensitive than CT in the detection of metastases that involve the brain, liver and musculoskeletal system [15], and results in alteration in the treatment plan in nearly one quarter of the patients. Still, MRI would not be a first – line investigation for staging of melanoma, and it is most useful as an adjunctive method of investigating indeterminate lesions found in previous imaging studies.

1.1.5. Sentinel Lymph Node Biopsy – Nuclear Medicine Imaging Modalities

The reference standard for the lymph node staging in melanoma patients with no clinical evidence of regional nodal metastasis, is sentinel lymph node biopsy (SLNB), a technique that was developed by Morton more than 20 years ago [16], typically performed following intraoperative lymphatic mapping. Formal regional lymphadenectomy is now reserved for patients with clinical suspicion of metastatic adenopathy, which is usually confirmed with ultrasound – guided fine needle aspiration (FNA).

In the event of a negative SLNB, patients are considered to have a clinical stage I/II disease, whereas patients with positive SLNB following a complete regional lymphadenectomy, will require further imaging in order to detect clinically occult metastases. Nuclear medicine imaging modalities, such as positron emission tomography (PET), with or without combination with computed tomography (PET/CT) are also becoming increasingly popular in the staging of melanoma. Their scientific basis lies on the fact that malignant cells have a higher metabolic rate, and this is detected by infusion of a radio-labeled glucose analogue, 18-fluoro-deoxy-D-gucose (18-FDG), which is taken up by tumor cells. However, a PET scan alone offers a limited spatial resolution, and small (< 1cm) or non-metabolically active lesions may be missed. Thus, PET alone is considered to be more accurate in stage III disease rather than stage I/II [17], while SLNB has been shown to have superior sensitivity in stage I/II melanoma patients (Table 2.2).

The addition of PET images to CT images acquired simultaneously has been the new revolution in Nuclear Medicine Imaging, and offers more accurate localization of 18-FDG uptake. The accuracy of PET/CT is increased compared to PET alone, even in patients with early stage melanoma [18, 19]. PET/CT has the potential of covering the whole body, which is not easy to accomplish with other imaging techniques, as well as an increased spatial resolution compared to PET alone (6mm vs 10mm).

Table 2.2. Selected studies comparing nodal status detection by SLNB and PET in Stage I/II melanoma patients

Author	No of patients	PET positive (%)	SLNB positive (%)
Wagner et al., 1999	70	3	16.7
Hafner et al., 2000	100	2	26
Wagner et al., 2005	144	9	43

However, some limitations still exist: its specificity is still low, as lesions with increased metabolic rate such as inflammatory on infectious can be falsely considered positive, and there are a small proportion of low – metabolic rate lesions that PET/CT will not detect. Finally, its increased cost and limited availability pose another drawback to this technique, and its use is mostly reserved for patients with high risk of recurrence after successful resection or response to systemic treatment.

1.2. Assessment of Skin Burns

Burn wounds are a common clinical entity a plastic surgeon has to face in everyday clinical practice. Since burn wounds that heal within a short time (e.g., 2-3 weeks) have an acceptable aesthetic and functional outcome, it is critical that the burn depth is assessed accurately early, in order to better stratify patients that are deemed to undergo surgery that involves excision and grafting, in order to achieve healing within this 2-3 week timeframe.

The initial clinical assessment is usually effective when it comes to burns that are classified as superficial or full thickness, however, in partial thickness skin burns the depth is not well defined and the clinical estimation of the depth is often inaccurate. Studies have shown that in the case of an indeterminate depth burn, the clinical assessment has an accuracy ranging between 65-70%, even when the burn depth is assessed by experienced plastic surgeons [20, 21]. For this reason, much research has focused on potential imaging adjuncts that will assist the clinician in making a correct burn depth assessment.

The foremost among these techniques, that has met great approval among plastic surgeons, was the laser Doppler technique [22]. The laser Doppler technique utilizes the Doppler Effect in order to assess burn depth, as laser light is directed at the moving blood cells in the sampled tissue, and the frequency change of the waves of laser light is proportional to the amount of perfusion in the tissue.

The correlation between burn depth and perfusion has been documented since as early as 1984, when Micheels and colleagues showed that superficial or partial – thickness burns result in supranormal dermal perfusion, whereas deep or full – thickness burns display significantly reduced dermal blood flow [23, 24].

The current evidence in the evaluation of skin burns with laser Doppler is growing [22], and recent studies show that a new technique, the Laser Doppler Imaging is more efficient than LD flowmetry, superseding the latter one. The LDI is usually applied within 48 – 72 hours, and provides a significant aid to the clinical evaluation, predicting the possibility of healing within 21 days, and this has been validated in both adult and pediatric patients. Current limitations of the technique include its increased cost, the topographical artifacts when curved areas of the body are assessed, its difficulty in the assessment of tattooed areas of the body and possible ambiguous results in patients with concurrent infections, peripheral vascular disease or anemia.

Furthermore, there is no current consensus on the cut – off points of perfusion values, and burn centers still have to evaluate their devices independently and find the most suitable cut - off points and levels of burn wound depth stratification. However, the objective benefit of LDI, when used as an adjunct to clinical assessment, has now been well documented, and its use improves the prediction of burn healing and reduces ensures a timely decision to operate.

1.3. Scar Evaluation Using Modern Imaging

Skin scars are the end result of a cutaneous injury, iatrogenic or not, following a series of events that are involved in the wound healing process [25]. Cutaneous scarring is affected by a plethora of genetic, physiologic, environmental and biochemical factors, and all these produce a continuum of scar types (keloid, hypertrophic, atrophic, contracted, fine line, etc.), with up to 70% of the scars being symptomatic, aesthetically unsatisfactory, physiologically distressing or functionally restrictive to the individual [26].

The accurate assessment of the scar allows for better quantification of the scar inflammatory state, its morphology and evolution, as well as its response to interventional or conservative treatments [26]. In the quest of objective adjuncts in scar evaluation, a number of imaging techniques have been evaluated, such as laser Doppler and ultrasonography, along with a bunch of, mostly experimental, other techniques.

Laser Doppler Flowmetry is based on the fact that the blood perfusion in the cutaneous tissue correlates with the extent of the vascularization. Laser Doppler has been extensively used in burn assessment, and when applied to scars, it can act as a predictor during scar maturation, as hypertrophic scars tend to have increased blood flow [27]. The increased cost and low availability is currently the method's main drawback, but as this technology further disseminates, the cost is expected to decrease, increasing its clinical use.

Ultrasound is also a useful method in the assessment of cutaneous problems, and many devices have been used for scar depth quantification [28-30]. Ultrasound has been shown to be able to discriminate between hypertrophic scar and normal scar with good sensitivity and specificity, both in burn and surgical scars.

2. Image – Based Preoperative Planning in Plastic and Reconstructive Surgery

Since the evolution and access to sophisticated imaging techniques has increased in the past decades, plastic surgery is one of the fields that has benefited most.

The detailed information that is acquired by modern imaging techniques allows plastic surgeons to have precise preoperative data related to the actual clinical status of the patient, allowing them to plan flaps in a refined and precise way, selecting the best option for the patient. In the current era of anatomically predefined flaps, preoperative imaging is now a routine method, not only to study the donor and recipient area, but also to improve the surgical outcome and ensure minimal morbidity.

Almost all kinds of available imaging modalities have been used in the preoperative evaluation of vessels in microvascular plastic surgery. These include Doppler ultrasound, angiography, computed tomographic angiography (CTA) and magnetic resonance imaging angiography (MRA) (Table 3.1). Although the latter two methods are nowadays being increasingly used, there is no consensus on which imaging modality should be used, and, as research in this field is ongoing, this chapter will focus on the use of CTA and MRA in preoperative planning of plastic surgery operations. CTA uses computer – analyzed x-ray images in combination with the infusion of a contrast agent, in order to produce highly accurate reconstruction images of the vasculature [31].

Table 3.1. Overview of pros and cons of imaging modalities in the preoperative evaluation of the vascular anatomy

Method	US Doppler	CTA	MRA
Pros	Low cost	High sensitivity and specificity	High sensitivity and specificity
	Easily accessible	Higher perforator detection ratc	No exposure to ionizing radiation
	Simple use	Currently the gold standard	Better depiction of intramuscular vessels
	No contraindications		
Cons	Operator dependent	Exposure to ionizing radiation	Contraindications (severe obesity, metal or cochlear implants)
	Variable sensitivity and specificity	Medium – to –high cost	High cost
	May be time consuming	Contrast – related risks	Risk of nephrogenic systemic fibrosis
			Inferior to CTA (using 1.5T magnetic field)

CTA: Computed Tomographic Angiography, MRA: Magnetic Resonance Imaging Angiography.

CTA produces more accurate images than Doppler or color Doppler, providing detailed information regarding the intramuscular course of perforating vessels, and may give additional information on incidental findings or anatomic variations [32, 33], and has been used in the preoperative evaluation of both free and perforator flaps.

There is a plethora of studies that have demonstrated the effectiveness of CTA in accurately assessing perforating vessels, most of them in planning Deep Inferior Epigastric Perforator (DIEP) flaps [34-39].

While CTA is often criticized for the high radiation exposure, the benefits of its preoperative use include shortened dissection and operative times, reduced complication rates and, eventually, reduced overall cost. CTA can effectively depict perforators greater than 1mm in caliber and, in several international centers is considered as the gold standard in preoperative imaging of DIEP flaps.

On the other hand, Magnetic Resonance Imaging has also evolved from an initial use for solid organ study to an effective and feasible technique for vascular study.

Even small caliber vessels, including perforator vessels, can now be evaluated with MRA, without the need of exposure to radiation, maintaining high sensitivity and specificity in the evaluation of vessel course and size. Most studies available in the current literature report a sensitivity of 97-100% in the identification of perforators of the DIEA, which is similar to that of CTA [40-42].

However, in the study by Rozen et al., MRA is reported to have a lower perforator detection rate compared to CTA, particularly in perforators < 1mm [41]. These results are likely to be due to the fact that CTA has a better contrast in depicting the vessel course within fatty tissue, whereas, on the other hand, MRA can better depict the intramuscular vessel course.

Finally, a recent study by Hartung et al., suggests that the sensitivity of MRA can be improved when 3.0T magnetic fields are used, compared to 1.5T, offering increased spatial resolution, decreased acquisition time and better visibility of the vessels [42].

REFERENCES

[1] Balch, C. M., Soong, S. J., Murad, T. M., Smith, J. W., Maddox, W. A., Durant, J. R. A multifactorial analysis of melanoma. IV. Prognostic factors in 200 melanoma patients with distant metastases (stage III). *Journal of clinical oncology: official journal of the American Society of Clinical Oncology*. 1983;1(2):126-34.

[2] Lee, M. L., Tomsu, K., Von Eschen, K. B. Duration of survival for disseminated malignant melanoma: results of a meta-analysis. *Melanoma research*. 2000;10(1):81-92.

[3] Patel, J., Didolkar, M., Pickren, J., Moore, R. Metastatic pattern of malignant melanoma: a study of 216 autopsy cases. *The American Journal of Surgery*. 1978;135 (6):807-10.

[4] Terhune, M. H., Swanson, N., Johnson, T. M. Use of chest radiography in the initial evaluation of patients with localized melanoma. *Archives of dermatology*. 1998;134(5): 569-72.

[5] Hofmann, U., Szedlak, M., Rittgen, W., Jung, E. G., Schadendorf, D. Primary staging and follow-up in melanoma patients--monocenter evaluation of methods, costs and patient survival. *British journal of cancer*. 2002;87(2):151-7.

[6] Bessoud, B., Lassau, N., Koscielny, S., Longvert, C., Avril, M. F., Duvillard, P., et al., High-frequency sonography and color Doppler in the management of pigmented skin lesions. *Ultrasound in medicine and biology*. 2003;29(6):875-9.

[7] Harland, C. C., Kale, S. G., Jackson, P., Mortimer, P. S., Bamber, J. C. Differentiation of common benign pigmented skin lesions from melanoma by high-resolution ultrasound. *The British journal of dermatology*. 2000;143(2):281-9.

[8] Dancey, A. L., Mahon, B. S., Rayatt, S. S. A review of diagnostic imaging in melanoma. *Journal of plastic, reconstructive and aesthetic surgery: JPRAS*. 2008;61 (11):1275-83.

[9] Garbe, C., Schadendorf, D. Surveillance and follow-up examinations in cutaneous melanoma. *Onkologie*. 2003;26(3):241-6.

[10] Machet, L., Nemeth-Normand, F., Giraudeau, B., Perrinaud, A., Tiguemounine, J., Ayoub, J., et al., Is ultrasound lymph node examination superior to clinical examination in melanoma follow-up? A monocentre cohort study of 373 patients. *The British journal of dermatology*. 2005;152(1):66-70.

[11] Saiag, P., Bernard, M., Beauchet, A., Bafounta, M. L., Bourgault-Villada, I., Chagnon, S. Ultrasonography using simple diagnostic criteria vs palpation for the detection of regional lymph node metastases of melanoma. *Archives of dermatology*. 2005;141(2): 183-9.

[12] Chai, C. Y., Zager, J. S., Szabunio, M. M., Marzban, S. S., Chau, A., Rossi, R. M., et al., Preoperative ultrasound is not useful for identifying nodal metastasis in melanoma

patients undergoing sentinel node biopsy: preoperative ultrasound in clinically node-negative melanoma. *Annals of surgical oncology*. 2012;19(4):1100-6.

[13] Halton, K. P. Radiological considerations in diagnosis of metastatic melanoma. *The Mount Sinai journal of medicine*, New York. 1992;59(3):211-6.

[14] Heaston, D. K., Putman, C. E., Rodan, B. A., Nicholson, E., Ravin, C. E., Korobkin, M., et al., Solitary pulmonary metastases in high-risk melanoma patients: a prospective comparison of conventional and computed tomography. *AJR American journal of roentgenology*. 1983;141(1):169-74.

[15] Muller-Horvat, C., Radny, P., Eigentler, T. K., Schafer, J., Pfannenberg, C., Horger, M., et al., Prospective comparison of the impact on treatment decisions of whole-body magnetic resonance imaging and computed tomography in patients with metastatic malignant melanoma. *European journal of cancer* (Oxford, England: 1990). 2006;42 (3):342-50.

[16] Morton, D. L., Wen, D. R., Wong, J. H., Economou, J. S., Cagle, L. A., Storm, F. K., et al., Technical details of intraoperative lymphatic mapping for early stage melanoma. *Archives of surgery*. 1992;127(4):392-9.

[17] Prichard, R. S., Hill, A. D., Skehan, S. J., O'Higgins, N. J. Positron emission tomography for staging and management of malignant melanoma. *The British journal of surgery*. 2002;89(4):389-96.

[18] Reinhardt, M. J., Joe, A. Y., Jaeger, U., Huber, A., Matthies, A., Bucerius, J., et al., Diagnostic performance of whole body dual modality 18F-FDG PET/CT imaging for N- and M-staging of malignant melanoma: experience with 250 consecutive patients. *Journal of clinical oncology: official journal of the American Society of Clinical Oncology*. 2006;24(7):1178-87.

[19] Iagaru, A., Quon, A., Johnson, D., Gambhir, S. S., McDougall, I. R. 2-Deoxy-2-[F-18]fluoro-D-glucose positron emission tomography/computed tomography in the management of melanoma. *Molecular imaging and biology: MIB: the official publication of the Academy of Molecular Imaging*. 2007;9(1):50-7.

[20] Hoeksema, H., Van de Sijpe, K., Tondu, T., Hamdi, M., Van Landuyt, K., Blondeel, P., et al., Accuracy of early burn depth assessment by laser Doppler imaging on different days post burn. *Burns: journal of the International Society for Burn Injuries*. 2009;35 (1):36-45.

[21] Monstrey, S., Hoeksema, H., Verbelen, J., Pirayesh, A., Blondeel, P. Assessment of burn depth and burn wound healing potential. *Burns: journal of the International Society for Burn Injuries*. 2008;34(6):761-9.

[22] Khatib, M., Jabir, S., Fitzgerald O'Connor, E., Philp, B. A systematic review of the evolution of laser Doppler techniques in burn depth assessment. *Plastic surgery international*. 2014;2014:621792.

[23] Micheels, J., Alsbjorn, B., Sorensen, B. Laser doppler flowmetry. A new non-invasive measurement of microcirculation in intensive care? *Resuscitation*. 1984;12(1):31-9.

[24] Micheels, J., Alsbjorn, B., Sorensen, B. Clinical use of laser Doppler flowmetry in a burns unit. *Scandinavian journal of plastic and reconstructive surgery*. 1984;18(1):65-73.

[25] Bayat, A., McGrouther, D. A. Spectrum of abnormal skin scars and their clinical management. *British journal of hospital medicine*. 2006;67(10):527-32.

[26] Perry, D. M., McGrouther, D. A., Bayat, A. Current tools for noninvasive objective assessment of skin scars. *Plastic and reconstructive surgery*. 2010;126(3):912-23.

[27] Oliveira, G. V., Chinkes, D., Mitchell, C., Oliveras, G., Hawkins, H. K., Herndon, D. N. Objective assessment of burn scar vascularity, erythema, pliability, thickness, and planimetry. *Dermatologic surgery: official publication for American Society for Dermatologic Surgery* [et al.,]. 2005;31(1):48-58.

[28] Lau, J. C., Li-Tsang, C. W., Zheng, Y. P. Application of tissue ultrasound palpation system (TUPS) in objective scar evaluation. *Burns: journal of the International Society for Burn Injuries*. 2005;31(4):445-52.

[29] Nedelec, B., Correa, J. A., Rachelska, G., Armour, A., LaSalle, L. Quantitative measurement of hypertrophic scar: interrater reliability and concurrent validity. *Journal of burn care and research: official publication of the American Burn Association*. 2008; 29(3):501-11.

[30] Fong, S. S., Hung, L. K., Cheng, J. C. The cutometer and ultrasonography in the assessment of postburn hypertrophic scar--a preliminary study. *Burns: journal of the International Society for Burn Injuries*. 1997;23 Suppl. 1:S12-8.

[31] Pratt, G. F., Rozen, W. M., Chubb, D., Ashton, M. W., Alonso-Burgos, A., Whitaker, I. S. Preoperative imaging for perforator flaps in reconstructive surgery: a systematic review of the evidence for current techniques. *Annals of plastic surgery*. 2012;69(1):3-9.

[32] Rozen, W. M., Palmer, K. P., Suami, H., Pan, W. R., Ashton, M. W., Corlett, R. J., et al., The DIEA branching pattern and its relationship to perforators: the importance of preoperative computed tomographic angiography for DIEA perforator flaps. *Plastic and reconstructive surgery*. 2008;121(2):367-73.

[33] See, M. S., Pacifico, M. D., Harley, O. J., Francis, I., Smith, R. W., Jones, M. E. Incidence of 'Incidentalomas' in over 100 consecutive CT angiograms for preoperative DIEP flap planning. *Journal of plastic, reconstructive and aesthetic surgery: JPRAS*. 2010;63(1):106-10.

[34] Masia, J., Clavero, J. A., Larranaga, J. R., Alomar, X., Pons, G., Serret, P. Multidetector-row computed tomography in the planning of abdominal perforator flaps. *Journal of plastic, reconstructive and aesthetic surgery: JPRAS*. 2006;59(6):594-9.

[35] Masia, J., Kosutic, D., Cervelli, D., Clavero, J. A., Monill, J. M., Pons, G. In search of the ideal method in perforator mapping: noncontrast magnetic resonance imaging. *Journal of reconstructive microsurgery*. 2010;26(1):29-35.

[36] Masia, J., Kosutic, D., Clavero, J. A., Larranaga, J., Vives, L., Pons, G. Preoperative computed tomographic angiogram for deep inferior epigastric artery perforator flap breast reconstruction. *Journal of reconstructive microsurgery*. 2010;26(1):21-8.

[37] Alonso-Burgos, A., Garcia-Tutor, E., Bastarrika, G., Cano, D., Martinez-Cuesta, A., Pina, L. J. Preoperative planning of deep inferior epigastric artery perforator flap reconstruction with multislice-CT angiography: imaging findings and initial experience. *Journal of plastic, reconstructive and aesthetic surgery: JPRAS*. 2006;59(6):585-93.

[38] Rozen, W. M., Phillips, T. J., Ashton, M. W., Stella, D. L., Gibson, R. N., Taylor, G. I. Preoperative imaging for DIEA perforator flaps: a comparative study of computed tomographic angiography and doppler ultrasound. *Plastic and reconstructive surgery*. 2008;121(1 Suppl.):1-8.

[39] Pacifico, M. D., See, M. S., Cavale, N., Collyer, J., Francis, I., Jones, M. E., et al., Preoperative planning for DIEP breast reconstruction: early experience of the use of computerised tomography angiography with VoNavix 3D software for perforator navigation. *Journal of plastic, reconstructive and aesthetic surgery: JPRAS*. 2009;62 (11):1464-9.

[40] Newman, T. M., Vasile, J., Levine, J. L., Greenspun, D. T., Allen, R. J., Chao, M. T., et al., Perforator flap magnetic resonance angiography for reconstructive breast surgery: a review of 25 deep inferior epigastric and gluteal perforator artery flap patients. *Journal of magnetic resonance imaging: JMRI*. 2010;31(5):1176-84.

[41] Rozen, W. M., Stella, D. L., Bowden, J., Taylor, G. I., Ashton, M. W. Advances in the pre-operative planning of deep inferior epigastric artery perforator flaps: magnetic resonance angiography. *Microsurgery*. 2009;29(2):119-23.

[42] Hartung, M. P., Grist, T. M., Francois, C. J. Magnetic resonance angiography: current status and future directions. *Journal of cardiovascular magnetic resonance: official journal of the Society for Cardiovascular Magnetic Resonance*. 2011;13:19.

In: The Role of Imaging Technology …
Editor: Georgios Tsoulfas

ISBN: 978-1-63483-490-2

Chapter 13

Wrist Fractures in Adults: What Should a Medical Student Know?

Fares E. Sayegh*, MD, PhD

Aristotle University of Thessaloniki, Thessaloniki, Greece

Abstract

Wrist fractures are common fractures and are seen frequently in the emergency department. They mainly occur in the elderly as a result of a fall on an outstretched hand. Wrist fractures are also seen in high-energy mechanism injuries such as road traffic accidents or a fall from a height. Those fractures are always accompanied with other injuries. The ability to detect the different types of wrist fractures requires an adequate understanding of the anatomy of the wrist, the mechanism that causes that type of injury, and the accurate interpretation of different imaging processes of the bony and articular structures of the wrist. Therefore, appropriate evaluation of the radiological x-rays is important for therapeutic intervention, surgical or conservative, and for the complete restoration of normal wrist function after an injury.

Bony Anatomy

The wrist is composed of the distal parts of the radius, the ulna, the proximal and distal carpal rows, and the bases of five metacarpals. The distal extraarticular part of the radius is broadened 2-3 cm proximal to the radio-carpal joint and this small area of metaphyseal widening is characterized by a decrease of the amount of cortical bone and increase in the amount of cancellous bone that is weaker and easily predisposed to fracture if an injury of the wrist occurs [5, 6, 7]. On the lateral surface of the distal radius, one can also palpate the radial styloid, a strong cone shaped cortical projection. The Lister tubercle is a bony prominence that is found over the dorsal aspect of the distal radius.

* Corresponding author: Fares E. Sayegh, MD, PhD. Associate Professor in Orthopaedics, Aristotle University of Thessaloniki, Thessaloniki, Greece. E-mail: fsayegh@auth.gr.

The intra-articular surface of the distal radius has a fossa for the scaphoid carpal bone where it sits, it is named scaphoid facet or fossa, and another fossa where the lunate carpal bone sits and it is named lunate facet or fossa [5, 6]. A narrow, concave, smooth depression is also found on the medial side of the distal radius. This is called the sigmoid notch and it acts as a seat for the distal ulna. The sigmoid notch facilates the rotation and provide relative stability to the distal radio-ulnar joint [6] (Figure 1). The carpal bones of the wrist are eight in number and lie in two rows. From the radial to ulnar side, the proximal row consists of the scaphoid (navicular), lunate, triquetrum, and the pisiform carpal bones. Similarly, the distal row, from radial l to ulnar, includes the trapezium, trapezoid, capitate, and hamate carpal bones that normally articulate with the bases of the metacarpals. It is important to remember that the proximal carpal bone row is considered and named as intercalated segment as the forces acting on its proximal and distal articulations determine its position [5, 6, 7] (Figure 2). The collapse of this bony anatomy after a wrist injury is an indication of wrist instability. The surfaces of the distal and proximal rows carpal bones are joined together with intrinsic ligaments. As a result, the wrist is separated into different articular compartments; the radiocarpal compartment, the midcarpal, the pisiform-triquetal, the common carpometacarpal, intermetacarpal and the distal radioulnar compartments [6, 7].

IMAGING EVALUATION

In cases where a patient with a wrist injury is presented to the emergency room, a series of radiological views are to be requested. As a start, the standard x-rays; the postero-anterior (PA), and the lateral x-ray should be included. In many cases the detailed clinical examination of the injured wrist may require more radiological imaging in order to better describe the fracture. The therapeutic doctor should recognize (Figure 3, 4):

a) The location of the fracture. Is the fracture extra or intraarticular?
b) The configuration of the fracture. Is the fracture transverse, oblique, or comminuted?
c) The displacement. Is there a change in the radial tilt, length and angle
d) Are there any signs of joint instability? (radiocarpal, radioulnar, intercalated)
e) Is there any suspicious for an unrecognized underlying fracture of carpal bones? (scaphoid, hamate, triquetrum, …)

Postero-Anterior Wrist View

This is a standard view of the wrist and one can distinguish the many normal interosseous relationships [5, 6, 7].

In this poster-anterior view one should appreciate;

a) The three smooth arcs of the wrist
b) The scapholunate joint space
c) The ulnar length
d) The carpal height

a. Arcs of the Wrists

Three carpal arcs are distinguished along the radiocarpal and midcarpal joints. A line that follows the proximal articular surfaces of the scaphoid, lunate and the triquetrum carpal bones forms arc 1. A line drawn over the distal articular surfaces of the same carpal bones forms arc 2. The arc 3 is formed from a line that follows the proximal articular surfaces of the capitate and hamate carpal bones. In a normal x-ray of a wrist, the 3 carpal arcs are not disrupted and shown to be almost equal in size, smooth, and parallel to each other (Figure 5).

It is important to note that the interosseous carpal and intercarpal spaces are nearly equal in size. However, normal variants of step-off carpal arcs are described.

b. Scapholunate Joint Space

The normal size of scapholunate joint space does not differ from the size of the other joint spaces that lie between pairs of the other carpal bones.

There is a kind of parallelism between the carpal joint spaces. Normally the width of the intercarpal joint space at its midportion measures 2 mm or less and its width does not alter with the wrist in either radial or ulnar deviation.

c. Ulnar Variance (Known As Hulten Variance)

This refers to the change in the length of the ulna relative to the length of radius. This change in length can be found by drawing a line on the distal articular surface of the radius toward the ulna, and another line on the distal articular surface of the ulna. The distance measured between those 2 drawn lines is named the ulnar variance.

Normally both ulnar and radial articular surfaces are at the same level. If the ulna projects more distally than the radius the ulnar variance is considered to be positive. If the ulna projects more proximally, then the ulnar variance is negative.

d. Radial Inclination

It represents the angle formed between a line that connects the radial tip to the ulnar aspect of the distal radius and a second line drawn perpendicular to the long axis of the radius. This angle of radial inclination ranges from 13-30° (Figure 6).

e. Radial Length or Height

It can be measured along the longitudinal axis of the radius, and it is the distance between a line that passes through the distal tip of the radial styloid and a second line passing through the distal articular surface of the ulna. Normally, the radial length measures 11-13mm (Figure 7).

f. Carpal Height

This is a radiological concept that helps in the quantification of the carpal collapse in a patient over time. The height can be found by measuring the distance between the base of the 3rd metacarpal and the distal articular surface of the radius (Figure 8).

Lateral Wrist View

A true lateral x-ray of the wrist is considered when there is parallelism of the long axis of the 3rd metacarpal with the long axis of the radius, and the pisiform carpal bone overlie the distal pole of the scaphoid carpal bone [5, 6, 7].

a. The Longitudinal Axes of Radius, Lunate, Capitate

On a lateral x-ray of the wrist the longitudinal axes through the 3rd metacarpal, the capitate, the lunate, and the radius all fall on the same line.

b. The Capitolunate Angle

It is where the axes of the radius, lunate, and capitate should superimpose with 0-30° angle.

c. The Scapholunate Angle

It is the angle formed between the longitudinal axis of the scaphoid and the log axis of the radius, lunate, and the capitate carpal bones. Normally it ranges between 30-60°.

d. The Palmar or Volar Tilt of Distal Radius

This is the angle that is formed between a line that is drawn tangentially to the most distal articular surface and a perpendicular line to the midshaft of the radius. A normal wrist has a range of 11° of volar or palmar tilt to 4° of dorsal tilt.

Oblique Wrist View

In this view the fractures of the waist of the scaphoid and the tuberosity are better seen [5, 6, 7]. Fractures of the dorsal part of the triquetrum can be also detected.

Moreover, the scaphotrapezial, scaphotrapezoidal, trapezotrapezoidal, capitolunate, and the first carpometacarpal joints are well visualized [5, 6].

Radial and Ulnar Deviation Wrist Views

In both wrist projections, the scaphoid carpal bone is better visualized.

Common Distal Wrist Fractures

Fractures of the distal end of the radius are the most common fracture-injuries seen and treated by orthopaedic surgeons in the emergency room [2]. Looking at the x-ray of such fractures, the therapeutic doctor should be able to interpret and to describe the pattern and the characteristics of such fractures [1, 2, 3, 4]. Therefore, one should understand the location of the fracture; is the fracture line only located in the metaphysis of the radius and does not involve the radial articular surface? (extraarticular fracture).

Does the fracture line extend to the radiocarpal joint? (intraarticular fracture) [1, 2, 5].

It is also important to recognize the configuration of the fracture, is the fracture transverse, oblique, or comminuted? One should recognize if the fracture is unstable, and look for type of displacement of the fracture and if there is any change in the normal radial tilt, length or angle [5, 6].

Moreover, any signs of joint instability and the coexistence of other accompanied fractures of carpal bones or ulnar styloid should be interpreted and described.

1. Colles' Fracture

This is a fracture of the distal end of the wrist. It is one of the most common fractures seen at the emergency department. The incidence of this fracture is increased in the elderly due to osteoporosis. The mechanism of injury is usually a fall on an outstretched hand.

A colles' fracture is usually a transverse extraarticular fracture, but it could be comminuted and intraarticular. In this fracture, there is impaction and dorsal angulation of the distal fracture fragment (Figure 9).

Therefore beside the recognition of the presence of a transverse metaphyseal fracture of the distal radius, the doctor should look and describe the presence of other fracture features [3, 4, 5, 6]:

1. Extension of the fracture line to the radiocarpal joint
2. Extension of the fracture line medially to the distal radioulnar joint
3. Is there radial shortening due to fracture impaction?
4. Is there a loss of radial inclination?
5. Degree of dorsal angulation in relative to the proximal fracture fragment?

2. Smith Fracture

This is an extraarticular fracture of the metaphysis of the distal radius. It is also called the reverse colles, as the distal fracture fragment is displaced and angled volarly (palmar direction) relative to the proximal radial fracture fragment. This fractures mainly occurs in younger patients, and the mechanism of injury is a fall on a flexed wrist [2, 4, 5, 6] (Figure 10).

3. Barton Fracture

This is an intraarticular fracture of the distal radial articular surface. The intraarticular fracture fragment is displaced together with the carpus.

This translation or displacement of the distal fracture fragment with the carpus may be in a palmar (volar) or dorsal direction in relation to the shaft of the radius [1, 2] (Figure 11).

4. Hutchinson (Chauffeur) Fracture

This is an oblique intraarticular fracture of the radial styloid. It is rarely displaced and it is better distinguished on a PA view of the wrist [5, 6]. The fracture line may extend to the space between the scaphoid and the lunate fossae causing scapholunate ligamentous injuries that may lead to scapholunate instability or dissociation. The term "chauffeur" fracture was originally described in the early 20th century as an injury that occurred while using the starting automobile crank that suddenly reversed during an engine backfire (Figure 12).

5. Die-Punch Fracture

This is an intraarticular fracture of the distal radius. It is a depressed fracture of the lunate fossa of the articular radial surface as a result of a transverse load transmitted through the lunate carpal bone (Figure 13). Sometimes this type of fracture can be easily missed on a PA wrist view. A good understanding of the carpal arcs of a wrist as seen on a PA wrist view, will help in noticing the disturbance of the smooth carpal arc I that connects the outer proximal convexities of the scaphoid, lunate, triquetrum.

This finding should arouse suspicion of the existence of such a fracture [3, 5, 6].

Common Carpal Bone Fractures

1. Scaphoid Fracture

It is the most common fractured carpal bone. It usually occurs in young males after a fall on an outstretched hand while the wrist is extended and radially deviated. If an injury to the scaphoid carpal bone is suspected, a PA, lateral and oblique views of the wrist are the routine x-rays that are required to visualize the scaphoid bone. Views with the wrist in an ulnar deviation (the scaphoid view) will better illustrate the waist of the scaphoid carpal bone [4, 5]. Anatomically, the scaphoid bone has a waist, a proximal and a distal pole. The most common fractures of the scaphoid occur through the waist. Early recognition of the scaphoid fracture is important, as early immobilization of the wrist with a cast is essential for achieving bone union. It should be emphasized that the blood supply of the scaphoid carpal bone is unique as the entire blood supply of this carpal bone enters from its distal pole. Therefore, fractures of the scaphoid and especially of the distal pole may predispose to avascular necrosis [3, 4, 5] (Figure 14 a, b).

2. Triquetrum Fracture

The triquetrum fracture is considered the 2nd most commonly injured carpal bone. The dorsal avulsion fracture of the triquetrum could be easily missed on conventional x-rays of the wrist. In cases where there is a clinical suspicion of such fracture, a CT tomography is the method of choice (Figure 15).

3. Hamate and Hook of the Hamate Fracture

Usually the fracture of the hamate may be detected on a plain x-ray. Fractures that involve the hook of the hamate are difficult to notice on standard views. Beside the use of using a carpal tunnel view, CT, or MRI to detect a clinically suspicion fracture of the hamate or hook of the hamate, a bone scan is another option to locate the fracture site [5, 6, 7] (Figure 16).

4. Pisiform Fracture

This fracture is usually the result of a direct blow to the pisiform carpal bone. Pisiform fractures occur in 1-3% of all the carpal bone fractures and are difficult to detect on standard x-rays. A carpal tunnel view, a lateral oblique, or a radial deviation view is sometimes necessary to show the fracture. MRI, and CT scan may also help in detecting the fracture [6] (Figure 17).

Conclusion

Fractures of the distal radius and the carpal bones are common and complex fractures that are seen routinely in the emergency room. This chapter provides the medical students with a concise and complete understanding of some of the common wrist fractures that they should know during their medical studies.

References

[1] Catalano, L. W. III, Cole, R. J., Gelberman, R. H., Evanoff, B. A., Gilula, L. A., Borrelli, J. Jr. Displaced intra-articular fractures of the distal aspect of the radius. *J. Bone Joint Surg. Am.* 1997; 79:1290–1302.

[2] DePalma, A. F. Comminuted fractures of the distal end of the radius treated by ulnar pinning. *J. Bone Joint Surg. Am.* 1952; 34:651–662.

[3] Cohen, M. S. Fractures of the carpal bones. *Hand Clin.* 1997; 13:587–599.

[4] Dobyns, J. H., Linscheid, R. L. Fractures and dislocations of the wrist. In: Rockwood, C. A. Jr, Green, D. P., eds. *Fractures in adults.* 3rd ed. Philadelphia, Pa: Lippincott, 1984; 411–509.

[5] Goldfarb, C. A., Yin, Y., Gilula, L. A., Boyer, M. I. Wrist Fractures: What the Clinician Wants to Know. *Radiology* 2001; 219:11–28.

[6] Loredo, R. A., MD, Sorge, D. G., et al., Radiographic Evaluation of the Wrist: A Vanishing Art. *Semin. Roentgenol.* 2005 Jul;40(3):248-89.

[7] Scalcione, L. R., Gimber, L. H., A. M. Ho et al., Spectrum of Carpal Dislocations and Fracture-Dislocations: Imaging and Management. *AJR* 2014; 203:541–550.

INDEX

#

A

B

C

D

E

R

S

T

U

V

W